T0293188

CONJUNCTIVITIS: SYMPTOMS, TREATMENT AND PREVENTION

EYE AND VISION RESEARCH DEVELOPMENTS

Books in this series can be found on Nova's website at:

https://www.novapublishers.com/catalog/index.php?cPath=23_29&seriesp=
Eye+and+Vision+Research+Developments

E-books in this series can be found on Nova's website at:

https://www.novapublishers.com/catalog/index.php?cPath=23_29&seriespe=
Eye+and+Vision+Research+Developments

EYE AND VISION RESEARCH DEVELOPMENTS

CONJUNCTIVITIS: SYMPTOMS, TREATMENT AND PREVENTION

ANNA R. SALLINGER
EDITOR

Nova Biomedical Books
New York

For permission to use material from this book please contact us:
Telephone 631-231-7269; Fax 631-231-8175
Web Site: http://www.novapublishers.com

NOTICE TO THE READER

LIBRARY OF CONGRESS CATALOGING-IN-PUBLICATION DATA
Available upon request

ISBN: 978-1-61668-321-4

Published by Nova Science Publishers, Inc. ✴ *New York*

CONTENTS

PREFACE

Conjunctivitis (commonly called "pink eye" or "Madras eye" is an inflammation of the conjunctiva (the outermost layer of the eye and the inner surface of the eyelids), most commonly due to an allergic reaction or an infection (usually viral, but sometimes bacterial). In this book, the authors discuss allergic disorders of the conjunctiva as well as novel drug delivery approaches in dry eye syndrome therapy. Allergic contact conjunctivitis caused by ophthalmic preparations is explored and examined also are the clinical signs of conjunctivitis.

Chapter I - The allergic response is an over-reaction of the body's immune system to innocuous foreign substances or allergens, such as airborne pollen, animal dander, house dust mite, that the body perceives as a potential threat or undesirable. It is a malady that is estimated to affect approximately 20 % of the population. Of this subset, at least 20% suffer from a specific subset of signs and symptoms known as ocular allergy. Both systemic allergy and ocular allergy have a significant impact on the quality of life of the individual. Allergic diseases involve antibody- and/or T-lymphocyte mediated mechanisms.

Allergic disorders of the conjunctiva are characterized by specific responses such as: 1) an IgE-mast cell mediated response, as seen in allergic conjunctivitis and 2) chronic mast cell activation and eosinophil/T-lymphocyte mediated response, as seen in giant papillary conjunctivitis, vernal keratoconjunctivitis and atopic keratoconjunctivitis. Traditionally, the signs and symptoms of ocular allergy include itching, tearing, redness, chemosis and eyelid edema. The mechanism of allergic eye disease includes: 1) allergen-induced immunoglobulin E (IgE) production and mast cell sensitization; 2) IgE-mediated mast cell degranulation and the release of preformed mediators and chemotactic factors; and 3) persistent mast cell activation and Th2-mediated delayed-type hypersensitivity (DTH) reaction, involving the actions of newly formed mediators and chemotactic factors that incite the recruitment of additional inflammatory cells, which then leads to the allergen-induced late phase allergic response.

The management of allergic disorders of the conjunctiva is aimed at avoiding exposure to allergen, preventing the release of mediators of allergy, controlling the allergic inflammatory cascade and preventing ocular surface damage. The clinician should recommend non-pharmacologic and pharmacologic therapeutic regimens that address the acute presentation of ocular allergy and provide prophylaxis aimed at providing long-term maintenance therapy. The clinician may use pharmaceutical agents that prevent mast cell degranulation; block the histamine receptors; inhibit the arachidonic acid cascade; inhibit T-lymphocyte activation; inhibit IgE production by activated B-lymphocytes; and block the action of cyclooxygenase and/or inhibit Lipoxygenase.

Chapter II - Dry eye syndrome or the *keratoconjunctivitis sicca* is a common disease of tear film and ocular surface developed in numerous aetiologies. Tear film instability and ocular surface disturbances that subsequently influence the tear film are among the primarily causes of this disease, but many other factors are involved in tear film disorders. Clinical manifestations commonly include eye discomfort, feeling of a foreign body in the eye, itching or even visual disturbance; inflammation and damage of ocular surface may follow. The therapeutic approaches are based on the dry eye symptoms relief, increasing the patient's comfort and preventing further damage to ocular surface. This can be achieved by renewing the normal function of tear film and ocular surfaces. Although eye surface is easily reached by classical ocular dosage forms, novel drug delivery systems for ocular administration offer advantages in terms of increased residence time on eye surface and/or controlled release of the drug, with enhanced therapeutic effectiveness. Patient's acceptance can also be improved by developing formulations that do not require frequent application, or cause blurred vision, and having a more pleasant appearance. Biodegradable, biocompatible, non-toxic, and mucoadhesive materials are being used for the design of colloidal carriers. Novel polymers for hydrogels suitable for ocular administration are reviewed in this chapter, giving overview on their potential benefits and limitations in dry eye syndrome management and reported successful formulations.

Chapter III - Novel strategies for ocular anti-inflammatory therapies are extensively being investigated to increase drug bioavailability and decrease adverse side effects of common treatments. Colloidal carriers based on lipid materials are becoming a suitable alternative due to several advantages, including solubilization of hydrophobic/lipophilic anti-inflammatory drugs followed by bioavailability enhancement, modification of pharmacokinetic parameters, and protection of sensitive drugs from physical, chemical or biological degradation. Furthermore, by modulating the surface properties e.g. with viscosity-enhancing agents or mucoadhesive polymers may also improve drug bioavailability since the carriers are maintained in the target area for longer time. Likewise, submicron meter particles allow efficient crossing of biological barriers protecting the eye and transport enabling efficient drug delivery to the target tissues and fluids of the anterior segment (cornea, conjunctiva, sclera, anterior uvea) or posterior segment (uveal region, vitreous fluid, choroids and retina). Lipid-based colloidal carriers broadly comprise micro and nanoemulsions, liposomes and lipid nanoparticles (Solid Lipid Nanoparticles and Nanostructured Lipid Carriers). These have been already tested for ocular delivery of several anti-inflammatory drugs including corticosteroids and non-steroidal anti-inflammatory drugs, revealing a great potential discussed herein. Novel drug delivery systems are being improved on a daily basis since they are considered a promising strategy to enhance the ocular bioavailability of topically administered drugs.

Chapter IV - Both preservatives and active ingredients of ophthalmic preparations may produce allergic contact conjunctivitis. The number of potential ophthalmic allergens is destined to increase. According to a recent review of the literature, an additional 15 allergenic ingredients were reported between 1997 and 2007.

Preservatives, such as benzalkonium chloride, chlorhexidine and thimerosal, are well-known, frequent sensitizers in eyedrops and in contact lens solutions. Other less frequently reported allergenic ophthalmic preservatives include disodium EDTA, polyquaternium 1, phenylmercuric nitrate, chlorobutanol, parabens, and sorbic acid. Preservative-free monodose containers are now available for the most important ophthalmic preparations.

Active ingredients of the ophthalmic products that may produce contact sensitization include beta-blockers, mydriatics, antibiotics, antiviral drugs, anthistamines, anti-inflammatory drugs, corticosteroids and anesthetics.

Symptoms may be limited to the conjunctiva or may more frequently also involve the periocular skin and the eyelids. Ophthalmologic examination reveals pronounced vasodilation and chemosis of the conjunctiva. Lacrimation and papillary reaction can be present. Corneal involvement is usually limited to punctuate epithelial keratitis. Eyelid dermatitis is not a constant finding.

Allergic contact conjunctivitis may be caused by type IV allergy, although type I allergy, other hypersensitivity mechanisms, or irritation cannot be excluded. Conventional patch testing is sometimes a poor detector of contact allergy from ophthalmic preparations. Some authors have suggested that patch tests should be performed on stripped or scarified skin, or after pricking the skin, and by intradermal testing. Pre-treatment with sodium lauryl sulphate has recently been found to be another effective method of patch testing. The diagnosis of allergic contact conjunctivitis may be confirmed by a conjunctival challenge test with the ophthalmic preparation believed to be responsible for the allergy.

If correctly diagnosed and managed, allergic contact conjunctivitis has a good prognosis as it clears spontaneously when use of the offending allergen is discontinued, without the need in many cases of any other therapy.

Chapter V - Stevens-Johnson syndrome (SJS) and toxic epidermal necrolysis (TEN) are acute inflammatory vesiculobullous reactions of the skin and mucous membranes. Drugs are the suspected etiologic factor in SJS/TEN. SJS/TEN patients often experience the prodromata, including nonspecific fever, coryza, and sore throat, that closely mimics upper respiratory tract infections treated with antibiotics.

IκBζ, is important for Toll-like receptor (TLR)/IL-1 receptor signaling and essential for innate immune responses; knockout (KO) mice exhibit severe, spontaneous ocular surface inflammation with the loss of goblet cells, and perioral inflammation.

As findings in IκBζ-KO mice suggested that dysfunction/abnormality of innate immunity can result in ocular surface inflammation, we posited that it may play a role in human ocular surface inflammatory disorders. Under the hypothesis of a disordered innate immune response we performed gene expression analysis of CD14$^+$ cells from peripheral blood of SJS/TEN patients with ocular complications. We found that IL-4R gene expression differed between SJS/TEN patients and the controls; upon LPS stimulation, it was down-regulated in patients and slightly up-regulated in the controls. We also found that the expression of 2 genes, IκBζ and IL-1α, was significantly down-regulated in SJS/TEN. Single nucleotide polymorphism (SNP) association analysis of candidate genes associated with innate immunity, allergy, or apoptosis revealed that TLR3 SNP (rs.3775296 and rs.3775290), IL4R SNP Gln551Arg (rs.1801275), IL13 SNP Arg110Gln (rs.20541), and FasL SNP (rs.3830150 and rs.2639614) were significantly associated with SJS/TEN with ocular complications.

SJS/TEN may be different from allergic diseases since in both Arg110Gln of IL-13- and Gln551Arg of IL-4R polymorphisms the ratio of each allele was the inverse of that reported for atopy and asthma. IL-4R and FasL may play a role in innate immunity which reportedly able to regulate allergy and apoptosis.

We hypothesized that viral infection and/or drugs may trigger a disorder in the host innate immune response and that this event is followed by aggravated inflammation of the mucosa, ocular surface, and skin.

Ophthalmologists and dermatologists documented that the HLA-B12 (HLA-Bw44) antigen was significantly increased in Caucasian SJS patients; in our Japanese study population there was no such association. Although HLA-A*0206 was strongly associated with SJS/TEN with ocular complications in the Japanese, it is absent in Caucasian populations, suggesting strong ethnic differences in the HLA-SJS/TEN association.

Genetic and environmental factors may play a role in an integrated etiology of SJS/TEN and there may be an association between SJS/TEN with ocular complications and disordered innate immunity.

Chapter VI- Although the involvement of systemic malignant lymphoma in the ocular region is rare, primary ocular lymphoma and reactive lymphoid hyperplasia (pseudo-lymphoma) have been increasing recently. These lymphoproliferative diseases in the ocular region exist in ocular adnexa such as conjunctiva, the adjoining orbit, and the lachrymal gland [1,2]. In conjunctiva, lymphocytes and plasma cells are found in the layer of substantia propria, which is designated mucosa-associated lymphoid tissue (MALT). When a long-standing inflammatory condition, such as toxic reaction, allergy, or infection, appears in the MALT, true follicles with visible germinal centers will be provoked [3]. Especially, the palpebral conjunctiva has lymphoid tissues containing components for immune responses, suggesting the term 'conjunctiva-associated lymphoid tissue' (CALT) [4]. In contrast, the orbit that mainly consists of fat, extrinsic muscles, and the lachrymal gland, has no distinct lymph node. Since the lachrymal gland, located in the lachrymal fossa in the anterior lateral portion of the roof of the orbit, possesses migrating lymphocytes and plasma cells in the interstitium of lobes after inflammatory stimulation, reactive pseudo-tumors (Figure 1), pseudo-lymphomas, and malignant lymphomas (Figure 2) are often observed there. In the current article, we discuss the incidence, etiology, diagnosis, and treatment of ocular adnexal MALT lymphoma, and focus on the possibility of microorganisms as pathogenetic factors in ocular adnexal MALT lymphoma, especially chlamydial infections.

Chapter VII - Conjunctivitis is the inflammation of conjunctiva, which is manifested as vasodilatation/hyperemia, edema and exudation. Conjunctivitis may arise due to bacterial or viral infections or due to allergy or injury by chemical or physical agents. A number of chemical mediators like prostaglandins and leukotrienes derived from arachidonic acid cascade, histamine released from mast cells, and cytokines from lymphocytes, monocytes and macrophages have been implicated in the mediation of inflammatory response. Topical management of conjunctivitis involves the treatment of underlying cause and associated inflammation. The differential clinical diagnosis of bacterial and viral conjunctivitis is very difficult. Acute bacterial conjunctivitis is self-limiting, but the use of topical antibiotics improves the rate of clinical recovery. Conventionally topical corticosteroids were employed in management of inflammation but because of their tendency to raise the intraocular pressure, facilitate infection and cataract formation, they have been replaced by the safer non-steroidal anti-inflammatory drugs (NSAIDs). Current treatment modalities for allergic conjunctivitis include topical mast cell stabilizers / antihistaminic, and NSAIDs.

In: Conjunctivitis: Symptoms, Treatment and Prevention   ISBN: 978-1-61668-321-4
Editor: Anna R. Sallinger, pp. 1-73   © 2010 Nova Science Publishers, Inc.

Chapter I

ALLERGIC DISORDERS OF THE CONJUNCTIVA

De Gaulle I. Chigbu and *Andrew S. Gurwood*

Pennsylvania College of Optometry at Salus University, Elkins Park, PA 19027, USA.

ABSTRACT

The allergic response is an over-reaction of the body's immune system to innocuous
foreign substances or allergens, such as airborne pollen, animal dander, house dust mite,
that the body perceives as a potential threat or undesirable. It is a malady that is estimated
to affect approximately 20 % of the population. Of this subset, at least 20% suffer from a
specific subset of signs and symptoms known as ocular allergy. Both systemic allergy
and ocular allergy have a significant impact on the quality of life of the individual.
Allergic diseases involve antibody- and/or T-lymphocyte mediated mechanisms.

Allergic disorders of the conjunctiva are characterized by specific responses such as:
1) an IgE-mast cell mediated response, as seen in allergic conjunctivitis and 2) chronic
mast cell activation and eosinophil/T-lymphocyte mediated response, as seen in giant
papillary conjunctivitis, vernal keratoconjunctivitis and atopic keratoconjunctivitis.
Traditionally, the signs and symptoms of ocular allergy include itching, tearing, redness,
chemosis and eyelid edema. The mechanism of allergic eye disease includes: 1) allergen-
induced immunoglobulin E (IgE) production and mast cell sensitization; 2) IgE-mediated
mast cell degranulation and the release of preformed mediators and chemotactic factors;
and 3) persistent mast cell activation and Th2-mediated delayed-type hypersensitivity
(DTH) reaction, involving the actions of newly formed mediators and chemotactic
factors that incite the recruitment of additional inflammatory cells, which then leads to
the allergen-induced late phase allergic response.

The management of allergic disorders of the conjunctiva is aimed at avoiding
exposure to allergen, preventing the release of mediators of allergy, controlling the
allergic inflammatory cascade and preventing ocular surface damage. The clinician
should recommend non-pharmacologic and pharmacologic therapeutic regimens that
address the acute presentation of ocular allergy and provide prophylaxis aimed at

---

* Correspondence concerning this article should be addressed to: Dr. De Gaulle I. Chigbu, Pennsylvania College
of Optometry at Salus University, 8360 Old York Road, Elkins Park, PA 19027, USA.

providing long-term maintenance therapy. The clinician may use pharmaceutical agents that prevent mast cell degranulation; block the histamine receptors; inhibit the arachidonic acid cascade; inhibit T-lymphocyte activation; inhibit IgE production by activated B-lymphocytes; and block the action of cyclooxygenase and/or inhibit Lipoxygenase.

1. INTRODUCTION[1]

Allergy is an over-reaction of the body's immune system to harmless foreign substances or allergens, such as airborne pollen, animal dander, house dust mite, that the body perceives as undesirable. It is a malady that is estimated to affect approximately 20 % of the population, of which, at least 20 % suffer from ocular allergy (Leonardi 2005; Pavesio and Decory 2008). The incidence of ocular allergy may vary by geographical location; however, it is more widespread in individuals that suffer from allergic disorders such as atopic dermatitis and asthma (Manzouri, Flynn et al. 2006). Ocular allergy is a disease that affects the ocular surface and its adnexa (Leonardi, De Dominicis et al. 2007; Leonardi, Motterle et al. 2008; Uchio, Kimura et al. 2008). It ranges in severity from mild forms, which can interfere with one's quality of life, to severe cases with increased potential for causing visual impairment (Leonardi, Motterle et al. 2008).

Allergic disorders of the conjunctiva include perennial allergic conjunctivitis (PAC), seasonal allergic conjunctivitis (SAC), giant papillary conjunctivitis (GPC), vernal keratoconjunctivitis (VKC), atopic keratoconjunctivitis (AKC), and contact dermatoconjunctivitis (CDC). These conditions have a significant impact on the quality of life and wellbeing of the individual. An allergic eye condition can affect learning performance in school-aged individuals and work productivity in adults. Allergic disease imposes a significant burden on the economy of countries in the form of rising healthcare costs and reduced productivity through lost man-days (Pawankar 2007). Seasonal allergens include tree pollen (early spring), grass pollen (May-July), weed (ragweed) pollen (August-October) and outdoor molds such as Cladosporium, Alternaria, epicoccum, aerospora, and basidiospores (Reiss, Abelson et al. 1996). The perennial allergens include house dust mites (Dermatophagoides farinea and D. pteronyssinus), indoor molds [aspergillus species (A. flavis and A. fumigates) and penicillium species], feather, cockroaches, and animal dander (dog and cat dander) (Reiss, Abelson et al. 1996).

Allergic eye diseases encompass antibody-mediated disorders and/or T-lymphocyte-mediated disorders. Ocular allergy is an adaptive immune response mounted against the presence of allergens on the eye. The key cellular components of ocular allergy are mast cells, eosinophils and T-lymphocytes (Manzouri, Flynn et al. 2006). The pathophysiological mechanism of acute ocular allergy involves acute antibody (Immunoglobulin E [IgE]-)mediated mast cell degranulation and minimal presence of migratory inflammatory cells. In

---

[1] Portions of this chapter appeared in Chigbu DI. The pathophysiology of ocular allergy: a review. Contact Lens Anterior Eye. 2009 Feb; 32(1): 3-15 with permission; and Chigbu DI. The Management of Allergic Eye Diseases in Primary Eye Care. Contact Lens Anterior Eye. 2009 Dec; **32**(6): 260-272 with permission.

chronic ocular allergy, the pathophysiology consists of persistent activation of mast cells and eosinoiphil-T-lymphocyte-mediated delayed-type hypersensitivity (DTH) response (McGill, Holgate et al. 1998; Berdy 1999; Leonardi 1999; Stahl, Cook et al. 2002).

In allergic disorders of the conjunctiva, the ocular allergic response results from the exposure of the conjunctiva to an environmental allergen and the allergen-induced cross linking of IgE to specific IgE receptors on the surface of the conjunctival mast cells (Leonardi, De Dominicis et al. 2007). This triggers mast cell activation and subsequent release of preformed and newly synthesized mediators, as well as cytokines and chemotactic factors (Rosenwasser, Mahr et al. ; Leonardi, De Dominicis et al. 2007). The release of these mediators leads to the development of clinical manifestations of ocular allergy (Rosenwasser, Mahr et al.).

Most individuals with signs and symptoms of ocular allergy present with complaints of itchy, red watery eyes. Others have chemosis and eyelid edema. Skin prick testing or the radioallergosorbent (RAST) test can be used to confirm the diagnosis of allergy and identify the offending allergen (Manzouri, Flynn et al. 2006). A skin prick test examines the existence of sensitization to given allergens whereas RAST evaluates the amount of specific IgE antibodies in serum (Lambiase, Minchiotti et al.). Skin prick test or RAST are of limited use in diagnosing chronic ocular allergies since it has been reported that more than 40% of these patients have negative results on these tests (Bonini, Lambiase et al. 2003; Bonini 2004; Bonini, Coassin et al. 2004). Tear cytology or conjunctival scrapping is useful in assessing the type and number of cells involved in the conjunctival inflammation (Bonini 2004; Leonardi, De Dominicis et al. 2007).

The treatment options for allergic disorders of the conjunctiva range from non-pharmacological to pharmacological management using supportive, prophylactic and pharmaceutical therapy. Although removal or avoidance of the offending allergens that incite allergy is the only absolute cure for allergic eye disease, when this is impossible, the clinician should recommend any of the above mentioned treatment options. When non-pharmacologic management fails to mitigate an allergic reaction, the next step is to prescribe specific pharmacological agents, basing the selection on a comprehensive case history and the diagnostic classification and disease process. The clinician may use pharmaceutical agents that prevent mast cell degranulation, block the histamine receptors, inhibit the release of arachidonic acid, inhibit T–lymphocyte activation, block the action of cyclooxygenase and inhibit Lipoxygenase pathway or combinations.

In this chapter, the basic concepts of immunology with emphasis on adaptive immunity, and lymphocyte activation as well as the components of the immune system that are relevant to ocular allergy will be discussed. Moreover, a detailed review of the clinical features, immunopathogenesis and histopathological manifestations of allergic disorders of the conjunctiva will be discussed, since such knowledge is critical to achieving success in the treatment and management of ocular allergy. The antibody- and cell-mediated immune hypersensitivity reaction will also be discussed, with particular emphasis on the different phases of ocular allergic immune response involved in allergic disorders of the conjunctiva. The treatment and management options including the preventative measures, as well as the complications and prognosis of the allergic disorders of the conjunctiva will be discussed in detail.

2. IMMUNOLOGY RELEVANT TO ALLERGIC EYE DISEASE

2.1. Introduction

The main function of the response mounted by the immune system is to discriminate between self and non-self and thereby eliminate what it considers to be foreign (Goodman 1991). The two levels of defense against invasion by foreign agents are innate immunity (antigen-non-specific defense mechanism) and adaptive immunity (antigen- specific defense mechanism) (Goodman 1991).

Innate immunity is present from birth. The surfaces of the body (skin, mucous membranes) provide a physical barrier against foreign substance and infections, which is reinforced by secretions (Goodman 1991). The monocytes, macrophages, basophils, mast cells, eosinophils, natural killer cells (NK cells) and cytokines meditate the innate immune system (Male and Roitt 1989; Goodman 1991; Siminovitch 1992).

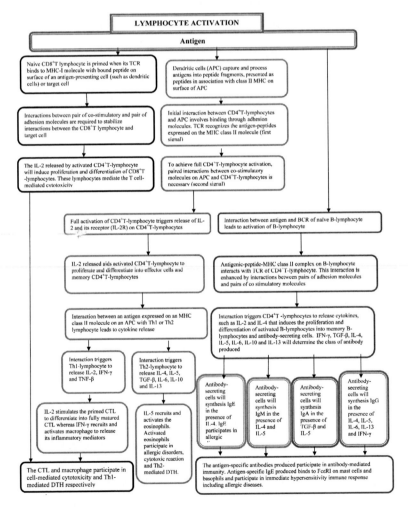

Figure 1. Lymphocyte Activation.

The adaptive immune response is composed of humoral immunity mediated by B-lymphocytes and cell-mediated immunity mediated by T-lymphocytes. Humoral immunity is an adaptive immune response that involves the production of $CD4^+$T-lymphocyte-derived cytokines, which act to signal the B-lymphocytes to produce antibodies in response to an antigen. Cell-mediated immunity is an adaptive immune response that involves the production of antigen-specific cytotoxic T-lymphocytes and effector $CD4^+$T-lymphocytes along with cytokines in response to antigen (Del Prete, Maggi et al. 1994).

The adaptive (acquired) immune system is designed to react with and remove specific antigens. It improves upon repeated exposure to a given antigen and involves antigen presenting cells; the activation and proliferation of lymphocytes; differentiation of lymphocytes into effector cells and memory cells and cytokines (Figure 1) (Male 1989 ; Goodman 1991; Lanier 1991; Siminovitch 1992). The characteristics of the adaptive immune system includes the ability to distinguish one antigen from another (specificity); cells with antigen receptors that have the ability to recognize antigen (diversity); the ability to produce immune cells that can recognize and/or eliminate the antigen (amplification); the ability to produce an immune response to a specific antigen upon re-exposure of the host to the antigen (memory); and the ability to distinguish between self and non-self (tolerance) (Siminovitch 1992)

2.2. Lymphocyte Activation

The first step in the adaptive immune pathway is the process of activating the naïve $CD4^+$T-lymphocytes. These lymphocytes require activation, expansion and differentiation signals for clonal expansion and differentiation of naïve T-lymphocytes to occur. The first (activation) signal is triggered by recognition of peptide- major histocompatibility complex (MHC) by T-lymphocyte Antigen Receptor (TCR) on $CD4^+$T-lymphocyte. The second (co-stimulatory) signal involves co-stimulatory interactions. The third (differentiation) signals involve directing T-lymphocyte differentiation (Murphy 2008). Antigen-presenting cells (APC), such as dendritic cells, capture and process the allergens into peptide fragments, which are presented as peptides in association with class II major histocompatibility complex (MHC) on the surface of the APC. This results in the formation of class II MHC-allergen complex on the APC. The initial interaction between $CD4^+$T-lymphocytes and APCs involves non-specific binding through adhesion molecules such as intercellular adhesion molecule -1 (ICAM-1) on the APC and lymphocyte function-associated antigen-1 (LFA-1) on $CD4^+$T-lymphocytes. This non-specific binding allows the T cell Antigen Receptor on naïve $CD4^+$T-lymphocytes to fully interact with MHC-peptide complex on the APC. This interaction of specific peptide-MHC complex with the TCR on T-lymphocyte activates naïve T-lymphocytes but it is not enough to promote T-lymphocyte differentiation and proliferation into effector cells. The specificity of the APC- $CD4^+$ T-lymphocytes interactions occurs, once the TCR recognizes the allergen-peptides expressed on the MHC class II molecule (this is the first or activation signal) (Male 1996; Akbar 2006; Delves 2006; Trowsdale 2006.). To achieve full $CD4^+$T-lymphocyte activation, interactions between co-stimulatory molecules or ligands on the APC and co-stimulatory receptors on the $CD4^+$T-lymphocytes (co-stimulatory signals involve interactions of CD28 on T-lymphocytes with B7 (B7.1 or B7.2) molecules on APC) is necessary. B7 on APC is the most potent co-stimulator (Benjamin 2000; Delves 2006; Taylor 2007). This signal is involved in promoting the survival and proliferation of naïve T-lymphocytes (this is the co-stimulatory or survival and expansion signal). Cytotoxic T-Lymphocyte Antigen 4 (CTLA-4) is another CD28-related protein that has a high affinity for B7 molecules. The interaction between CTLA-4 (CD152) and B7 molecules will inhibit the proliferation of activated T-lymphocytes (Murphy 2008). Co-stimulatory interactions between CD28 and B7 molecules contribute to the production of IL-2. CD4$^+$T-lymphocyte releases IL-2 and its receptor (IL-2R) on the CD4$^+$T-lymphocytes. IL-2 produced by the activated T-lymphocyte drives the differentiation of activated T-lymphocytes into effector T-lymphocytes (differentiation signal). The third (differentiation) signal is primarily involved in directing T-lymphocyte differentiation into effector T-lymphocytes. When a T-lymphocyte recognizes specific antigen in the absence of co-stimulation through its CD28 molecule, little IL-2 is produced and the T-lymphocyte does not proliferate. Thus, the most important function of the co-stimulatory signal is to promote the synthesis of IL-2 (Murphy 2008). The activated CD4$^+$T-lymphocyte proliferate into identical CD4$^+$T-lymphocytes, and subsequently differentiate into Th1-lymphocytes and Th2-lymphocytes, as well as memory CD4$^+$T-lymphocytes (Figure 1) (Hendricks 1996; Streilein 1996; Ashrafzadeh and Raizman 2003) CD4$^+$T-lymphocyte induces the activation and maturation of B-lymphocytes and cytotoxic T-lymphocytes. Th1-derived cytokines promote macrophage activation; antibody-dependent cell-mediated cytotoxicity; and Th1-mediated delayed-type hypersensitivity (DTH). Th2-lymphocytes release cytokines that are responsible for mucosal immunity, IgA synthesis, eosinophils accumulation (Interleukin (IL)-5), IgE antibody production by B-lymphocytes (IL-4 and IL-13), mast cells growth (IL-4 and IL-10), and mucus hyperproduction (IL-9, IL-13) (Uchio, Ono et al. 2000; Bonini, Lambiase et al. 2003; Delves 2006; Marini 2006). Th2-lymphocyte derived-cytokines play an important pathophysiological role in ocular allergic conditions (Leonardi 1999; Uchio, Ono et al. 2000).

The development of the antibody-mediated immunity usually involves the action of CD4$^+$T-lymphocytes, B-lymphocytes, CD4$^+$T-lymphocytes-derived cytokines, and antigen. Antigen-specific activation of B-lymphocytes occurs, when an antigen binds to antigen receptors of a resting B-lymphocyte, and the antigen is subsequently processed and presented as peptides in association with MHC class II molecules on the B-lymphocyte. B-lymphocytes are involved in activating T-lymphocytes to provide antigen-specific help to B-lymphocyte. Resting B-lymphocytes become activated to proliferate and differentiate, when interactions between antigen peptide-MHC complex on B-cell receptors (BCR) and TCR of the CD4$^+$T-lymphocyte is accompanied by interactions of pairs of adhesion molecules (ICAM-1 on B-lymphocytes and LFA-1 on CD4$^+$T-lymphocyte) and pairs of co-stimulatory molecules (CD40 on B-lymphocytes and CD40L [CD 154] on the CD4$^+$T-lymphocyte) on the B-lymphocyte and CD4$^+$T-lymphocytes. The co-stimulation signals through CD40-CD40L interactions are essential for efficient B-lymphocyte activation, as well as promoting B-lymphocyte proliferation and antibody synthesis. This pathway of antigen presentation allows B-lymphocytes to be targeted by antigen-specific CD4 T-lymphocytes, which drive their differentiation. The B-lymphocyte-CD4$^+$T-lymphocyte interaction triggers the CD4$^+$T-lymphocytes to release cytokines (IL-2 and IL-4) that will enable the activated B-lymphocytes to proliferate into identical B-lymphocytes, as well as differentiate into memory B-lymphocytes and antibody secreting cells (Lanier 1991; Benjamin 2000; Delves 2006; Marini 2006; Murphy 2008; Murphy 2008). Th1- and Th2-derived cytokines promote differentiation of activated B-lymphocytes into antibody-secreting cells, which are capable of secreting antibodies such as Immunoglobulin G (IgG), IgA, IgM, IgE and IgD. The products of the proliferation and differentiation of the B-lymphocytes mediate the antibody-mediated immunity (Figure 1) (Lanier 1991; Marini 2006; Lydyard 2006). TCR-MHC interactions and co-stimulatory molecule interactions are necessary signals for the proliferation and differentiation of naïve T-lymphocytes. Interaction of adhesion pairs plays a role in enhancing the bond between T-lymphocytes to APC. Co-stimulatory interactions are essential during the activation of unprimed T-lymphocytes, but they are less likely to play a central role in the activation of primed or memory T-lymphocytes. Antigen-driven differentiation of B-lymphocytes and T-lymphocytes will also result in the production of memory cells (Benjamin 2000; Delves 2006).

2.3. Immune Hypersensitivity Reaction in Allergic Eye Diseases

Antibody and cell-mediated immune hypersensitivity reaction occurs when the adaptive immune system overreacts in response to an antigen with consequential tissue damage (Schmid and Schmid 2000). The immune hypersensitivity mechanisms involved in allergic disorders include IgE-mediated hypersensitivity response, IgG-mediated hypersensitivity reactions and T-lymphocyte-mediated hypersensitivity response (Terr 1994). The immune hypersensitivity that will be discussed in this chapter are IgE-mediated immediate hypersensitivity and T-lymphocyte mediated hypersensitivity mechanisms.

2.3.1. Antibody-Mediated Hypersensitivity in Allergic Eye Diseases

Antibody-mediated hypersensitivity reactions are characterized by allergen-induced mast cell activation and include IgG- and IgE-mediated hypersensitivity reactions. Antigen-mediated mast cell activation plays an important role in the initiation of cellular reaction in ocular allergy (Tkaczyk, Okayama et al. 2004).

2.3.1.1. IgG-Mediated Hypersensitivity Immune Reactions

Human mast cells treated with interferon gamma (IFN-γ) up-regulate the high affinity IgG receptor (FcγR) (Woolhiser, Brockow et al. 2004). Interactions between IgG and FcγR are crucial to the initiation of hypersensitivity immune responses (Sibéril, Dutertre et al. 2006). The activation of FcγR on the surface of the mast cells regulates Th2-dependent inflammatory responses. Allergen-specific IgG plays a role in Th2-lymphocyte-mediated disease (Bandukwala, Clay et al. 2007).

IgG, particularly of the IgG1 subtype complexed to soluble protein antigen binds to FcγR on APC with subsequent development of IgG-antigen-FcγR APC complex (Hjelm, Carlsson et al. 2006). The antigen is processed and presented as antigen peptides on MHC-II to specific CD4$^+$T-lymphocytes, which undergo clonal expansion and differentiation. The activated CD4$^+$T-lymphocytes interact with antigen-specific B-lymphocyte resulting in an antibody response. Antigen specificity is provided by antibodies that happen to be present in the environment and bind to FcγR (Hjelm, Carlsson et al. 2006; Malbec and Daëron 2007). When a previously sensitized eye is re-exposed to the same allergen later, a hypersensitivity reaction will be initiated, as the allergen binds to the IgG1 molecules on the FcγRI on the surface of the sensitized mast cells. This leads to cross linking of the FcγRI on sensitized mast cells. Aggregation of FcγRI on mast cells leads to degranulation and generation of preformed and newly formed mediators (prostaglandins, thromboxaness, and leukotrienes) as well as the release of both cytokines and chemotactic factors. The biologic consequence of recruiting mast cells into the site of inflammation through IgG-dependent activation is similar to those observed following IgE-dependent activation (Woolhiser, Okayama et al. 2001; Tkaczyk, Okayama et al. 2002; Woolhiser, Brockow et al. 2004).

IgG1 was the only IgG isotype that mediated significant mast cell activation (Woolhiser, Okayama et al. 2001). Minimal degranulation was observed when mast cells were incubated with IgG2, IgG3 and IgG4 followed by the appropriate antibody to aggregate the IgG bound receptors (Tkaczyk, Okayama et al. 2002). IgG1 antibodies are capable of activating the classic complement cascade leading to production of anaphylatoxins, e.g., C3a and C5a, and the release of vasoactive amines from mast cells (Ballow, Mendelson et al. 1984).

2.3.1.2. IgE-Mediated Hypersensitivity Immune Reactions

The phases of *IgE-mediated hypersensitivity* reactions include 1] antigen-driven IgE antibody production and the binding of antigen-specific IgE to the high affinity IgE receptors (FcεRI) on mast cells (*sensitization phase*); 2] re-exposure of the ocular surface to allergen induces mast cell degranulation with release of allergic mediators, a physiologic/biochemical process mediated by antigen-driven cross-linking of IgE bound to FcεRI on sensitized mast cells (*activation phase*); and 3] the clinical manifestations of the early and late phase response, reactions which are attributable to the effects of the mediators released following mast cell activation (*effector phase*) (Benjamin, Coico et al. 2000).

The mechanism of the IgE-mediated ocular allergic response occurs in three phases: the sensitization process, the early phase response, and the late phase response. The early-phase reaction lasts for 20-40 minutes following ocular allergen challenge, while the late phase response occurs approximately 4-6 hours after the early phase response (Solomon, Pe'er et al. 2001). The late phase response leads to persistence of the allergic expression and chronic inflammation of the ocular surface. The early phase response (EPR) is mediated by histamine whereas the late phase is mediated by the newly-formed mediators of mast cell activation and inflammatory cells. The phases of the ocular allergic response are discussed below.

Sensitization Phase of Ocular Allergy: This occurs on initial exposure of the ocular surface to allergens, and there are no ocular manifestations of allergic response in this phase (Epstein 2002). When deposited on the conjunctival mucosal epithelium, the environmental allergens are captured and processed by the APC into peptide fragments, which are displayed on the surface of the APC by MHC class II molecules (Abelson 2002). The peptide fragment/MHC II complex on the APC interacts with the TCR on the naïve CD4+-lymphocytes. The TCR-MHC interaction in conjunction with paired interactions between costimulatory molecules on the APC and naïve CD4+T-lymphocytes leads to the activation of the naïve CD4+T-lymphocytes, and its subsequent differentiation into Th2-lymphocytes

(Hendricks and Tang 1996; Leonardi 1999). The interaction between the Th2-lymphocytes and the B-lymphocytes triggers the release of Th2 cytokines (IL-4, IL-5, IL-6, IL-10, and IL-13). The B-lymphocytes, which recognized the same allergen that induced the Th2-lymphocyte differentiation, will in the presence of IL-4 and other signals from accessory molecules differentiate into antibody-producing plasma cells, with subsequent production of antigen-specific IgE antibodies (Hendricks and Tang 1996; Leonardi 1999; Butrus and Portela 2005). The antigen-specific IgE antibodies produced becomes specific for that particular antigen and binds to the high affinity IgE receptors (FcεRI) located on the surface of mast cells, a step that primes the mast cell for subsequent allergen exposure, completing the process of sensitization (Figure 2) (Goodman 1991).

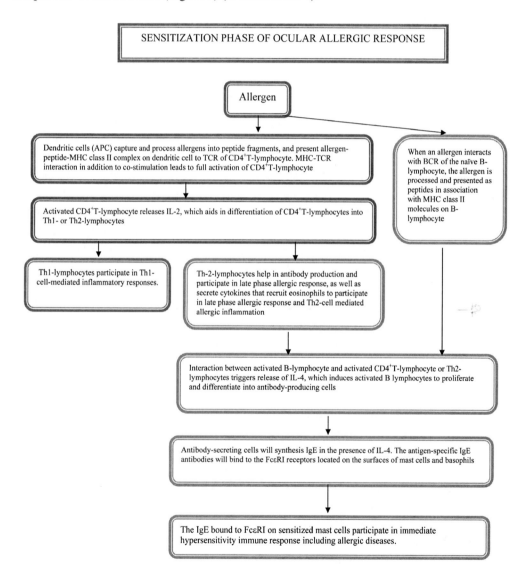

Figure 2. Sensitization Phase of Ocular Allergic Response.

Figure 2

Early Phase Response (EPR) of Ocular Allergy: When a previously sensitized eye is re-exposed to the same allergen later, an allergic reaction will be initiated as the allergen binds to the IgE molecules on the FcεRI receptors on the surface of the sensitized mast cells leading to cross linking of FcεRI on sensitized mast cells (Butrus and Portela 2005). This triggers a change in the affected mast cell outer membrane, which renders it more permeable to calcium ions with subsequent mobilization of intracellular calcium (Berdy 1999; Tabbara 2003). The influx of calcium ion into the mast cells initiates the biochemical process that results in the degranulation of the mast cell (Terr 1991; Reiss, Abelson et al. 1996). Mast cell degranulation leads to the following: 1] immediate release of preformed mediators such as biogenic amines (histamine), neutral proteases (chymase, tryptase), proteoglycans (heparin), chemotactic factors, and acid hydrolases, which set in motion the allergic response; 2] activation of phospholipase A2, which causes the release of arachidonic acid (AA) metabolites from membrane phospholipids (occurs within minutes of mast cell activation); 3] release cytokines (IL-4, IL-5, IL-6, IL-9, IL-13, TNF-α, and granulocyte macrophage-colony-stimulating factor [GM-CSF]) within minutes to hours following mast cell activation; and 4] activation of vascular endothelial cells by mast cell-derived cytokines triggers the expression chemokines (RANTES, monocytes chemotactic protein-1, IL-8, eotaxin) and adhesion molecules (intercellular adhesion molecule (ICAM)-1, vascular cell adhesion molecule (VCAM)-1 and so on (Brown, Wilson et al. 2008; Irani 2008). The preformed mediators are primarily responsible for the early phase symptoms, which last for approximately 40 minutes following initial exposure. The histamine released stimulates the blood vessels (when histamine binds to H1 and H2 receptors on endothelial smooth muscles), nerves (when histamine binds to H1 receptors on nerves), and mucous-producing glands resulting in the hallmark signs and symptoms of ocular allergy (redness, itching, tearing, chemosis and eyelid edema) (Leonardi 1999; Abelson, Smith et al. 2003). The AA metabolites are then biosynthesized via the cyclooxygenase pathway into prostaglandins (PGD2, PGE1, PGE2) and thromboxanes; and via the lipoxygenase pathway into leukotrienes (LTB4, LTC4, LTD4) (Howarth 2002). The products of arachidonic acid metabolism are referred to as the newly-formed mediators. The adhesion molecules and chemokines released by the activated vascular endothelial cell recruits and activates eosinophils and other inflammatory cells to the site of allergic exposure (Abelson, Smith et al. 2003). Cytokines activate ocular surface (conjunctival and corneal) epithelial cells and fibroblasts to express cytokines, chemokines and adhesion molecules. The chemokines (e.g. eotaxins and TARC) and adhesion molecules (e.g. VCAM-1 and ICAM-1) mediate the recruitment of eosinophils and other inflammatory cell types to the site of late phase reaction (LPR). Thymus- and activation-regulated chemokine (TARC), a potent chemoattractant for Th2-lymphocytes, mediate the recruitment of Th2-lymphocytes to the site of allergic inflammation (Brown, Wilson et al. 2008; Irani 2008). The newly-formed mediators and chemotactic factors contribute to the inflammatory reaction, and incite recruitment and activation of inflammatory cells, leading to the late phase of the allergic response (Figure 3) (Lemanske 1983; Cousins and Rouse 1996). The release of preformed and newly formed mediators in the EPR represents the immunopathophysiology of ocular allergy (Bonini 2006).

Late Phase Response (LPR) of Ocular Allergy: The late phase of the allergic reaction commences 4 to 6 hours after the mast cells releases their pre-formed and newly formed mediators (Epstein 2002). This response is characterized by T-lymphocyte activation, the production of Th2-lymphocyte-derived cytokines and infiltration of the conjunctiva by eosinophils, neutrophils, and basophils (Durham 1998). The chemotactic factors released during the EPR mediate the recruitment and activation of inflammatory cells to the site of allergic reaction, resulting in the infiltration of the conjunctiva by eosinophils, neutrophils, T-lymphocytes, monocytes, and basophils (Hendricks and Tang 1996; Durham 1998; Leonardi 1999; Askenase 2000; Abelson, Smith et al. 2003; Leonardi 2005). The eosinophils release their granule products, such as eosinophil major basic protein, which are capable of inducing a chronic allergic inflammatory response typical of a Th2-mediated DTH/LPR (Romagnani 1994; Cousins and Rouse 1996; Askenase 2000; Abelson, Smith et al. 2003).

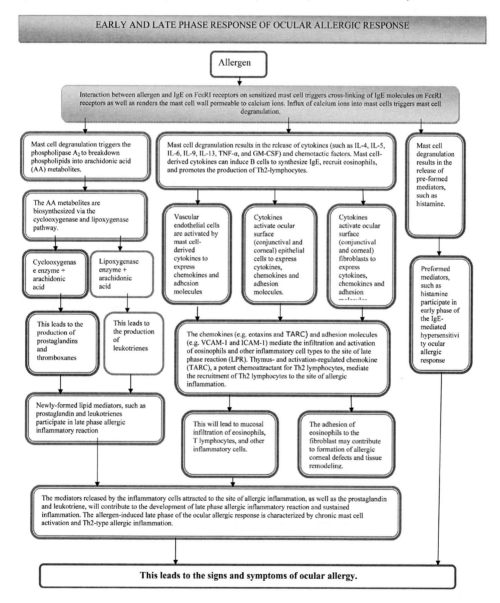

Figure 3. The Early and Late Phase Response of IgE-mediated hypersensitivity in Ocular Allergy.

The mediators released by the inflammatory cells attracted to the site of allergic inflammation, as well as the prostaglandin and leukotriene, will contribute to the continued symptomatology and the development of late phase allergic inflammatory reaction (Figure 3) (Leonardi 1999). The late phase reaction is a persistent process that intensifies the allergic inflammation and heightens the entire allergic mechanism, thus prolonging the allergic expression (Leonardi 1999). The release of histamine by both mast cell and basophil in late phase response by histamine-releasing factors, and the activation of vascular endothelial cells, epithelial cells and fibroblasts are other mechanisms that may intensify the allergic inflammation (Leonardi 1999; Abelson, Smith et al. 2003). Co-stimulatory molecular interactions affect the induction of Th2 immunity and the late phase response in allergic eye diseases (Niederkorn 2008). The LPR is an essential aspect of the immunopathophysiology of chronic ocular allergy. The LPR effects are the major cause of ocular surface damage, such as keratitis, limbal infiltration, tissue remodeling, and corneal ulceration that occurs in the ocular allergic diseases (Abelson 2002).

2.3.2. T-Lymphocite-Mediated Hypersensitivity in Allergic Eye Diseases

T-lymphocyte mediated hypersensitivity response occurs when allergen react with antigen-specific sensitized Th1 or Th2-lymphocytes with consequential release of cytokines. The IFN-gamma (Th1-derived cytokine) and IL-5 (Th2-derived cytokine) will recruit and activate macrophage and eosinophil to the site of allergic inflammation respectively. The process occurs in two phases – the sensitization phase and elicitation phase. The *sensitization phase* occurs when APC, such as Langerhans' cells present processed haptenic peptide-MHC class II complex to T-lymphocytes with consequential differentiation of $CD4^+T$-lymphocytes into effector $CD4^+T$-lymphocytes and memory T-lymphocytes. The *elicitation phase* occurs when memory T-lymphocytes recognize the allergen peptide together with MHC class II molecules on Langerhans cells. This interaction between the TCR on the memory $CD4^+T$-lymphocytes and MHC on the Langerhans cells stimulates the memory T-lymphocyte to proliferate and release cytokines that mediate T-lymphocyte mediated hypersensitivity response (Delves, Martin et al. 2006; Griffiths 2006). Th1-derived cytokines, such as IFN-γ induces recruitment and activation of macrophage leading to Th1-mediated delayed-type hypersensitivity (Akbar 2006). It plays a role in contact dermatitis (Romagnani 1994). Th2-derived cytokines, such as IL-5 stimulates the chemotaxis and activation of eosinophil to the site of inflammation leading to Th2-mediated delayed-type hypersensitivity (Akbar 2006). Th2-lymphocyte mediated DTH is characterized by chronic IgE production, as well as mast cell and eosinophil activation. It plays a role in atopic dermatitis and late phase response of allergic diseases (Romagnani 1994).

3. Cells and Mediators in Allergic Eye Disease

3.1. Antigen

Antigen is a substance or molecule, foreign to the host that can induce an immune response following interaction with lymphocytes (Adkinson 1990).

3.2. Antibodies

Antibodies are immunoglobulins produced by B-lymphocytes in response to antigenic stimulation. They have the ability to react with the specific antigens that stimulated their production (Male 1996; Chigbu 2009). The five classes of antibodies are IgG (Immunoglobulin G), IgM (Immunoglobulin M), IgA (Immunoglobulin A), IgD (Immunoglobulin D), and IgE (Immunoglobulin E). Immunoglobulins participate in antibody-mediated hypersensitivity immune reactions.

3.3. B Lymphocytes

B-lymphocytes are cells, produced in the bone marrow, which become activated following a primary exposure to an antigen (Feldmann and Male 1989; Lanier 1991). They express immunoglobulin on cell surface membranes. These immunoglobulins act as antigen receptors (Lanier 1991). The majority of B-lymphocytes carry MHC class II antigens (Lydyard P 1989). Th2-lymphocytes interact with B-lymphocytes and help them to proliferate, differentiate and secrete antibodies (Male 2006.; Chigbu 2009).

3.4. Antigen Presenting Cells

Antigen presenting cells (APC) are cells (macrophages, B-lymphocytes and dendritic cells) that are capable of taking up antigen, processing it and then presenting it to the lymphocytes in a form they can recognize (Revillard ; Turner 1989; Cousins and Rouse 1996). They link the innate and adaptive immune systems by producing cytokines, which enhance innate immunity and contribute to lymphocyte activation and function. They display antigen peptide-MHC complexes on their surface as well as express co-stimulatory signals that are necessary for initiating immune responses. B-lymphocytes and macrophages present antigen primarily to previously sensitized T-lymphocytes, whereas dendritic cells are involved in triggering primary T-lymphocyte responses as well as secondary responses of resting memory T-lymphocytes (Male 1996; Chigbu 2009).

3.5. Dendritic Cells

Dendritic cells are the principal antigen presenting cells involved in the induction and maintenance of Th2-mediated allergic responses (Lambrecht 2001; Chigbu 2009). These cells function to: 1] present antigen to naïve T-lymphocytes in primary immune response; 2] trigger antigen-driven secondary responses of resting memory T-lymphocytes and 3] stimulate allergen-specific memory Th2-lymphocytes to produce Th2 cytokines, which can contribute to allergic inflammation (Kamani NR 1991; Cousins and Rouse 1996; Streilein 1996; Rissoan, Soumelis et al. 1999; Moser and Murphy 2000; Lambrecht 2001).

3.6. Major histocomapibility complex (MHC)

MHC is a cell surface recognition structure that plays a role in the transporting processed antigen in the form of a complex to T-lymphocytes (Owen 1989).

3.7. Tryptase

Tryptase, a major protease released by mast cells, is a specific marker of mast-cell activation. It is capable of cleaving C3 and C3a (Solomon, Pe'er et al. 2001; Leonardi 2002).

3.8. Histamine

Histamine, a major vasoactive mediator stored in mast cells and basophils, is the foremost pro-inflammatory allergic mediator that accounts for the majority of signs and symptoms of the allergic reaction (Deschenes, Discepola et al. 1999; Tabbara 2003). Histamine is released by activated mast cells and basophils (Kumar 2009). Histamine exerts its biological effects by interacting with four G-protein coupled receptors, classified as H1-H4. The binding of histamine at the H1 receptor on blood vessels and nerve cells induces the vasodilation and itching of allergy respectively. The stimulation of H2 receptors also contributes to vasodilation (Leonardi 1999; Abelson 2002). It also modifies the behavior of the conjunctiva epithelium and fibroblasts (Kumar 2009).

3.9. Langerhans Cells (LC)

Langerhans cells are involved in exogenous antigen recognition, antigen processing and activation of T-lymphocytes (Zhan, Smith et al. 2003). They express numerous receptors for IgE, IgG, IL-2 and C3 on their cell surface. Allergen binding to IgE on epidermal LC results in T-lymphocyte proliferation (Casey and Abelson 1997; Zhan, Smith et al. 2003). Clinical studies have suggested that interaction of CD86 on Langerhans cells with T-lymphocytes mediates the development of the Th2-type immune response and plays a major role in regulating the inflammatory reaction seen in chronic ocular allergy (Abu-El-Asrar, Al-Kharashi et al. 2001).

3.10. Mast Cells

Mast cells originate from hematopoietic stem cells and differentiate under the influence of stem cell factor (Irani 2008). In the normal conjunctiva, the mast cells are concentrated in the conjunctival substantia propria (Leonardi 1999; Howarth 2002; Leonardi 2002). Mast cells are important effector cells in the conjunctiva (Galatowicz, Ajayi et al. 2007). They play a pivotal role in initiating the inflammatory cascade in allergic eye disease (Kumar 2009). Mast cells express Fe (epsilon) RI and Fcγ (gamma) R on their cell surface, which enables them to bind IgE and IgG respectively (Malbec and Daëron 2007; Kumar 2009). Mast cell FcγR include activating and inhibitory receptors (Malbec and Daëron 2007). Human mast cells have been shown to chemoattract C3a (Woolhiser, Brockow et al. 2004). Mast cells are involved in allergy and autoimmunity (Malbec and Daëron 2007).

The mast cell plays a fundamental role in releasing pro-allergy (e.g. histamine) and pro-inflammatory mediators, leading to the clinical presentation of ocular allergy (Solomon, Pe'er et al. 2001). Basophils are the blood borne equivalent of the tissue-bound mast cell (Cousins and Rouse 1996). Activated mast cells can release cytokines such as IL-4, IL-6, IL-8, IL-13, tumour necrosis factor (TNF)-α and transforming growth factor (TGF)-b, which have profound effects on the mucosa. They also release chemokines and adhesion molecules that contribute to the recruitment of **inflammatory** cells (Leonardi, Motterle et al. 2008).

Immunohistochemical studies have demonstrated the presence two types of mast cells. Tryptase-positive (MC_T) mast cells contain tryptase. Chymase-positive (MC_{TC}) mast cells contain both tryptase and chymase (Elhers and Donshik 2008). Immunohistochemical phenotyping of mast cells (MC) in the normal human conjunctiva has demonstrated that the MC_{TC} (tryptase and chymase-positive MC) phenotype is predominant (Donshik, Ehlers et al. 2008; Leonardi, Motterle et al. 2008). The MC_T mast cell appears to be dependent on functional T-lymphocytes, whereas MC_{TC} mast cells are not dependent on functional T-lymphocytes (Donshik, Ehlers et al. 2008). MC_{TC} mast cells expresses IL-4, a cytokine that plays a key role in allergy promoting T-lymphocyte growth, inducing IgE production from B-lymphocytes, upregulating the adhesion molecules and regulating T helper type 2-lymphocyte differentiation (Leonardi, De Dominicis et al. 2007).

Specific allergen-induced mast cell degranulation results in the release of pro-inflammatory mediators, including histamine, proteases, prostaglandin D2 and leukotriene C4. These mediators are responsible for causing the clinical manifestation of ocular allergy (Kumar 2009).

3.11. Prostaglandins

Prostaglandin, a potent inflammatory mediator, is formed from the cyclooxygenase pathway of arachidonic acid metabolism (Cousins and Rouse 1996; Howarth 2002). Prostaglandins D2 (PGD2), a major prostaglandin, is produced by connective tissue mast cells (Terr 1997). An increase in the production of PGD2 has been observed by human mast cells via both IgG1- and IgE-dependent mechanisms (Woolhiser, Okayama et al. 2001). Prostaglandins E1 (PGE1) and Prostaglandins E2 (PGE2) induces vasodilation, redness, swelling, and pain (Howarth 2002).

3.12. Leukotrienes

Leukotriene, a potent inflammatory mediator formed from the lipoxygenase pathway of the arachidonic acid metabolism, plays an important role in the pathogenesis of allergic disorders (Terr 1997). Leukotriene D4 (LTD4) and Leukotrienes E4 (LTE4) are chemotactic only for eosinophils, whereas Leukotriene B4 (LTB4) is chemotactic for eosinophils and neutrophils (Cousins and Rouse 1996; Solomon, Pe'er et al. 2001). LTC4, LTB4, LTD4 and LTE4 are released by mucosal mast cells (Terr 1997). Although studies have shown an increase in the production of LTC4 following FcγRI and FcεRI aggregation, there was significant generation of LTC4 with IgE cross linking (Woolhiser, Okayama et al. 2001). The biological activities of leukotrienes on the conjunctiva may contribute to the presence of the characteristic manifestations of ocular allergy, such as excessive mucous secretion, conjunctival hyperemia and chemosis. They also play a role in papillary formation (Bonini, Coassin et al. 2004; Bielory, Katelaris et al. 2007; Elhers and Donshik 2008).

3.13. Adhesion Molecules

Adhesion molecules play a pivotal role in the recruitment of leukocytes to the site of inflammation. It has been demonstrated that over expression of cell adhesion molecules promotes the recruitment of inflammatory cells. It is a key player in the pathogenesis of chronic ocular allergies, such as VKC (Abu el-Asrar, Geboes et al. 1997).

The cell adhesion molecules are classified into three major families: 1] the integrins; 2] the immunoglobulin gene superfamily; and 3] the selectins. Very late activation antigen-4 (VLA-4) and lymphocyte function associated antigen-1 (LFA-1) are members of the integrin family. Intercellular adhesion molecule -1 (ICAM-1), ICAM-3 and vascular cell adhesion molecule-1 (VCAM-1) are members of the immunoglobulin gene superfamily. E-selectin, L-selectin and P-selectin are members of the selectin family. It has been shown that interferon gamma (IFN-γ), interleukin-1 beta (IL-1β) and tumor necrosis factor-alpha (TNF-α) can induce the expression of ICAM-1. In the normal conjunctiva, the expression of endothelial leukocyte adhesion molecule-1 (ELAM-1) and VCAM-1 was virtually non-existent. It has been reported that ELAM-1 mediates adherence of neutrophils, monocytes and some memory T-lymphocytes to vascular endothelium in the early phase of inflammatory reactions (Abu el-Asrar, Geboes et al. 1997). ICAM-1 may play an important role in homing and migration of neutrophils and eosinophils that are involved in the inflammatory process or reaction (Zhan, Smith et al. 2003).

3.14. Neutrophils

Neutrophils, also called polymorphonuclear leukocytes (PMNs), are efficient phagocytes and act as important effector cells through the release of granule products and cytokines. They are the predominant cells in ocular inflammations and play a role in acute T-lymphocyte-mediated delayed hypersensitivity reactions of the conjunctiva (Cousins and Rouse 1996). It has been reported that neutrophils play a role in tissue destruction of the cornea. Reactive oxygen metabolites, a toxic mediator produced by neutrophils, are capable of tissue destruction during inflammation (Shimmura, Igarashi et al. 2003). Neutrophils and Neutrophil-derived mediators (Neutrophil myeloperoxidase, elastase) are also increased in chronic ocular allergies such as VKC and AKC (Cook 2004).

3.15. Complement

Complement plays a vital role in immune hypersensitivity reactions. Activation of the complement system leads to generation of C3a, a potent pro-inflammatory mediator and marker for complement activation. C3a is capable of triggering mast cell degranulation with subsequent release of pro-inflammatory and pro-allergic mediators (Meijer, Pogany et al. 1993).

3.16. Matrix Metalloproteinases (MMP)

MMPs are extracellular endopeptidases that selectively degrade components of the extracellular matrix (Kumar 2009). MMP are key enzymes for normal extracellular matrix (ECM) turnover and for breakdown of ECM associated with inflammatory reactions and wound healing (Abu El-Asrar, Van Aelst et al. 2001).

MMP-9 can be produced by many inflammatory cells, such as macrophages, neutrophils, mast cells, eosinophils, epithelial cells, conjunctival fibroblasts, T-lymphocytes, and monocytes (Leonardi, Brun et al. 2007; Kumar 2009). Double immunohistochemical analysis has shown that 90% of gelatinase B is expressed by eosinophils whereas 10% of monocytes/macrophages express gelatinase B. Gelatinase B (MMP-9) also plays a role in extracellular matrix remodeling in VKC (Abu El-Asrar, Van Aelst et al. 2001). It is predominantly secreted by eosinophils and functions with EMBP and ECP to cause corneal epitheliopathy and ulcer (Leonardi, De Dominicis et al. 2007).

The presence and activation of MMP-9 as well as MMP-2 is characteristic of allergic inflammation in the conjunctiva (Kumagai, Yamamoto et al. 2002).

Kumagai et al demonstrated in their study that the prevalence of active forms of MMP-2 and MMP-9 was significantly higher in patients with VKC than those with allergic conjunctivitis. Although, non-allergic conjunctivae contained the proform of the MMP-2 and MMP-9, the active forms of MMP-2 and MMP-9 were absent. It has been demonstrated that the marked presence of the active forms of MMP-2 and MMP-9 plays a role in the pathogenesis of corneal lesions in VKC (Tuft, Cree et al. 1998; Kumagai, Yamamoto et al. 2002).

3.17. Growth Factors

Growth factors, such as epidermal growth factor (EGF), fibroblast growth factor (FBF), and transforming growth factor beta 1 (TGFβ-1) induce fibroblast growth and procollagen. These growth factors participate in the pathogenesis of chronic ocular allergy such as VKC (Kumar 2009).

3.18. Eosinophils

Eosinophils are predominantly found on mucosal epithelial surfaces exposed to the external environment (Srivastava, Sur et al. 2003). They cause profound changes in the conjunctival mucous, as well as play a role in the development and progression of ocular allergic disease (Leonardi, Brun et al. 2003).

The presence of a high percentage of eosinophils in tear fluid and in conjunctival tissues is a characteristic feature of chronic ocular allergy [(Leonardi and Secchi 2003)]. Chemokines, adhesion molecules and cytokines are involved in the recruitment of eosinophils to the site of inflammation (Abu El-Asrar, Struyf et al. 2000; Abu El-Asrar, Struyf et al. 2001).

It has been demonstrated that eosinophils are involved in keratopathy and tissue remodeling in ocular allergy (Cook, Stahl et al. 2006). Activated eosinophils release strong basic cytotoxic proteins such as eosinophils major basic protein (EMBP), eosinophil cationic protein (ECP), eosinophil peroxidase (EPO) and eosinophil derived neurotoxin (EDN). These cytotoxic proteins are released in the conjunctiva and tear fluid, and damage the conjunctival and corneal epithelium (Abu El-Asrar, Struyf et al. 2000; Abu El-Asrar, Struyf et al. 2001). The cytotoxic effect of eosinophilic mediators has been shown to have an adverse effect on the epithelium wound healing in VKC patients with corneal ulcer (Leonardi and Secchi 2003).

Eosinophil major basic protein is toxic to corneal epithelial cells. EMBP, a cytotoxic mediator, is capable of inhibiting wound healing of the corneal epithelium as well as causing superficial keratitis and corneal ulceration in patients with severe VKC (Cameron, Antonios et al. ; Gupta, Sharma et al. 1999).

Eosinophil Chemotactic Factor (ECF) released from mast cells is a potent chemo-attractant for eosinophil migration into the conjunctiva (Reiss, Abelson et al. 1996).

3.19. Epithelial Cells

Ocular surface epithelial cells act as mechanical barrier to prevent entry of foreign particles including bacteria and virus into the eye (Irkeç and Bozkurt 2003; Calonge and Enríquez-de-Salamanca 2005). Several studies have demonstrated the ability of epithelial cells to produce chemokines and cytokines upon stimulation. Ocular surface epithelial cells, upon stimulation by mast cell-derived cytokines, will express cytokines, chemokines and adhesion molecules (Hingorani, Calder et al. 1998; Calonge and Enríquez-de-Salamanca 2005). They play a role in the pathogenesis of ocular allergic inflammatory disorders via expression of cytokines, adhesion molecules and chemokines. These chemoattractants promote eosinophilia. They also promote the proliferation, differentiation, activation and chemotaxis of various inflammatory cell types to the site allergic inflammation (Hingorani, Calder et al. 1998; Irkeç and Bozkurt 2003; Calonge and Enríquez-de-Salamanca 2005).

3.20. Fibroblast

Fibroblasts are the immune modulators of ocular allergic disorders. IL-4 and IL-13 stimulates corneal fibroblasts to express chemokines (eotaxins and thymus- and activation-regulated chemokine [TARC]) and adhesion molecules (VCAM-1 and ICAM-1). TARC is a potent chemoattractant for Th2-lymphocytes, and eotaxins and adhesion molecules mediate the infiltration and activation of eosinophils. Conjunctival fibroblasts produce extracellular matrix (ECM) and tissue inhibitor of matrix metalloproteinase that contribute to excessive deposition of ECM that is characteristic of giant papillae in chronic ocular allergy (Fukuda 2005; Fukuda, Kumagai et al. 2006). Corneal and conjunctival fibroblasts contribute to tissue remodeling [(Kumar 2009)]. TGF-β, IL-1 and Th2-derived cytokines stimulates conjunctival fibroblasts to produce vascular endothelial growth factor (VEGF), which may play a crucial role in neovascularization and formation of giant papillae in chronic ocular allergy (Asano-Kato, Fukagawa et al. 2005).

Fibroblasts can modulate the functions of mast cells and eosinophils through the membrane form of stem cell factor and granulocyte macrophage colony-stimulating factor (GM-CSF), respectively (Solomon, Puxeddu et al. 2003).

3.21. T-Lymphocytes

T-lymphocytes are cells, developed in the thymus, which have definite cell markers called T cell antigen receptors (TCR). T-lymphocytes initiate the immune response, mediate antigen-specific effector responses and regulate the activity of other leukocytes by secreting cytokines (Lanier 1991). The interaction between dendritic cells and naïve T-lymphocytes leads to the production of cytotoxic T-lymphocytes, Th2-lymphocytes and Th1-lymphocytes (Rook 1989; Romagnani 1994; Ashrafzadeh and Raizman 2003). Memory T-lymphocytes are capable of initiating a second immune response against an antigen, when the host is re-exposed to the same antigen (Lanier 1991).

Activated T-lymphocytes play a vital role in the pathogenesis of chronic allergic inflammation. Th2-lymphocytes are responsible for increased production of IgE, recruitment and activation of mast cells and eosinophils (Kumar 2009). Th2-lymphocytes play a pivotal role in the development of allergic disorders by producing regulatory and inflammatory cytokines such as IL4, IL-5 and IL-13 (Leonardi, Fregona et al. 2006). Th2-type cytokines IL-4 and IL-13 stimulate the migration, proliferation and collagen production from conjunctival fibroblasts (Leonardi, De Dominicis et al. 2007; Leonardi, Motterle et al. 2008).

CD4+CD25+ regulatory T-lymphocytes constitute about 5%-10% of peripheral CD4+T-lymphocytes in humans and play a pivotal role in preventing or controlling immune-mediated inflammations and autoimmune reactions (Lydyard P 1989; Akbar and Cook 2006; Chen 2006; Wraith 2006). CD4+CD25+ regulatory T-lymphocytes sustain the normal immunosuppressive ocular microenvironment through their production of immunosuppressive cytokines such as TGF-β and suppression of inflammatory T-lymphocyte activity (Calder and Lackie 2004). It may play a beneficial role in controlling allergic diseases, since it has the ability to suppress both Th1 and Th2 responses (Akbar and Cook 2006; Wraith 2006).

3.22. Co-Stimulatory Molecules and Receptors

B7 (B7.1 [CD80] AND B7.2 [CD86]) are co-stimulatory molecules or ligands. They are cell surface proteins on antigen presenting cells (APC) that interact with cell surface (co-stimulatory) receptors on naïve T-lymphocytes, to transmit a signal that is required along with antigen stimulus to T-lymphocyte activation (Leonardi, De Dominicis et al. 2007; Murphy 2008). Co-stimulatory molecule CD86 is essential for the successful antigen presentation and the development of the Th2-lymphocyte-mediated immune response. It is expressed by Langerhans cells in conjunctiva. Thus, antigen-presenting cells provide an important mechanism for Th2-lymphocyte activation (Kumar 2009). Studies have shown that blockade of CD86 co stimulatory molecules on APC at the time of initial sensitization to allergens will result in reduced T-lymphocyte production of IL-5, a key Th2-derived cytokine necessary for recruitment of eosinophils (Niederkorn 2008).

CD28 is a co-stimulatory receptor on the surface of all naïve T-lymphocytes and binds to co-stimulatory ligands or molecules B7 molecules (CD80 and CD86), which are expressed mainly on antigen-presenting cells such as dendritic cells (Leonardi, De Dominicis et al. 2007; Murphy 2008).

Immunohistochemical studies have suggested that the CD28/CD86 co-stimulatory pathway may be involved in the pathogenesis of VKC. Several studies have demonstrated that the CD28/CD86 costimulatory pathway is required for antigen-induced eosinophil recruitment, Th2-derived cytokine production and local production of IgE in allergic inflammation (Leonardi, De Dominicis et al. 2007).

Cytotoxic T-Lymphocyte Antigen 4 (CTLA-4) is another CD28-related protein that has a high affinity for B7 molecules. The interaction between CTLA-4 (CD152) and B7 molecules will inhibit the proliferation of activated T-lymphocytes. CD28 interaction with co-stimulatory ligands on APC will enhance T cell receptor signaling whereas CTLA-4 interaction with the same co-stimulatory ligand will cause an inhibition of the T- cell receptor signaling (Leonardi, De Dominicis et al. 2007; Murphy 2008).

3.23. Cytokines

Cytokines are small secreted proteins that mediate and regulate immunity and inflammation (Kumar 2009). Cytokines are potent inflammatory mediators produced by lymphocytes and mast cells in response to an antigen (Oppenheim, Ruscetti et al. 1991; Terr 1997). They mediate or signal interactions between cells,as well as function as chemical messengers for regulating the immune system (Oppenheim, Ruscetti et al. 1991). Interleukins (ILs) are the cytokines that are made by leukocytes and act on other leukocytes (Kumar 2009). Activated helper T-lymphocytes, mast cells and eosinophils are the main cytokine-producing cell types infiltrating the conjunctiva in chronic ocular allergy (Kumar 2009). Th1-lymphocytes secrete IL-2, IFN-γ and TNF-β while Th2-lymphocytes secrete IL-4, IL-5, IL-6, IL-9, IL-10, and IL-13 (Romagnani 1994; Chandler 1996.; Ashrafzadeh and Raizman 2003).

Interleukin-2 (IL-2), produced mainly by CD4$^+$T-lymphocytes, promotes the differentiation and proliferation of activated CD4$^+$T-lymphocytes and CD8$^+$T-lymphocytes, as well as driving B-lymphocyte proliferation (Abu El-Asrar, Struyf et al. 2003; Leonardi and Secchi 2003).

Interleukin-4 (IL-4) is the chief cytokine involved in the secretion of immunoglobulins, particularly IgG and IgE in response to T-dependent antigens (Rook 1989; Delves, Martin et al. 2006). IL-4 plays a critical role in switching of B-lymphocytes to produce IgE, promoting T-lymphocyte growth, and up-regulating Th2-lymphocyte subset differentiation, and as such, they may play an important role in the pathogenesis of ocular allergy (Uchio, Ono et al. 2000; Kumar 2009). IL-4 may be produced by mast cells in allergic conjunctivitis and is predominantly produced by Th2-lymphocytes in chronic ocular allergy (Ozcan, Ersoz et al. 2007). IL-4 is localized to MC_{TC} mast cell phenotype (Abelson, Smith et al. 2003).

Interleukin-5 (IL-5) is produced mainly by Th2-lymphocytes and is localized to the MC_T mast cell (Abelson, Smith et al. 2003). It activates mature eosinophils, prolongs their survival and contributes to their accumulation at sites of inflammation (Uchio, Ono et al. 2000). Additionally, it is capable of stimulating the proliferation and differentiation of antigen-activated B-lymphocytes (Feldmann and Male 1989).

The Interleukin-10 (IL-10), produced by the Th2-lymphocytes, is an immunosuppressive cytokine that inhibits Th1-derived cytokine production by reducing the ability of macrophages to present antigens to Th1-lymphocytes (Mosman 1992). IL-10 has recently been shown to stabilize mast cells and reduce their degranulation in vitro and as a result attenuate allergic conjunctivitis (Li, Tripathi et al. 2008).

Interleukin-12 (IL-12), produced mainly by macrophages and dendritic cells, is an inducer of cell-mediated immunity. It stimulates the synthesis of IFN-γ and the differentiation of naive T4-lymphocytes into IFN-γ producing Th1-lymphocytes (Park 2001).

Interleukin-13 (IL-13), produced mainly by Th2-lymphocytes, is involved in the production of IgE by B-lymphocytes (Feldmann and Male 1989; Bonini, Lambiase et al. 2003). Like IL-4, it is also localized to MC_{TC} mast cell phenotype (Abelson, Smith et al. 2003).

Interferon-gamma (IFN-γ), produced primarily by Th1-lymphocytes, T8-Lymphocytes, and NK cells, is the principal cytokine for activating macrophages (Rook 1989). IFN-γ is an important mediator in the delayed type-hypersensitivity (DTH) reaction (Romagnani 1994).

Alpha-melanocyte stimulating hormone (α-MSH), an immunosuppressive cytokine and anti-inflammatory neuropeptide, stimulates the activation of regulatory T-lymphocytes and suppresses the induction of T-lymphocyte-mediated DTH response (Calder and Lackie 2004; Taylor 2007).

TGF-beta, an immunosuppressive or immunoregulatory cytokine, is involved in the regulation of the immune response (Chen 2006). In the ocular microenvironment, it acts to alter APC (macrophages and dendritic cells) production, prevents DTH reactions and contributes to aqueous humor induction of regulatory T-lymphocytes (Taylor 2007). It also depresses the proliferation of T-lymphocytes, B-lymphocytes and NK cells (Male 1996).

3.24. Chemokines

Chemokine, a chemotactic cytokine (CC), is a potent activator and chemoattractant (Kumar 2009). Chemokines are produced by inflammatory cells, stimulated epithelial cells, fibroblasts and vascular endothelial cells in the conjunctiva (Leonardi and Secchi 2003). Chemokines transport and recruit leukocytes during inflammation by inducing chemotaxis and inflammatory cell activation at site of inflammation (Kumar 2009). The four subfamilies of chemokines include CXC subfamily, CC subfamily, C subfamily and the CX3C subfamily. CC chemokines include monocyte chemotactic protein (MCP), regulated upon activation, normal T cells expressed and secreted (RANTES), macrophage inhibitory protein (MIP), thymus and activation-regulated chemokine (TARC) and eotaxin. The CC-chemokines act on eosinophils, basophils, monocytes and lymphocytes, suggesting their important role in the pathogenesis of ocular allergy (Abu El-Asrar, Struyf et al. 2000; Kumar 2009).

Exotaxin is a potent and selective eosinophil chemoattractant. It has the ability to induce the release of reactive oxygen species, which have been shown to be damaging to the tissue (Abu El-Asrar, Struyf et al. 2000).

RANTES is a potent chemoattractant for eosinophils, basophils, monocyte/macrophages and CD45RO/CD4$^+$ memory T-lymphocytes (Abu El-Asrar, Struyf et al. 2000)

The chemokine IL-8 actively secreted by macrophages and epithelial cells is a chemoattractant as well as an activator of neutrophils. It plays a crucial role in inflammatory cell migration (Kumar 2009).

4. PHARMACOLOGIC THERAPY OF ALLERGIC EYE DISEASE

The primary treatment for allergic eye conditions in general is removal of the offending agent. To that effect, a non-pharmacological approach is typically the first step in the management of allergic disorders of the conjunctiva. The secondary treatment algorithm includes the addition of pharmacological agents with anti-allergic and anti-inflammatory properties (Manzouri, Flynn et al. 2006).

4.1. Vasoconstrictors

Antihistamine/vasoconstrictor combinations contain both an antihistamine (e.g. antazoline phosphate) and vasoconstrictor (e.g. naphazoline or phenylepherine). The antihistamines in these topical agents help to decrease the itch associated with allergic conjunctivitis. The vasoconstrictors in these agents are adrenergic agonists that stimulate α-adrenoreceptors. They are capable of reducing the chemosis, redness and eyelid edema resulting from tissue congestion (Bielory 2008). Antihistamine/vasoconstrictor combination agents are indicated for relieving the symptoms and signs of allergic conjunctivitis. The antihistamine/vasoconstrictor combination agents are relatively fast acting but the duration of action last only 2 to 4 hours. Dosing more frequently has the potential to cause adverse effects (Leonardi 2005; Bielory 2008; Bielory 2008). These agents have a limited duration of action, and as such, they may not provide all day coverage for prevention of allergy signs and symptoms (Abelson and Greiner 2004). The adverse effects of these agents include burning and stinging on instillation; mydriasis, especially in patients with lighter irides; follicular conjunctivitis; eczematoid blepharoconjunctivitis and rebound hyperemia or conjunctivitis medicamentosa (an allergic reaction to the agent itself) with long-term use (Bielory 2008). The clinician should use caution when prescribing vasoconstrictors to patients with cardiovascular disease, hyperthyroidism or angle-closure glaucoma. The non-specificity of the pharmacologic action of antihistamine/vasoconstrictors combination agents in dealing with the ocular allergic response and its adverse ocular effects makes them inappropriate for long term use (Leonardi 2005; Bielory, Katelaris et al. 2007).

4.2. Antihistamines

In general, older or first-generation oral H1 receptor antagonists, such as chlorphenamine or cyclizine were agents with both symptom relieving and sedating effects. Today, new, second-generation agents are non-sedating. The sedative effect is due to their lipophilic nature, which enables first-generation agents to cross the blood–brain barrier and inhibit the central neurotransmitter effects of histamine. The most serious adverse side effect of the first generation antihistamines is cardiotoxicity in the form of an increase in the QT interval with potential for cardiac arrhythmia. The newer second-generation drugs (such as cetirizine, desloratidine, fexofenadine and loratidine) have safer cardiac side effect profiles (Manzouri, Flynn et al. 2006).

Oral antihistamines have a slower onset of action than topical agents and may cause ocular and systemic adverse effects. Topical treatment is, therefore, preferable for isolated allergic disorders of the conjunctiva. Topical H1 antagonists have much lower systemic absorption, and as such, they have fewer side effects than their oral counterparts. The second-generation topical H1 receptor antagonists have little or no effect on dopaminergic, adrenergic or serotonin-mediated receptors, and have a prolonged clinical effect (Manzouri, Flynn et al. 2006).

The new generation topical antihistamines such as levocabastine 0.05% and emedastine 0.05% are superior to the first generation topical antihistamines (pheniramine and antazoline) and work by competitively blocking histamine receptors on the ocular mucosal surface (Bielory 2008). The first generation topical antihistamines have limited potency whereas the newer antihistamines have longer duration and are well tolerated (Leonardi 2005). Levocabastine HCl ophthalmic suspension 0.05 %, a cyclohexy-3-methylpiperidine derivative, is a potent topical selective H1-receptor antihistamine suspension with rapid onset of action. On average, it exerts an effect within 15 minutes of administration and has a prolonged clinical effect lasting up to 4 hours (Noble and McTavish 1995). It has been shown, in an ocular allergen challenge model, to downregulate intracellular adhesion molecules by almost 50%. Clinical studies have shown the duration of action of levocabastine to exceed 4 hours with a recommended dose of four times a day as needed

(Manzouri, Flynn et al. 2006). Emedastine difumarate 0.05% ophthalmic solution is a safe and effective selective histamine H1-receptor antagonist with no apparent effects on adrenergic, dopaminergic or serotonin receptors (Kumar 2009). It is indicated for the temporary relief of the signs and symptoms associated with allergic conjunctivitis (Discepola, Deschenes et al. 1999). It is also recommended at a dosage of four times a day as needed. Clinical studies comparing ketotifen and emedastine suggested that emedastine and ketotifen are not significantly different with respect to anti-itching efficacy in the CAC model of acute allergic conjunctivitis (D'Arienzo, Leonardi et al. 2002; Horak, Stübner et al. 2003).

4.3. Mast Cell Stabilizers

Topical mast cell stabilizers prevent the release of allergic mediators from mast cells by suppressing mast cell degranulation. The blockade of mast cell degranulation inhibits the release of preformed and newly formed mediators of allergy. It also inhibits the release of chemokines and cytokines (Abelson, Smith et al. 2003; Bielory 2008). They also achieve their clinical effect by preventing calcium influx across the cell membrane (Katelaris, Ciprandi et al. 2002; Leonardi 2002). Mast cell stabilizers are safe and effective for the long term therapeutic management of allergic eye diseases. They require a loading time of up to two weeks since it has no effect on acute allergic reactions induced by histamine already released on the ocular surface (Bonini, Lambiase et al. 2003; Bielory, Katelaris et al. 2007). All mast cell stabilizers are dosed four-times-daily, except nedocromil, which is dosed twice-daily.

Sodium cromoglycate is a mast cell stabilizer that is suitable for long term prophylaxis and therapeutic management of ocular allergy. It is not as effective at inhibiting the degranulation of mucosal mast cells. This may explain the poor response of chronic ocular allergies to sodium cromoglycate (Leonardi 2002). The efficacy of the medication seems to be dependent on the concentration of the solution used (Manzouri, Flynn et al. 2006). The major adverse effect is burning and stinging. The 4% formulation is dosed four to six times daily, and tapered to twice daily when symptoms subside (Bielory 2008).

Lodoxamide Tromethamine 0.1% ophthalmic solution possesses mast-cell stabilizing properties that are considered to be 2500 times more potent than that of sodium cromolyn (Bielory 2008). Better efficacy of lodoxamide was linked to significantly decreased CD4[+]T-lymphocytes and inflammatory cells, especially eosinophils in conjunctiva (Kumar 2009). It is safe for use in children and adults on a four-times-daily dosing for up to 3 months. The most common side effects are burning or stinging (Bielory 2008).

Pemirolast potassium 0.1% ophthalmic solution, a pyridopyrimidine compound, is a mast cell stabilizer that is used for the treatment of seasonal allergic and vernal conjunctivitis. It is dosed four-times-daily and it is safe for use in children as young as 2 years of age (Bielory 2008).

Nedocromil sodium 2% ophthalmic solution, a pyranoquinoline dicarboxylic acid, is a potent stabilizer of both connective and mucosal type mast cells (Leonardi 2005; Bielory 2008). It has been reported that mast cell stabilization by Nedocromil sodium may be due to its ability to inhibit chloride ion flux in mast cells, epithelial cells and neurons (Manzouri,

Flynn et al. 2006). The inhibition of IgE production by B-lymphocytes may be an alternative mechanism of this action (Solomon, Pe'er et al. 2001; Manzouri, Flynn et al. 2006). In patients with chronic ocular allergies, nedocromil sodium has been shown to be very effective at preventing release of allergic mediators from the mucosal type mast cell. Nedocromil sodium ophthalmic solution is an effective and well tolerated anti-allergic agent for the long-term management of ocular allergies (Alexander, Allegro et al. ; Verin 1998). It is associated with ocular stinging or burning upon instillation and a distinctive taste (Bielory 2008).

4.4. Multimodal or Dual Acting Agents

Antihistamine/Mast cell Stabilizing combinations are multimodal action anti-allergic agents that act as both a histamine receptor antagonist and a mast cell stabilizer. Olopatadine ophthalmic solution, epinastine ophthalmic solution, ketotifen ophthalmic solution, and azelastine ophthalmic solution are topical anti-allergic pharmaceutical agents that are readily available. These agents reduce the allergic cascade by providing immediate symptomatic relief by blocking histamine receptors and inhibiting the release of allergic mediators via stabilization of mast cells. Multimodal agents with both antihistamine and mast cell stabilizing properties have been tested within the conjunctival allergen challenge (CAC) model and have proven to be efficacious for up to 8 hours (Abelson, Gomes et al.).

Olopatadine HCL (0.1% and 0.2%) ophthalmic solution is a multimodal anti-allergic agent that possesses selective H1-receptor antagonism and mast cell stabilizing features. It inhibits the release of allergic mediators from mast cells and prevents histamine from producing its effects on the eye (Bielory 2008). It has a rapid onset of action and prolonged clinical effect (Berdy, Stoppel et al. 2002). The prolonged clinical effect of olopatadine could be attributed to its ability to suppress the release of allergic mediators and inhibit inflammatory cell recruitment. It reduces all signs and symptoms of allergic conjunctivitis, including redness, itching, chemosis, tearing and eyelid edema. Olopatadine is approved for the treatment of the signs and symptoms of allergic conjunctivitis (Berdy, Stoppel et al. 2002; Abelson and Gomes 2008). The olopatadine 0.1% formulation is dosed twice daily whereas the olopatadine 0.2% formulation is dosed once daily. The safety of olopatadine along with tolerability and efficacy has been well established. Multiple clinical studies have shown that olopatadine has exceptional duration of action, efficacy, and tolerability (Abelson, Gomes et al.). The agent demonstrates clear efficacy for relief from ocular pruritus and has the advantage of having a more neutral PH with lower surface activity (Bielory, Buddiga et al. 2004). Another clinical study demonstrated that olopatadine 0.2% reduced the signs and symptoms of allergic conjunctivitis, both at onset of action and 16 hours after medication instillation, demonstrating significant length of action. Data produced by June et al, in their study, suggested that olopatadine does not interfere with allergy skin testing making discontinuation in preparation for skin prick testing unnecessary (Jones, Temino et al. 2008)(Abelson, Gomes et al.). Several studies have shown that olopatadine 0.2% is effective for up to 24 hours after instillation when dosed once daily with a well tolerated safety profile in adults and children of 3 years of age and older. Finally, olopatadine has been reported to have the ability to decrease the mucus discharge in VKC by reducing the goblet cell density in the conjunctiva (Corum, Yeniad et al. 2005; Kumar 2009).

Azelastine HCl 0.05% ophthalmic solution, a phthalazinone derivative, is a twice-a-day dosed multiple-action anti-allergic agent. It has a rapid onset of action and is capable of inhibiting release of allergic mediators. Azelastine ophthalmic solution is indicated for the treatment or relief of ocular itching associated with allergic conjunctivitis. It has a noticeable bitter taste and can cause ocular stinging upon instillation (Ciprandi, Buscaglia et al. 1997; Spangler, Bensch et al. 2001; Bielory 2008). This phthalazinone derivative functions as a topical ocular selective histamine H1-receptor antagonist and an inhibitor of mast cell mediator release and other pro-inflammatory mediators. It has duration of action of up to 8 hours. It is approved for use in adults and children 3 years of age and older. It has demonstrated histamine H1 and H2 receptor antagonist activity and also inhibits histamine release from mast cells following antigen and non-antigenic stimuli. Its anti-inflammatory properties appear to stem from its ability to inhibit mast cell mediator release, as well as inhibit leukotriene (LT) production (Bielory, Buddiga et al. 2004). Topical azelastine has been shown to be a potent suppressor of itching and conjunctival hyperemia after conjunctival provocation with an allergen (Manzouri, Flynn et al. 2006). Azelastine reduces antigen induced production of LTC4 and LTD4. It can inhibit the 5-lipoxygenase pathway of arachidonic acid metabolism without much impact on the cyclooxygenase pathway (Bielory, Buddiga et al. 2004).

Ketotifen fumarate 0.025% ophthalmic solution, a benzocycloheptathiophene derivative, is a twice-a-day dosed multi-modal anti-allergic agent. It possesses both mast cell stabilizing and strong H1 receptor antagonism. It is approved for the temporary prevention of ocular itching due to allergic conjunctivitis (Greiner, Michaelson et al. ; Bielory 2008). It is now available as an over-the-counter anti-allergic agent. The medicine works through selective non-competitive blocking of the H1 receptor. Besides mast-cell stabilization and H1 receptor antagonism, it prevents eosinophil accumulation (Kumar 2009). It is also able to inhibit leukotriene formation thereby reducing eosinophil activation and cytokine release (Manzouri, Flynn et al. 2006).

Epinastine 0.05% ophthalmic solution is an antihistamine with mast cell stabilizing and anti-inflammatory properties certified for use as a twice-daily dosed multimodal anti-allergic agent. It is indicated for the prevention of itching associated with allergic conjunctivitis. It has affinity for H1 and H2 receptors with prolonged therapeutic effect lasting up to 12 hours and onset of action within 3 minutes (Friedlaender 2006; Trattler, Luchs et al. 2006).

4.5. Nonsteroidal Anti-Inflammatory Drugs (NSAID)

NSAIDs may be useful, as an adjunct, in treating ocular allergy as they are effective in relieving pruritus and reducing conjunctival hyperemia. It has been shown that Prostaglandin E2 and I2 act to lower the threshold of human skin and conjunctiva to histamine-induced itching. They may be considered a valuable steroid-sparing therapeutic agent since they do not mask ocular infections, affect wound healing, increase intraocular pressure or contribute to the formation of cataracts (Manzouri, Flynn et al. 2006). Topical formulations, such as ketorolac 0.5% and diclofenac 0.1% have been shown to diminish ocular pruritus and conjunctival hyperemia associated with allergic conjunctivitis. The disadvantage of using these preparations is that they have weaker anti-inflammatory action than topical steroidal agents. While these medications reduce conjunctival hyperemia, they have little effect on papillary size (Kumar 2009). Although there may be limited concern over the phenomenon of NSAID-induced asthma (topically or orally), it seems to only be a problem in patients who have the triad of asthma, nasal polyposis and aspirin sensitivity (Verin 1998; Manzouri, Flynn et al. 2006).

4.6. Steroids

Topical corticosteroids are potent anti-allergic agents that are considered appropriate for the treatment of chronic ocular allergic conditions. They have the ability to suppress the recruitment and activation of pro-inflammatory allergic mediators during the late phase of ocular allergic response (Leonardi 2002; Melton and Thomas 2003). They work by blocking the action of mast cell phospholipase A2, an enzyme necessary for the hydrolysis of arachidonic acid, thereby reducing the production of late-phase allergic inflammatory mediators such as prostaglandins and leukotrienes. Steroids are incapable of blocking histamine receptors. However, they can inhibit histamine production in mast cells by blocking the action of histidine decarboxylase. Additionally, corticosteroids can reduce the amount of unbound histamine on the ocular surface by increasing the availability of histaminases. Corticosteroids are not effective in stabilizing mast cells due to their inability to prevent calcium influx into the mast cell. However, they are capable of inhibiting T-lymphocyte response and production of cytokines such as interleukin (IL) 4 and IL-5. Furthermore, corticosteroids can also inhibit neovascularisation and reduce capillary permeability (Durham 1998; Ilyas, Slonim et al. 2004; Butrus and Portela 2005; Bielory 2008). Topical mast cell stabilizers are less effective in controlling the acute exacerbations seen in T-lymphocyte dependent chronic ocular allergy. Topical corticosteroids are the T-lymphocyte-targeted therapeutic agents that are beneficial in treating chronic allergic disorders of the conjunctiva such as VKC and AKC, in which T-lymphocyte infiltration is a prominent feature. Topical steroids are likely to be useful in treating or repairing the ocular surface damage caused by the release of epithelial toxic mediators from eosinophils and neutrophils. It is advisable to start off with steroids with low absorption and enhanced therapeutic index (e.g., loteprednol) with the dosing being based on the state of inflammation of the eye. Rimexolone 1.0% and loteprednol (0.2% and 0.5%) are two modified corticosteroids with low absorption and improved efficacy (Manzouri, Flynn et al. 2006).

Rimexoline (a derivative of prednisolone) is quickly inactivated in the anterior chamber of the eye, thus leading to improved efficacy and decreased safety concerns. When these agents, with lower potency are proven to be ineffective, more potent steroids (prednisolone, dexamethasone, betamethasone) can be employed (Manzouri, Flynn et al. 2006).

Loteprednol etabonate ophthalmic suspension, a site-specific soft steroid, primarily targets the late phase inflammatory aspect of the ocular allergic response. It is site specific in view of the fact that the active drug resides at the site of allergic inflammation long enough to render its therapeutic effect without causing adverse drug reactions, such as raised intraocular pressure (IOP) and cataract (Ilyas, Slonim et al. 2004; Bielory 2008; Pavesio and Decory 2008). Loteprednol is more lipophilic than ketone corticosteroids such as prednisolone and it's highly lipophilic nature may contribute to its increased efficacy by enhancing penetration into target inflammatory cells. The long term use of loteprednol has demonstrated lower propensity to induce IOP elevation even when used in known steroid responders since its active form undergoes rapid transformation into an inactive carboxylic acid metabolite (cortienic acid). This rapid transformation reduces the possibility of toxicity and duration of exposure of the anterior segment including the anterior chamber to the active form of loteprednol. This rapid transformation at the site of inflammation after rendering its therapeutic effect is due to the effect of numerous esterases in the eye. Mainly due to the above mentioned reasons, loteprednol, unlike ketone corticosteroids that have the ketone group at C-20 position, rarely causes cataract formation. Loteprednol is a suitable long term therapeutic option for chronic ocular allergies due to their superior safety profile relative to the ketone corticosteroids. Clinical studies have shown that loteprednol etabonate is a safe treatment option for individuals with allergic ocular inflammation (Berdy, Stoppel et al. 2002; Ilyas, Slonim et al. 2004; Bielory 2008; Pavesio and Decory 2008). It has been demonstrated to be effective in treating allergic conjunctivitis and giant papillary conjunctivitis (Leonardi 2005). Loteprednol etabonate was shown to be safe and effective when used for 12 months or more for the treatment of seasonal or perennial allergic conjunctivitis (Ilyas, Slonim et al. 2004).

Prednisolone acetate 1.0% is a an excellent choice for treating severe inflammatory disorders due to its good ocular penetrability while prednisolone sodium phosphate (0.125% and 1.0%) may be considered a suitable drug for moderate inflammatory disorders of the ocular surface due to its reduced ocular penetrability when compared to prednisolone acetate (Melton and Thomas 2003).

The fluorometholone-based steroids are used for treating mild to moderate ocular surface inflammatory conditions and chronic inflammatory condition requiring prolonged steroidal therapy. They have reduced propensity to induce an IOP rise. The acetate form of fluorometholone-based steroids has greater anti-inflammatory activity than the alcohol form (FML) due to their enhanced bioavailability (Melton and Thomas 2003). Clinical studies have shown that fluorometholone-based steroids reduces the clinical expression of VKC, including discharge, conjunctival redness, papillary hypertrophy and Tranta's dots (Abelson, Smith et al. 2003; Leonardi 2005).

Cream-based steroid such as triamcinolone and hydrocortisone are useful for treating periocular inflammation in contact ocular allergy (Melton and Thomas 2003).

4.7. Anti-Metabolites

Mitomycin C is an inhibitor of fibroblast proliferation. Mitomycin C 0.01% eye drops were shown to decrease the mucous discharge, conjunctival hyperemia and limbal edema in VKC patients refractory to topical steroids and mast-cell stabilizers (Kumar 2009). Despite some evidence of promise, these preparations are not generally considerd in ophthalmic practice.

4.8. Immunomodulators

Immunomodulators, such as cyclosporine and tacrolimus, have the potential to play a vital role in the treatment of allergic eye diseases due to their ability to inhibit calcineurin, a phosphate that is essential to the FcεRI-mediated release of preformed mediators from mast cells (Leonardi 2005). They are capable of blocking mast cell proliferation, inhibiting histamine release, blocking release of cytokines from T-lymphocytes, and reducing eosinophil chemotaxis (Abelson, Smith et al. 2003). The calcineurin inhibitors, cyclosporin A and tacrolimus, are used to induce systemic immunosuppression following organ transplantation. The enzyme calcineurin plays an important role in T-cell receptor signaling following antigen presentation. Cyclosporine A and tacrolimus inactivate calcineurin, thereby inhibiting IL-2 production and T-lymphocyte activation (Manzouri, Flynn et al. 2006).

Tacrolimus is a potent macrolide immunosuppressor in ocular allergy. It exerts its action by inhibiting IgE production by activated B-lymphocytes as well as by inhibiting T-lymphocyte activation and associated pro-inflammatory cytokine production. Tacrolimus also interferes with mast cell degranulation; suppresses antigen presentation by down-regulating FcεRI in epidermal dendritic Langerhans' cells and inflammatory dendritic epithelial cells; and suppresses late phase responses in ocular allergy. It has been shown to be well tolerated with an excellent safety profile for long-term management of dermatitis. Tacrolimus could be therapeutically beneficial for patients with atopic keratoconjunctivitis (AKC), vernal keratoconjunctivitis, atopic eyelid disease and atopic dermatitis (Donnenfeld and Pflugfelder ; Cheer and Plosker 2001; Manzouri, Flynn et al. 2006; Paller, Eichenfield et al. 2008; Katsarou, Armenaka et al. 2009). Transient burning sensation and recurrent herpetic lesions are reported side effects of tacrolimus (Miyazaki, Tominaga et al. 2008). Tacrolimus (0.1 and 0.03%) has been approved for topical use in atopic dermatitis. There are concerns regarding the topical use of tacrolimus. It can induce local immune suppression with the attendant risk of increasing a patient's susceptibility to local infections. Additionally, there is concern that topical tacrolimus may be carcinogenic. The FDA has advised that tacrolimus should be used as labeled since it has the potential to cause cancer (Manzouri, Flynn et al. 2006). Additional side effects of tacrolimus include pancytopenia, hyperglycemia, hyperkalemia, tremor, headache, insomnia, hypertension, dyspnea, pleural effusion, diarrhea, nausea and vomiting, pruritus, muscle cramps, nephropathy and arthalgia (Stumpf, Luqmani et al. 2006). In eyelid dermatitis, tacrolimus ointment was found to be effective and safe without causing skin atrophy, telangiectasia or increased intraocular pressure. Drug concentrations in the systemic circulation are low with topical use (Katsarou, Armenaka et al. 2009). Tacrolimus ointment, unlike steroids, does not reduce collagen synthesis or skin thickness, and as such, it can be used safely on the face and neck (Reitamo, Harper et al. 2004).

Cyclosporine (CsA) is a cyclic undecapeptide produced by the fungi Tolypocladium inflatum and Beauveria nevus. Inhibition of T-lymphocyte activation occurs when cyclosporine binds to cyclophilin A to form a cyclosporine-cyclophilin A complex. The interaction between the cyclosporine-cyclophilin A complex and serine/threonine phosphatase calcineurin results in the inhibition of serine/threonine phosphatase calcineurin. Cyclosporine-mediated inhibition of calcineurin blocks dephosphorylation of NF-AT in the cytoplasm, thereby preventing its transport to the nucleus and preventing increased transcription of the IL-2 gene and other genes involved in T-lymphocyte activation. There is evidence to suggest that calcineurin/NF-AT signaling is involved in cytokine and chemokine production by mast cells and eosinophils (Donnenfeld and Pflugfelder). CsA is quite effective in controlling ocular inflammation by blocking Th2-lymphocyte proliferation and IL-2 production. It also inhibits histamine release from mast cells. It also reduces eosinophil chemotaxis via inhibition of IL-5 production. Furthermore, it inhibits Th2-lymphocyte proliferation and IFN-γ with consequential modulating effect on Th1-lymphocyte-mediated DTH (Keklikci, Soker et al. ; Bonini, Coassin et al. 2004; Bielory 2008). Cyclosporine is prescribed, when steroids are contraindicated or deemed unsafe, for treating the severe form or steroid resistant cases of chronic ocular allergy (Leonardi 2005). A clinical study found that topical 0.05% cyclosporin A, dosed 4 – 6 times daily was effective in alleviating signs and symptoms of severe AKC refractory to topical steroid treatment (Manzouri, Flynn et al. 2006). Ozcan et al showed that topical CsA 0.05% has a significant beneficial effect on patients with VKC and AKC (Keklikci, Soker et al.). Unfortunately, the unavailability of commercial preparations of topical cyclosporine in higher concentrations makes its use in ocular allergy limited (Kumar 2009).

5. SPECIFIC ALLERGIC EYE DISEASES

5.1. Allergic conjunctivitis

Introduction: Allergic conjunctivitis is caused by an allergen-induced inflammatory response in which allergens interact with immunoglobulin E (IgE) bound to sensitized conjunctival mast cells resulting in mediator release and clinical manifestations of allergic conjunctivitis (Scoper, Berdy et al. 2007; Sanchis-Merino, Montero et al. 2008). Allergic conjunctivitis is caused by an IgE-mediated reaction to environmental airborne allergens, such as grass and tree pollens, ragweed, house dust mite, mould and animal dander (Leonardi, Motterle et al. 2008). Seasonal allergic conjunctivitis (SAC) is an intermittent IgE-mediated-condition and perennial allergic conjunctivitis (PAC) is a persistent IgE-mediated condition of the conjunctiva (Leonardi, De Dominicis et al. 2007). Allergic conjunctivitis is characterized by the absence of proliferative changes (Uchio, Kimura et al. 2008).

Approximately 15%-20 % of the population suffers from allergic conjunctivitis (Scoper, Berdy et al. 2007). The most common ocular allergies worldwide are SAC and PAC, with SAC being the most frequent form (Manzouri, Flynn et al. 2006). Allergic conjunctivitis can have a profound effect on the quality of life and wellbeing of an individual. It affects learning performance in school-aged individuals and work productivity in adults (Manzouri, Flynn et al. 2006; Pavesio and Decory 2008). Allergic conjunctivitis is a bilateral, self-limiting conjunctival inflammatory process that occurs in sensitized individuals of either sex. Individuals with allergic conjunctivitis usually have a personal or family history of atopic disease, such as allergic rhinitis, asthma, and/or atopic dermatitis (Manzouri, Flynn et al. 2006).

Pathophysiology and Histopathology: The pathogenesis of allergic conjunctivitis is predominantly an IgE-mediated hypersensitivity reaction. This occurs in three stages. The initial stage is referred to as the sensitization phase. The sensitization phase involves the initial exposure of the ocular surface to the allergens. This phase does not produce the ocular manifestations of allergic response (Epstein 2002). The antigen-specific IgE antibody produced becomes specific for that particular antigen. The antibodies bind to the high affinity IgE receptors (FcεRI) located on the surface of mast cells and basophils. This primes those mast cells for response upon subsequent allergen exposure, completing the process of sensitization.

The early phase response (EPR) of allergic conjunctivitis is an IgE-mediated reaction triggered by re-exposure to the same allergen that induced the sensitization of the mast cells. This involves allergen –induced cross-linking of allergen-specific IgE molecules bound to the FcεRI on the sensitized mast cells. This triggers a biological cascade that causes changes in membrane calcium transport. This leads to disruption of the cell membrane and mast cell activation. The activated mast cell undergoes degranulation with release of allergic mediators, such as histamine, into the extravascular space (Abelson and Greiner 2004). Histamine release following mast cell degranulation in the EPR is responsible for the signs and symptoms (itching, redness, chemosis, tearing and eyelid edema) of allergic conjunctivitis. Histamine is the primary mediator in allergic conjunctivitis (Abelson, Smith et al. 2003). The activation of histamine receptor on conjunctival neurons by histamine induces pruritus while binding of the histamine receptor on the vascular endothelium induces dilation (redness) and endothelial gapping (swelling) (Rosenwasser, Mahr et al.).

In allergic conjunctivitis, pathological changes such as increased mast cell activation, inflammatory cell migration, and early signs of cellular activation and modulation of T-lymphocyte function are not clinically significant. Eosinophil and Th2-lymphocytes do not play a major role in the pathogenesis of allergic conjunctivitis, as noted by the absence of corneal damage in SAC and PAC. IgE and mast cells play a major role in the disease mechanism of SAC and PAC (Leonardi, De Dominicis et al. 2007; Pavesio and Decory 2008).

The histopathological and laboratory findings in patients with allergic conjunctivitis revealed: 1] increased levels of mast cells in the conjunctival epithelium and substantia propria; and 2] increased levels of specific IgE antibody, histamine, and tryptase (Reiss, Abelson et al. 1996; Stahl, Cook et al. 2002). The serum levels of eosinophil cationic protein (ECP) are not significantly increased in allergic conjunctivitis (Leonardi 2005).

Clinical Presentation: The hallmark signs and symptoms of allergic conjunctivitis include itching, conjunctiva hyperemia, chemosis, mucoid or watery discharge, burning, redness, and eyelid swelling (Figures 4, 5 &6). In PAC, the non-specific signs and symptoms may persist with varying severity for months. The most bothersome symptom of allergic conjunctivitis is ocular itching and the most annoying sign is redness (Mah, Rosenwasser et al. 2007; Leonardi, Motterle et al. 2008).

Diagnosis: The diagnosis of allergic conjunctivitis is based on the constellation of clinical signs and symptoms. The skin prick testing or radioallergosorbent (RAST) test is used to identify offending allergens and for confirming the diagnosis of allergy (Manzouri, Flynn et al. 2006). Consulting with an allergist to assist in identifying the causative agents may be beneficial.

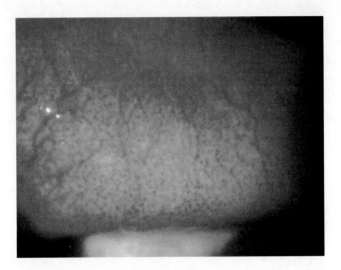

Figure 4. Fine papillary reaction in Allergic Conjunctivitis.

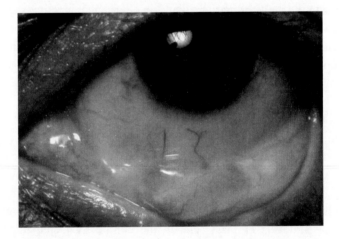

Figure 5. Chemosis in Allergic Conjunctivitis.

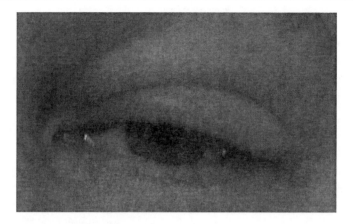

Figure 6. Eyelid Edema in Allergic Conjunctivitis.

Management: The first line of therapy for patients with allergic conjunctivitis is to avoid the offending allergens. The primary aim of a non-pharmacological management approach to ocular allergy is to prevent the onset of symptoms in the first place and to minimize the effect of allergens in general. It is considered the first-line treatment of ocular allergy and includes avoidance of known allergens; saline irrigation; avoid eye rubbing; and palliative therapy with cold compresses and preservative-free ocular lubricants.

Patients should be advised to stay indoors and keep the windows closed or wear a filter mask if it is necessary for them to stay outside on days when the pollen count is high. They should also be advised to be more aware of the pollen count through the weather forecast; avoid cutting grass on windy days and when the pollen count is high and avoid going near freshly cut grass during the height of the allergy season. Furthermore, the patient should be advised to avoid damp areas as these are potential breeding grounds for molds. They should be mindful to keep pets out of the bedroom, since their hair/fur can collect allergens (Kirkner 2001).

When avoidance fails, the clinician should recommend supportive and therapeutic anti-allergic therapy. It is good clinical practice to advise patients to use supportive therapies such as cool compresses, face washing and ocular lubricants as an adjunct to pharmacologic management. The clinician could advise the patient to keep preservative-free ocular lubricants in the refrigerator. The cold temperature of the refrigerated preservative-free ocular lubricants in conjunction with cool compresses induces vasoconstriction. This will counteract the allergen-induced vasodilatation effect that causes chemosis and eyelid swelling. Preservative-free ocular lubricants dilute and flush away allergens, histamine and other inflammatory mediators that may come into contact with the ocular surface without having any impact on the activity of inflammatory mediators. They also form a barrier to inhibit allergen contact with the ocular surface (Manzouri, Flynn et al. 2006; Chigbu 2009; Chigbu 2009).

Therapeutic agents used for treating allergic conjunctivitis include antihistamines, topical non-steroidal anti-inflammatory drugs (NSAIDs), topical corticosteroids, topical mast cell stabilizers and topical antihistamine/ mast cell stabilizer combinations. Prescription and over-the-counter oral antihistamine can also play a role in reducing the overall allergic sensitivity of the body.

Mild to moderate cases of allergic conjunctivitis will respond to antihistamine, topical multimodal anti-allergic agents, topical mast cell stabilizers and supportive therapies. Individuals that present with hyperacute expressions of allergic conjunctivitis, severe allergic conjunctivitis or allergic conjunctivitis that is refractory to conventional anti-allergic therapy would benefit from short term steroidal therapy aimed at suppressing the allergic inflammatory cascade (Butrus and Portela 2005). The pulse topical steroidal anti-inflammatory therapy can be tapered and discontinued, once the allergic inflammatory response is contained. However, it would be necessary to recommend the use of mast cell stabilizers or antihistamine/mast cell stabilizer combination agent for long-term management.

Patients who present with allergic rhinoconjunctivitis may benefit from using a nasal spray (e.g. azelastine hydrochloride nasal spray) or oral antihistamine (Clarityn or Zirtec) to provide therapeutic relief for the rhinitis and a topical multimodal anti-allergic ophthalmic agent to treat the allergic conjunctivitis (Crampton 2002; Butrus and Portela 2005; Leonardi 2005). The clinical features of rhino-conjunctivitis are nasal itching, irritation, sneezing, rhinorrhea and congestion. The ocular allergic component of rhinoconjunctivitis includes itching, chemosis, redness, tearing and lid swelling. A clinical study demonstrated the superiority of antiallergic ophthalmic medication over antiallergic nasal spray in treating allergic conjunctivitis (Rosenwasser, Mahr et al.).

If the clinician decides to recommend systemic antihistamines, they may advise the patient to use preservative-free ocular lubricants in view of the fact that systemic antihistamines can reduce the aqueous component of the pre-ocular tear film. Topical ophthalmic antihistamines offer rapid onset of relief but have a short duration of action. Systemic antihistamines have a long duration of action but have a delayed onset of action (Pavesio and Decory 2008). This is the reason clinicians are advised to treat allergic conjunctivitis with topical anti-allergic ophthalmic agents.

Antihistamines, mast cell stabilizers and multiple action anti-allergic agents are sufficient to control the clinical manifestations of allergic conjunctivitis. However, pulse therapy with topical steroids will become necessary in severe or hyperacute cases. The major advantage of using topical multiple action anti-allergic ophthalmic agents is that the antihistamine will provide immediate therapeutic effect aimed at resolving the effects of the released histamine, while the mast cell stabilizer provides long term prophylaxis. Mast cell stabilizers are not effective in treating acute allergic conjunctivitis; however, they are beneficial when used prior to the expected exposure to allergen or allergy season since they require a loading period of weeks before antigen exposure for maximal efficacy (Pavesio and Decory 2008).

Complications: Allergic conjunctivitis rarely causes permanent ocular surface damage. It responds well to supportive and topical pharmacotherapy (Manzouri, Flynn et al. 2006).

Prognosis: Allergic conjunctivitis has a very favorable prognosis. However, the condition tends to reoccur.

5.2. Vernal Keratoconjunctivitis

Introduction: Vernal keratoconjunctivitis (VKC) is a recurrent, bilateral, chronic allergic inflammation of the ocular surface affecting mainly children and young adult with a predominance in males (Abu El-Asrar, Van Aelst et al. 2001; Bremond-Gignac, Donadieu et al. 2008). VKC is characterized by persistent conjunctival inflammation with an over-expression of mast cells, eosinophils, basophils, neutrophils, macrophages and lymphocytes (Bonini, Coassin et al. 2004; Leonardi, Brun et al. 2007). There are three forms of the disease (Abu El-Asrar, Van Aelst et al. 2001):

- Palpebral
- Limbal
- Mixed.

The classification of VKC is based on the main site of the papillary reaction (Lambiase, Minchiotti et al. 2009). The palpebral form is seen predominantly in Caucasians, whereas the limbal variety is more typical in Black populations and Native Americans (Coutu 1991).

Patients with palpebral VKC present with giant papillae (i.e. >1mm) on the upper tarsal conjunctiva with no limbal infiltration (Cameron 1995). A variation of the palpebral or tarsal form of VKC may appear as diffuse upper tarsal conjunctival thickening, with fine and diffuse subepithelial fibrosis without papillae formation. The tarsal form is characterized by irregular sized hypertrophic papillae that lead to cobblestone appearance on the upper tarsal plate (Leonardi and Secchi 2003). It is characterized by giant papillary hypertrophy of the conjunctiva over the upper tarsal plate and corneal epithelial macroerosions. Vernal plaques are common complications. The palpebral form is most frequent in the temperate regions and is associated with a personal history of atopic disease. It is also more common in males and has a natural tendency to resolve after puberty (Tuft, Cree et al. 1998). Patients with limbal VKC present with gelatinous limbal infiltration and papillary reaction of the upper tarsal conjunctiva (i.e. papillae <1mm) (Cameron 1995). Visual loss from corneal complications is uncommon (Tuft, Cree et al. 1998; Kumar 2009). The purely or predominantly limbal form of VKC appears to be found more frequently in black populations (Holsclaw, Whitcher et al. 1996). Mixed VKC has both giant papillae on the upper tarsal conjunctiva and gelatinous infiltration of the limbus (Cameron 1995).

VKC is bilateral in 96%-98% of cases (Bonini, Lambiase et al. 2000). It has been reported that approximately 23% of patients have the perennial form of the disease, and more than 60% have recurrences during the winter (Keklikci, Soker et al. 2008). VKC is more of a perennial disease rather than a seasonal disease in most patients, with a tendency to become chronic and persistent over time (Bonini, Coassin et al. 2004). There is a variation in the geographic distribution of the disease (Collum 1999). VKC is more prevalent in warm climates, particularly in the Middle East, Mediterranean region, Africa, Central America, South America, Japan and Indian subcontinent (Bremond-Gignac, Donadieu et al. 2008; Keklikci, Soker et al. 2008). There is an increase in the prevalence of VKC in the Northern hemisphere and Australia which can be attributed to the migration of a susceptible population. This implicates genetic and environmental factors in its incidence (Bonini, Lambiase et al. 2003; Leonardi and Secchi 2003). The perennial form occurs more frequently in hot countries whereas the chronic seasonal patterns occur mostly in the temperate regions as atmospheric conditions promote flare-ups in the spring and summer (Bremond-Gignac, Donadieu et al. 2008). The predilection of VKC in Asian and African populations gives credence to the possibility of a genetic predisposition (Kumar 2009). The disease predominantly affects males; however, this disparity diminishes after puberty. The gender difference has been attributed to a possible role of hormonal factors in the development of VKC (Bonini, Lambiase et al. 2003; Leonardi and Secchi 2003; Bonini, Coassin et al. 2004; Kumar 2009). Approximately 50% of patients with VKC have a family history of allergic disorders such as asthma, rhinitis, eczema, and urticaria (Bonini, Lambiase et al. 2000). VKC is not associated with a positive response to skin tests and RAST in nearly 50% of patients, confirming that it is not solely an IgE mediated disease (Bonini, Coassin et al. 2004; Iovieno, Lambiase et al. 2008). Thus VKC patients that are positive to the standard allergen test, such as skin prick or RAST test often have a positive personal or family history of atopy (Leonardi and Secchi 2003). The over-expression of the cells and mediators of ocular allergy suggest that VKC may be a phenotypic model of up-regulation of the cytokine gene cluster on chromosome 5q. The cytokine gene cluster, through its products, which include interleukin (IL) IL-3, 4, 5 and granulocyte/macrophage-colony-stimulating factor, regulate the prevalence of T helper-lymphocyte type 2 (Th2) (Kumar 2009).

VKC has been associated with higher incidences of keratoconus, acute hydrops or sex-hormone related conditions such as polycystic ovary syndrome (Kumar 2009). Exacerbation of the chronic disease or acute episodic flare ups can be triggered by exposure to specific allergens or nonspecific stimuli such as wind, light, sun, dust and hot weather (Leonardi and Secchi 2003). This exaggerated hyper-reactivity to nonspecific stimuli may suggest some sort of neural involvement in the pathogenesis of the disease (Kumar 2009). It has been reported that VKC is strongly associated with atopy in temperate regions/climates with a less marked association in the tropical regions (Tuft, Cree et al. 1998).

Pathophysiology and Histopathology: The immunopathogenesis of VKC is multifactorial (Bonini, Lambiase et al. 2003). VKC could be an IgE-mast cell/Th2-lymphocyte-eosinophil or non-IgE-mast cell/Th2-lymphocyte-eosinophil mediated hypersensitivity reaction with additional nonspecific hypersensitivity responses (Leonardi and Secchi 2003). A variety of cells and mediators are responsible for the profound expression of Th2-derived cytokines in VKC encompassing both IgE- and non-IgE-mediated hypersensitivity immune reactions (Kumar 2009). It has been reported that climatic, environmental, hormonal, genetic, neural factors may influence the pathogenesis of VKC (Akinsola, Sonuga et al. 2008; Lambiase, Minchiotti et al. 2009), (Spadavecchia, Fanelli et al. 2006).

Cytological, challenge studies, immunohistochemical and biomolecular studies indicate that VKC is a Th2-lymphocyte-mediated allergic inflammatory disease with an over expression of Th2-drived cytokines, chemokines, adhesion molecules, eosinophils, growth factors, fibroblast, enzymes, and other cells and mediators within the conjunctiva (Leonardi and Secchi 2003), (Kumar 2009).

Studies have reported the involvement of neural factors such as substance P and neural growth factor (NGF) in the pathogenesis of VKC. The over-expression of nerve growth factor receptors in the conjunctiva coupled with high serum levels of NGF suggest a possible neural influence in the pathogenesis of VKC (Bonini, Coassin et al. 2004). There is an over expression of estrogen and progesterone receptors in the conjunctiva of VKC patients suggesting possible involvement of sex hormones in the pathogenesis of VKC (Bonini, Lambiase et al. 1995; Bonini, Coassin et al. 2004; Akinsola, Sonuga et al. 2008). These hormones may bind to conjunctival receptors and exert a proinflammatory effect through the recruitment of eosinophils to the conjunctival tissue (Bonini, Coassin et al. 2004).

The clinical, histological and biochemical features of VKC are related to the production of Th2–derived cytokines, which favor a local hyperproduction of IgE (IL-4, IL-9, IL-13), recruitment and activation of eosinophils (IL-5, GM-CSF) and differentiation and activation of mast cells (IL-3) (Leonardi and Secchi 2003; Bonini, Coassin et al. 2004).

Patients with VKC have demonstrated non-specific conjunctival hyper-reactivity to histamine (Bonini, Lambiase et al. 2003). It has been proposed that hyperreactivity of these tissues to specific and nonspecific stimuli are responsible for the abundant release of histamine and other pro-inflammatory mediators (Abelson, Leonardi et al. 1995). In one study, VKC patients complained of frequent conjunctival redness after exposure to these nonspecific stimuli. This finding supports previous reports acknowledging the presence of conjunctival hyperreactivity to the sun, dust, wind and other general climatic factors (Bonini, Coassin et al. 2004).

The histopathologic and clinical presentation of VKC correlates with the influence exerted by the cells and mediators in VKC (Abelson, Leonardi et al. 1995). Histopathological studies of conjunctival tissue from VKC patients show a prominent inflammatory cellular infiltration in the epithelium and substantia propria, as well as post inflammatory tissue remodeling (Kumar 2009). The influx of inflammatory cells and mediators into the conjunctiva leads to the clinical manifestations seen in VKC (Gupta, Sharma et al. 1999). Cytokines, chemokines, histamine, growth factors and metalloproteinase are mediators involved in the pathophysiology of VKC. Mast cells, T-lymphocytes, eosinophils and macrophages are seen in increased numbers among VKC patients (Kumar 2009).

The main histological feature of VKC consists of infiltration of the conjunctival epithelium and substantia propria by inflammatory cells, including eosinophils, basophils, mast cells, dendritic cells and dendritic cells bearing IgE, B-lymphocytes, plasma cells, CD4[+]T-lymphocytes expressing T-helper 2 (Th2)-lymphocyte-type cytokines, monocytes/macrophages, extracellular matrix hyperplasia, and remodeling caused by increased collagen deposition (Abu El-Asrar, Struyf et al. 2000; Abu El-Asrar, Van Aelst et al. 2001; Leonardi and Secchi 2003).

The histopathological findings in patients with VKC have also revealed 1] increased expression of adhesion molecules (Leonardi and Secchi 2003); 2] increased activity and expression of gelatinase B in the conjunctiva (Abu El-Asrar, Van Aelst et al. 2001); 3] increased production and activation of matrix metalloproteinases (MMP) (Leonardi, De Dominicis et al. 2007; Kumar 2009); 4] increased expression of chemokines, such as IL-8, eotaxin, MCP-1, MCP-3, and RANTES that induces massive eosinophil infiltration into the tissues (Leonardi and Secchi 2003); and 5] an over expression of Th2-derived cytokines, chemokines and mediators in both the tears and tissues of patients affected by VKC (Leonardi, Brun et al. 2005).

The increased tear levels of histamine have been reported to be associated with a defect in activity of the histaminases. This increase could explain why nonspecific histamine release occurs despite the absence of stimulation and exacerbating effects of chronic eye rubbing (Leonardi and Secchi 2003). Abelson et al in their study of the activity of histaminases activity in VKC demonstrated that a defect in histaminase activity in tears and serum may be responsible for the onset and maintenance of the allergic inflammation associated with VKC (Abelson, Leonardi et al. 1995).

VKC is also characterized by architectural remodeling of the conjunctival tissues. Tissue remodeling occurs secondary to excess extracellular matrix (ECM) deposition, subepithelial fibrosis, chronic cellular infiltrate and epithelial thickening [(Leonardi, Brun et al. 2007)]. Tissue-remodeling reactions produce giant papillae formation, hyperplasia of the epithelium with numerous epithelial ingrowths, extensive deposition of extracellular matrix components, peripheral corneal fibrovascular proliferation and superficial corneal changes (Abu El-Asrar, Al-Mansouri et al. 2006; Kumar 2009).

Elastase, serine proteases and MMPs initiate the tissue remodeling and collagen deposition that results in the changes that characterize VKC (Leonardi and Secchi 2003). In their study, Abu El-Asrar and colleagues demonstrated that epidermal growth factor receptor (EGFR), vascular endothelial growth factor (VEGF), transforming growth factor (TGFB), basic fibroblast growth factor (bFGF) and platelet-derived growth factor beta (PDGF) were involved in the immunopathogenesis of conjunctival remodeling in VKC. Vascular endothelial growth factor (VEGF) plays a central role in the process of angiogenesis and increases vascular permeability. In the presence of VEGF, plasma proteins can leak into the extravascular space leading to edema and profound alterations in the extracellular matrix. Epithelial cells and inflammatory cells including eosinophils, monocytes and macrophages are the major cellular sources of VEGF. Transforming growth factor beta (TGF-b) is able to stimulate fibroblast proliferation and increase the synthesis of VEGF by enlisting the fibroblasts of the extracellular matrix (Abu El-Asrar, Al-Mansouri et al. 2006).

Clinical presentation: The clinical features of VKC include itching, burning, tearing, blepharospasm, pseudoptosis due to heavy giant papillae on the upper tarsal conjunctiva or at the limbus, foreign body sensation, photophobia, mucus hyper-secretion resulting in mucous discharge, filamentous mucus discharge, eyelid edema, limbal conjunctival edema, perilimbal conjunctival pigmentation, neovascularization of the cornea, cicatrizing conjunctivitis, blepharitis, the presence of aggregates of epithelial cells and eosinophils at the limbus (Horner-Trantas dots) and superficial keratitis. The superficial punctate keratitis can evolve into corneal shield ulcers (Rao, Meenakshi et al. 2004; Corum, Yeniad et al. 2005; Keklikci, Soker et al. 2008; Kumar 2009).

Bonini et al proposed a clinical grading system to help physicians in the diagnosis and management of VKC (Bonini, Sacchetti et al. 2007; Kumar 2009). The *clinical manifestations of the mild form of VKC* includes occasional pruritus, mild tearing, mild discomfort including burning or foreign body sensation, mucoid discharge, mild photophobia, mild to moderate papillary reaction, mild corneal epithelial defects with or without corneal neovascularization, subepithelial fibrosis of the conjunctiva, mild hyperemia of the conjunctiva, and mild redness and edema of the eyelid (Bonini, Sacchetti et al. 2007; Keklikci, Soker et al. 2008). The *clinical manifestations of the moderate form of VKC* includes persistent itching, intermittent tearing, moderate discomfort, moderate mucoid discharge with the presence of crust upon awakening, moderate photophobia, moderate tarsal papillary hypertrophy and hyperemia with hazy view of the deep vessels, moderate bulbar conjunctival hyperemia, Horner-Trantas dots, moderate corneal epithelial defects with corneal neovascularization, moderate subepithelial fibrosis and moderate eyelid inflammation with Meibomian gland dysfunction. The *clinical manifestations of the severe form of VKC* includes constant itching and tearing, severe discomfort, marked mucoid discharge with agglutination of the eyelids upon awakening, extreme photophobia, severe tarsal papillary hypertrophy and hyperemia obscuring the visualization of the deep tarsal vessels, marked bulbar conjunctival hyperemia, severe corneal epithelial defects in the form of cornea erosion or ulceration with corneal neovascularization, numerous Horner-Trantas dots, the presence of symblepharon and severe inflammation of the eyelid (Bonini, Sacchetti et al. 2007; Keklikci, Soker et al. 2008).

A *circumcorneal or perilimbal pigment* described as fine, golden brown spotty pigmented limbal thickening is a consistent finding in VKC patients. The color varies from faint to dark brown and is most frequently found in the interpalpebral and inferior area of the bulbar conjunctiva around the limbus but not in the tarsal conjunctiva. There is an abundance of melanocytes around the limbus. Luk et al suggested that the perilimbal conjunctival pigmentation observed in VKC patients may be a by-product of complex immune interaction and pathways involving growth factors or interleukins that stimulates the melanocytes to produce the perilimbal pigment (Luk, Wong et al. 2008).

Conjunctival giant papillae in the superior tarsus and/or limbus are considered the hallmark of the disease (Figure 7) (Lambiase, Minchiotti et al. 2009). It has been reported that inflammation of the conjunctiva rather than mechanical factors plays a greater role in formation of giant papillae and exacerbation of VKC. Tissue remodeling is believed to be an important mechanism in giant papillary formation in VKC (Kato, Fukagawa et al. 2006). Investigations on the mechanisms leading to conjunctival giant papillae formation in VKC have pointed to the involvement of conjunctival resident cells (epithelium and fibroblasts) (Bonini, Lambiase et al. 2003). Leonardi and colleagues demonstrated that metalloproteinase may play a role in the structural changes seen in VKC (Leonardi, Brun et al. 2007).

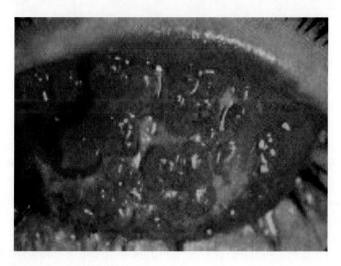

Figure 7. Giant papillae in Palpebral VKC.

The limbal form of the disease is characterized by multiple gelatinous yellow-gray limbal infiltrates (Figure 8). Limbal involvement in VKC includes limbal thickening or opacification, the presence on upper limbal papillae, Horner-Trantas' dots and pannus of the superior limbus (Leonardi and Secchi 2003).

Corneal involvement occurs in up to 25% of patients with VKC (Bremond-Gignac, Donadieu et al. 2008). The manifestations of corneal involvement in patients with VKC include punctate epithelial keratitis, epithelial macro-erosions, shield ulcer formation, plaque formation, corneal vascularization, secondary microbial keratitis, keratoconus, pellucid marginal degeneration (PMD), keratoglobus, superior corneal thinning, hydrops, pseudogerontoxon and corneal opacification (Cameron 1995; Kumar 2008; Kumar 2009). Punctate keratitis may be present in both limbal and palpebral forms but corneal shield ulcers are mostly seen in the tarsal form (Cameron, Al-Rajhi et al. 1989; Leonardi and Secchi 2003).

Pseudogerontoxon is a localized grey-white lipid deposition in the anterior stroma of the peripheral cornea. It resembles a small segment of arcus senilis or gerontoxon. It results from prolonged hyperemia, persistent limbal infiltration and altered limbal permeability secondary to limbal giant papillae (Leonardi and Secchi 2003; Jeng, Whitcher et al. 2004; Kumar 2009). It is seen in individuals with limbal vernal or atopic keratoconjunctivitis. It may be considered the only clinical evidence of previous allergic eye disease (Jeng, Whitcher et al. 2004).

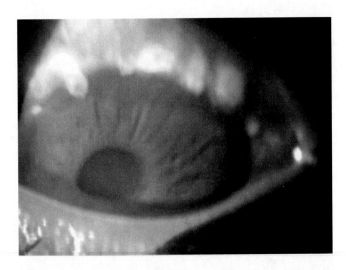

Figure 8. Gelatinous Limbal infiltration in Limbal VKC.

Shield ulcer is an oval or pentagonal shaped, superficial lesion located in the center of the superior third of the cornea (Cameron 1995; Gedik, Akova et al. 2006). A corneal shield ulcer (**Toby's** ulcer) is an uncommon but vision threatening complication that occurs in approximately 3%-11% of patients with VKC (Bonini, Coassin et al. 2004; Kumar 2009; Lambiase, Minchiotti et al. 2009). In a study by Lambiase and coworkers, corneal shield ulcer was reported more in patients with the tarsal form of VKC (Lambiase, Minchiotti et al. 2009).

The two hypotheses proposed to explain the pathogenesis of shield ulcer in VKC are the mechanical theory and the immune cytotoxic theory. The pathogenesis of shield corneal ulcers is believed to involve a combination of chronic mechanical abrading of the corneal epithelium by giant papillae on the upper tarsal conjunctiva and epithelial toxicity from inflammatory mediators secreted by eosinophils and mast cells (Cameron 1995; Cameron and Mullaney 1997; Solomon, Zamir et al. 2004). Eosinophil major basic protein (EMBP) is an inflammatory mediator that is capable of inhibiting corneal epithelial wound healing (Cameron 1995). The deposition of EMBP on the denuded Bowman's layer leads to the development of a dense plaque (Solomon, Zamir et al. 2004). Trocme reported that EMBP plays a pathogenic role in the formation and persistence of VKC-related shield ulcers (Trocme, Kephart et al. 1993). Kumar suggested that inflammatory cells, Th2-lymphocytes and tear film instability also plays a role in the pathogenesis of shield ulcer (Kumar 2008).

Shield ulcers are preceded by characteristic epithelial changes. Punctate epithelial erosion evolves into coarse epithelial keratopathy. Continued damage to the epithelium leads to the development of a frank corneal abrasion or macroerosion. An ulcer with a transparent base will form when the disease process extends through the epithelium and basement membrane into the Bowman's layer. As the disease progresses, inflammatory debris are deposited on the base of the ulcer giving the ulcer a translucent appearance. The filling of the ulcer cavity with inflammatory material eventually leads to the formation of an elevated plaque that extends above the level of the surrounding epithelium (Cameron 1995).

Cameron classified shield ulcers on the basis of their clinical characteristic, response to treatment and complications. Grade I corneal shield ulcers have a clear or transparent base. They have a favorable outcome and re-epithelialize with only mild scarring. Grade II corneal shield ulcers have a translucent base with inflammatory debris in the base. They respond poorly to medical therapy and exhibit delayed re-epithelialization. Grade III corneal shield ulcers have elevated plaques. They are resistant to medical therapy and frequently require surgical removal. Grade II and III corneal shield ulcers are prone to complications (Cameron 1995; Ozbek, Burakgazi et al. 2006; Pelegrin, Gris et al. 2008). Corneal plaques occur due to the continuous deposition of mucus and inflammatory products on the shield ulcer (Cameron 1995).

Diagnosis: The diagnosis of VKC is based on the constellation of clinical signs and symptoms. In difficult cases conjunctival scraping can be used to demonstrate the presence of eosinophils infiltrating the conjunctival epithelium. Conjunctival cytology is a fast and noninvasive diagnostic technique that can be performed. Tear cytology, conjunctival scraping, brush cytology or impression cytology may also be obtained (Bonini, Lambiase et al. 2003). Tear cytology or conjunctival scraping is useful in assessing the type and number of cells involved in the conjunctival inflammation in the active phase (Leonardi and Secchi 2003). Clinical and laboratory tests may be useful markers to monitor the disease's activity. Skin prick test or RAST are not considered useful in diagnosing VKC since it has been reported that approximately 50% of patients with VKC have negative results on these tests (Bonini, Lambiase et al. 2003; Bonini, Coassin et al. 2004).

Management: The goal of therapy is to suppress the allergic inflammatory process before the patient becomes symptomatic. The primary form of therapy for patients with VKC is identification and avoidance of allergens. The avoidance of allergens or exposure to nonspecific trigger factors such as sun, salt water, wind or dust with the use of sunglasses, hats, visors and swimming goggles may be beneficial. Frequent hand and face washing is also beneficial (Bonini, Lambiase et al. 2003; Leonardi and Secchi 2003).

The supportive therapy of VKC includes avoiding the trigger factors, avoiding eye rubbing, applying cool compress, saline irrigation to wash out allergens, and administering preservative-free ocular lubricants (Verin, Dicker et al. 1999). Preservative-free ocular lubricants aid in stabilization of the tear film, and dilute and flush away allergens and allergic mediators (Leonardi and Secchi 2003). Patients with a history of VKC should be started on prophylactic therapy with mast cell stabilizers prior to the allergy season or should remain on the therapy all year round, depending on the allergic exposure and duration of the allergic expression. Topical mucolytic agents such as Acetylcysteine (mucomyst) 10% could be beneficial when increased mucous production or thick, stringy discharge is problematic, as seen in chronic ocular allergies such as VKC, AKC and GPC. This agent could dissolve or loosen the thick stringy mucoid discharge (Brody 1996).

Educating patients and/or their parents about the disease process and the chronic, recurrent nature of VKC as well as about the possible trigger factors is an important aspect of management (Akinsola, Sonuga et al. 2008; Kumar 2009).

Therapeutic measures are required to avoid the longstanding permanent inflammatory sequelae that may lead to fibrovascular reaction, new collagen deposition, tissue inflammation, tissue remodeling and permanent visual damage (Bremond-Gignac, Donadieu et al. 2008). The chronicity and severity of the disease, warrants a combination of supportive and pharmacological treatment (Leonardi and Secchi 2003). Standard pharmacologic treatment of VKC is based on the use of topical mast cell stabilizer, anti-histamine, multimodal anti-allergic agents with mast cell stabilizer and antihistamine effects, steroid and immunosuppressive preparations (Lambiase, Minchiotti et al. 2009). Patients with mild VKC may benefit from supportive therapy as well as topical multimodal anti-allergic agents and/or mast cell stabilizers to provide symptomatic relief. However, a pulse topical steroidal therapy may be necessary to control the inflammation, if the anti-allergic therapy does not provide satisfactory therapeutic relief. Patients with moderate or severe VKC require concurrent use of topical steroids and mast cell stabilizers to achieve an adequate therapeutic effect. Topical corticosteroids with a proven safety profile such as loteprednol etabonate have been shown to be effective in controlling the chronic allergic inflammatory process in VKC. The maximum strength topical corticosteroid, such as prednisolone acetate 1.0% ophthalmic suspension could be considered when the moderate strength topical steroids or soft topical steroids are not effective in controlling the allergic inflammation. Topical cyclosporine A, a topical immunomodulator, has been proven to be effective for the long-term treatment of both limbal and tarsal VKC. It has been shown to significantly improve signs and symptoms without significant side effects (Leonardi and Secchi 2003). Keklikci et al in their clinical study noted that administration of topical cyclosporine A 0.05% for 3 months was remarkably effective at improving signs and symptoms in VKC. In their study, a low concentration of topical cyclosporine was used with no systemic adverse effects recorded (Keklikci, Soker et al. 2008). It has been reported that cyclosporine A 0.5%-2% used 4 times a day, may represent an alternative to steroidal therapy in severe forms of VKC (Bonini, Coassin et al. 2004). Spadavecchia et al also demonstrated the efficacy of 1.25% and 1.0% topical cyclosporine in the treatment of severe VKC with successful outcome. In their study, none of the patients had any major side effects or need for rescue topical steroid therapy (Spadavecchia, Fanelli et al. 2006). Although cyclosporine ophthalmic emulsion may be considered a suitable alternative to steroids, in the presence of corneal complications caused by epithelial toxic allergic mediators, such as eosinophil major basic protein (EMBP), topical steroidal therapy is the preferred choice. Treatment with systemic corticosteroids may become necessary when individuals present with severe VKC that does not respond to conventional topical therapy (Leonardi and Secchi 2003; Bonini, Coassin et al. 2004).

Holsclaw et al demonstrated the beneficial therapeutic effect of using supratarsal injection of corticosteroid in patient with refractory VKC. This therapeutic modality resulted in the resolution of large papillae, limbal edema and shield ulcer in their population study. They suggested that this therapeutic modality may also be beneficial for patients with AKC and refractory contact lens-induced GPC (Holsclaw, Whitcher et al. 1996).

Limbal gelatinous masses in VKC respond well to treatment with topical anti-inflammatory or immunomodulator. However, in recalcitrant cases, surgical interventions such as cryosurgery or surgical excision of the limbal lesion may be a viable therapeutic modality (Kobayashi, Nagata et al. 2002).

Patients with shield ulcer or corneal epithelial compromise secondary to VKC would benefit from the use of appropriate topical pharmaceutical agents and a therapeutic bandage contact lens. The objective of using a therapeutic bandage contact lens is to reduce the effect of the mechanical chafing between the papillae on the superior tarsal conjunctiva and corneal epithelial surface. The principal aim of using therapeutic bandage contact lens is to relieve pain, promote corneal epithelial healing and protect the fragile corneal epithelium during the healing process (Foulks, Harvey et al. 2003). The clinician could prescribe prophylactic antibiotics and recommend preservative-free ocular lubricants as essential adjunctive therapeutic strategies when therapeutic bandage contact lenses are used (Lemp and Bielory 2008). The complications associated with therapeutic bandage contact lenses use occur secondary to impaired corneal physiology and metabolism. The complications include infection, hypoxia, hypercapnia, tissue necrosis in the cornea, microcyst formation, decreased corneal sensation and pannus formation (Foulks, Harvey et al. 2003).

Grade I shield ulcer responds to medical therapy consisting of a topical steroid, topical antibiotic for prophylaxis and topical mast cell stabilizers with bandage contact lens to promote re-epithelialization. Grade II shield ulcers with translucent or opaque bases require medical therapy to control the active VKC and surgical intervention to remove the inflammatory material at the base of the ulcer. Grade III lesions (corneal plaques) with elevated plaque above the level of the surrounding epithelium respond well to surgical therapy (Cameron 1995). Grade II vernal shield ulcers and corneal plaques are potentially sight threatening, presenting a significant management problem for the clinician (Quah, Hemmerdinger et al. 2006). The rationale for surgical intervention is to remove the inflammatory material at the base and margins of the vernal corneal ulcer as it is mechanically preventing re-epithelialization as well as acting as a toxin to the epithelium. The inflammatory material at the base of the ulcer has been shown to be composed of several cationic proteins secreted from activated eosinophils. They have cytotoxic properties that hinder wound healing (Cameron 1995; Ozbek, Burakgazi et al. 2006).

Surgical excision of giant papillae is suggested if they protrude over the cornea (Bonini, Lambiase et al. 2003). The surgical interventions include excision of aggravating giant papillae with or without mitomycin C, surgical debridement of the ulcer base, amniotic membrane transplant, autologous conjunctival graft, excimer laser phototherapeutic keratectomy (PTK) and CO_2-assisted removal of giant papillae (Kumar 2008). Cameron et al demonstrated the benefit of using excimer laser PTK in treating shield ulcer and corneal plaque in VKC. They suggested that this procedure is an adjunctive therapy in treating serious sight-threatening corneal manifestations of VKC. The goal of excimer laser PTK is to promote re-epithelialization, remove residual toxic inflammatory products lodged in the base of the ulcer, and reduce or remove opacity present in conjunction with the corneal plaque (Cameron 1995).

Belfair et al demonstrated the use of CO_2 laser to safely remove giant papillae in patients with severe VKC with good outcomes (Belfair, Monos et al. 2005). Intraoperative topical mitomycin C treatment in conjunction with papillectomy has been used in the treatment of abnormal conjunctival proliferations (Leonardi and Secchi 2003). Nishiwaki-Dantas and colleagues were able to demonstrate the use of surgical resection of giant papillae with placement of autologous conjunctival graft in five patients with severe VKC refractory to conventional clinical treatment with good outcomes (Nishiwaki-Dantas, Dantas et al. 2000).

Sangwan et al reported the use of cultivated corneal epithelial transplantation to manage severe ocular surface disease in VKC with good outcome. They hypothesized that there is a potential for chronic limbal inflammation to lead to the development of limbal stem cell deficiency. This could be due to direct damage to stem cells by toxic allergic mediators or poor stromal support (Sangwan, Murthy et al. 2005).

Complications: Approximately 6% of patients develop a visual impairment secondary to corneal damage, corneal neovascularization, central corneal scars, irregular astigmatism, keratoconus, microbial keratitis, limbal tissue hyperplasia or steroid-induced cataract and glaucoma (Bonini, Lambiase et al. 2000; Bremond-Gignac, Donadieu et al. 2008; Kumar 2009)(Gupta, Sharma et al. 1999; Bonini, Lambiase et al. 2003).

Limbal infiltrates may cause transitory modifications of corneal astigmatism whereas keratoconus is the most frequent corneal ectasia associated with VKC. Eye rubbing and activation of metalloproteinase may play a role in the development of keratoconus in VKC (Leonardi and Secchi 2003).

Amblyopia seen among VKC patients may be caused by corneal opacity or refractive or meridional changes producing corneal curvature alterations or the development of keratoconus (Kumar 2009).

The risk factors for developing infective keratitis in VKC include environmental factors; frequent and vigorous eye rubbing that can induce mechanical microtrauma; tear film insufficiency; altered ocular immune response ; and history of steroid use (Gupta, Sharma et al. 1999).

Delays in treatment as well as under-treatment in moderate and severe cases of VKC may lead to the development of significant morbidity. Prompt diagnosis and appropriate treatment may prevent the development of permanent ocular complications and visual loss (Collum 1999; Gedik, Akova et al. 2006).

Prognosis: The long-term prognosis of patients with VKC is generally good. However 6% of patients develop visual complications. The majority of patients with VKC have spontaneous resolution of the disease after puberty without any further symptoms or visual complication (Bonini, Coassin et al. 2004). It has been reported that the bulbar form of VKC is said to have a worse long-term prognosis than the tarsal form (Bonini, Lambiase et al. 2000; Akinsola, Sonuga et al. 2008). Patients with shield ulcers without plaque formation usually undergo rapid re-epithelialization, resulting in an excellent visual outcome, whereas those patients with shield ulcers with plaque formation have a poor visual prognosis (Cameron 1995; Kumar 2008).

5.3. Giant Papillary Conjunctivitis

Introduction: Giant Papillary conjunctivitis (GPC) was initially described in 1974 by Spring as an allergic-type reaction on the upper tarsal conjunctiva (Chang, Tse et al. 2005). GPC is not strictly an allergic disease, but an inflammatory condition characterized by papillary hypertrophy on the superior tarsal conjunctiva in the absence of significant corneal involvement (Bartlett, Howes et al. 1993; Leonardi, De Dominicis et al. 2007). GPC may result from persistent mechanical conjunctival and corneal irritation or trauma secondary to the blink action, as the eyelid becomes raked by the rough surface of a contact lens, ocular prostheses, exposed sutures after ocular surgery, extruded scleral buckles, filtering blebs, band keratopathy, corneal foreign bodies, elevated corneal deposits, limbal dermoids or cyanoacrylate tissue adhesive (Allansmith and Ross 1988; Donshik 1994; Katelaris 1999; Leonardi, De Dominicis et al. 2007; Donshik, Ehlers et al. 2008). It may also occur as a result of hypersensitivity reaction to antigenic material adhering to the contact lens, ocular prostheses, exposed sutures or extruded scleral buckles (Allansmith and Ross 1988).

Contact-lens associated GPC may result from an immune-mediated hypersensitivity response to antigenic deposits on the contact lens surface (Suchecki, Donshik et al. 2003). The amount of protein deposition on the lens surface is dependent on the lens type, on the water content and the ionic properties of the lens (Katelaris 1999). A poorly fitted contact lens, coated contact lens or contact lens edge may cause tarsal conjunctiva irritation, allowing the antigens on the contact lens to come into contact with the conjunctival mucous surface, stimulating the mucosal immune system. Tears, cracks, and chips in the lenses can also lead to ocular surface irritation (Bartlett, Howes et al. 1993; Suchecki, Donshik et al. 2003). Studies have supported the irritative etiology for GPC since deposits and irregular edges on contact lens and prostheses are recognized as irritants to the upper tarsal conjunctiva providing an entry for the offending antigens (Meijer, Pogany et al. 1993). High oxygen permeable (Dk) silicone hydrogels can cause a generalized and localized form of GPC. The localized form is more common than the generalized form in wearers of high Dk silicone hydrogel contact lenses (Elhers and Donshik 2008). Silicone hydrogel lenses with higher modulus factors may induce focal GPC (Donshik, Ehlers et al. 2008).

GPC associated with ocular prosthetics was initially described in 1979 by Srinivasan et al (Chang, Tse et al. 2005). The papillary reaction associated with ocular prostheses is generalized whereas papillary reaction associated with filtering blebs or exposed sutures is usually localized (Elhers and Donshik 2008).

GPC may affect both atopic and non-atopic individuals (Katelaris 1999). GPC tends to develop earlier in patients wearing soft hydrogel contact lenses and later in wearers of rigid contact lenses (Elhers and Donshik 2008). Allansmith and associates reported an average development time of 10 months for soft lens wearers. In contrast, an average of 8.5 years was demonstrated for rigid gas permeable wearers. Data published by Donshik confirmed that GPC develops sooner in wearers of soft lens wearers than wearers of RGP lenses (Donshik

1994). Studies have reported that GPC tends to develop earlier in patients wearing silicone hydrogel materials followed by soft hydrogel contact lenses (Donshik, Ehlers et al. 2008; Elhers and Donshik 2008). In a study of 124 patients who developed GPC while wearing silicone hydrogels contact lenses, it was found that they were more likely to develop GPC sooner than HEMA-based hydrogel wearers (Skotnitsky, Naduvilath et al. 2006; Donshik, Ehlers et al. 2008). In a study of patients wearing planned frequent replacement soft contact lenses, who replaced their lens every 4 weeks, such individuals had a higher incidence of GPC than those who replaced their lenses every 2- 3 weeks (Donshik, Ehlers et al. 2008). Clinical studies have shown that FDA group IV, high water content, high porosity, ionic contact lenses are prone to protein deposition. Individuals wearing low and high porosity ionic soft contact lenses may also be prone to developing GPC with increased severity of signs and symptoms as well as a shorter time to onset or development of GPC (Porazinski and Donshik 1999). It has been reported that GPC patients who wore FDA group III low water content, ionic lenses had more severe signs and symptoms than those who wore FDA group I low water content, nonionic contact lens. Patients who wore FDA type III low water ionic contact lens are prone to developing more severe signs and symptoms with a shorter time to onset of GPC than those with FDA type I low water content non-ionic lens. There is no sex or age predilection (Donshik 1994). Clinical studies have shown that patients with GPC may have a history of allergies to environmental allergens or medications (Porazinski and Donshik 1999).

Pathophysiology and Histopathology: Clinical studies have reported that the immunopathologic process of GPC involves T-lymphocyte and humoral-mediated mechanisms (Katelaris 1999). The aetiopathogenesis of GPC is part immunologic and part mechanical. It has been shown that contact lenses tend to attract proteinaceous deposits on their surface (Donshik 2003). When the proteinaceous coating in the biofilm on the contact lens surface becomes antigenic it may stimulate the production of tear immunoglobulin IgE, IgG and in severe cases IgM, as well as activating the complement system to generate anaphylatoxin C3a, a potent pro-inflammatory mediator and a marker for complement activation. When the C3a, IgE and some IgG subtypes interact with mast cells, they trigger the release of mediators. The repeated mechanical trauma or irritation of the tarsal conjunctiva induced by the coated contact lenses, ocular prostheses, filtering bleb, scleral buckler, higher modulus silicone hydrogel contact lens or poorly fitted contact lens can trigger the release of neutrophil chemotactic factor (NCF) from injured conjunctival cells. The released NCF attracts inflammatory cells to the site of conjunctival trauma or irritation. The interaction of these recruited inflammatory cells with IgE, IgG and C3a results in the release of mediators that are responsible for the clinical manifestations of GPC (Donshik 1994; Donshik, Ehlers et al. 2008; Pavesio and Decory 2008).

The presence of locally produced immunoglobulins in the tears of patients with active GPC is suggestive of antigen-induced immune reaction. The presence of NCF on the ocular surface of GPC patients, which is released from injured conjunctival cells, is suggestive of a mechanical-induced GPC (Elhers and Donshik 2008). Elgebaly et al demonstrated in an experimental model that NCF is released from injured conjunctival tissues (Elgebaly, Donshik et al. 1991; Katelaris 1999).

The histologic appearance of the conjunctiva in VKC and GPC is almost identical. The main difference between the two is that the number of eosinophils and basophils is greater in VKC than in GPC (Allansmith and Ross 1988; Donshik 1994). The level of eosinophilic major basic protein (EMBP), which may be responsible for injury to the corneal epithelium, is increased in patients with VKC but not in those with GPC (Allansmith and Ross 1988). Histopathological examination of GPC reveals an epithelium infiltrated with mast cells, eosinophils, basophils, lymphocytes, and polymorphonuclear leukocytes. It also reveals the presence of eosinophils and basophils in the substantia propria of the conjunctiva (Donshik 1994; Chang, Tse et al. 2005). Although histopathologic studies of the conjunctiva of patients with GPC reveals the presence of eosinophils in the conjunctiva, they do not seem to play a major role in GPC pathogenesis, since eotaxin and ECP levels are not increased in affected patients. Additionally, it has been reported that eotaxin-mediated eosinophil recruitment and eosinophil activation do not seem to have a major role in the immunopathology of GPC (Leonardi, De Dominicis et al. 2007).

The histopathologic and laboratory findings in GPC also revealed elevated levels of Leukotriene C4 (LTC4) in tears even when minimal symptoms are present (Sengor, Irkec et al. 1995) as well as increased numbers of $CD4^+$T-lymphocytes in the conjunctiva (Metz, Bacon et al. 1996). It also revealed higher levels of NCF in the tears of individual with GPC to be 15 times the level found in the tears of normal individuals (Donshik, Ehlers et al. 2008).

The finding of elevated tear immunoglobulins, chemotactic factors and inflammatory mediators as seen in VKC, supports the hypothesis that GPC has an immunologic component to its pathogenesis (Donshik, Ehlers et al. 2008).

Clinical presentation: The normal tarsal conjunctiva has a satin appearance, in which the surface appears smooth and devoid of papillae. It is a pink mucous membrane with fine vessels radiating perpendicular to the tarsal margin (Donshik, Ehlers et al. 2008). The symptoms of GPC, which usually appear before the signs, include contact lens awareness, excessive lens movement, itching, and decreased lens tolerance (Donshik 1994; Porazinski and Donshik 1999). The early indications of GPC include itching immediately upon removal of the lens, excessive mucous and increased awareness of the contact lens associated with excessive movement, and mild blurring of vision from coatings on the lens after a few hours of wear (Allansmith and Ross 1988).

Donshik proposed a clinical grading system to guide clinicians in the diagnosis and management of GPC. The stages include preclinical, mild, moderate and severe GPC. The *preclinical stage of giant papillary conjunctivitis* is characterized by the presence of minimal to mild mucus discharge, minimal to mild hyperemia of the tarsal conjunctiva, mild coating of the contact lenses and occasional itching following contact lens removal. There is no obscuration of the normal conjunctival vascular pattern. The *mild stage of giant papillary conjunctivitis* is characterized by mild mucus production with associated itching, increased lens awareness and coating of the contact lenses. Mild papillary hypertrophy and mild-to-moderate hyperemia of the tarsal conjunctiva with partial obscurations of the normal vascular pattern are observed. Patients who present with the *moderate stage of giant papillary conjunctivitis* always complain of itching, increased mucoid discharge, reduced wearing time due to increased lens awareness and excessive lens movement noticed particularly upon blinking. Excessive lens movement results in fluctuating and blurred vision. Slit lamp examination will reveal moderate hyperemia and moderate papillary hypertrophy of the tarsal conjunctiva (Figure 9). There will be obscuration of the normal conjunctival vascular pattern. The apices of the papules may appear whitened from subconjunctival scarring and fibrosis. They may also stain with sodium fluorescein. In *severe giant papillary conjunctivitis*, the patient is completely intolerant to contact lens wear due to increased mucus production, discomfort upon contact lens insertion and excessive lens movement. There is eyelid agglutination upon awakening due to excessive mucus production. There is complete obscuration of the normal vascular pattern due to marked hyperemia and papillary hypertrophy of the tarsal conjunctiva. The papillae on the upper tarsal conjunctiva are large (sometimes 1 mm or larger) with flattened, scarred apices that stain positively with sodium fluorescein (Donshik 1994), (Katelaris 1999; Donshik, Ehlers et al. 2008).

Papillary reaction in the area along the medial and temporal aspect of the tarsal plate and along the superior border of the tarsal plate is not considered pathologic (Donshik, Ehlers et al. 2008). GPC is usually bilateral but may present unilaterally or asymmetrically (Donshik 1994). Korb and associates have shown that in soft contact lens wearers the papillae appear first in the zone of the tarsal conjunctiva nearest to the upper margin of the tarsal plate whereas in RGP wearers the papillae usually appear in the zone nearest the eyelid margin (Donshik 1994). Trantas dots and superficial punctate keratitis may also appear in GPC (Katelaris 1999).

Diagnosis: The presence of papillae 0.3 mm in diameter or larger on the superior tarsal conjunctiva in association with ocular pruritus, coated contact lenses, contact lens intolerance, increased mucus production and conjunctival injection is diagnostic of GPC (Katelaris 1999).

Management: The goal of therapy is to identify the offending agent, reduce the antigenic load and trauma to the conjunctiva, improve contact lens hygiene, modify the contact lens design or material, and modulate the immune hypersensitivity reaction with anti-allergic and/or anti-inflammatory agents (Bartlett, Howes et al. 1993; Donshik 1994).

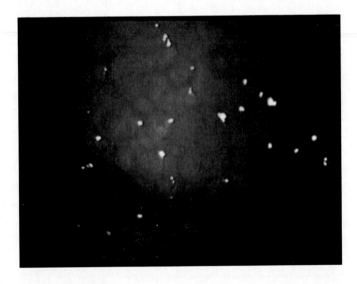

Figure 9. Papillary hypertrophy in GPC.

The goal of management in contact-lens induced GPC is to allow patients to recommence contact lens wear as soon as possible with the least obstructive therapeutic intervention. The initial step in managing contact lens-induced GPC is to discontinue contact lens wear until the inflammatory reaction subsides. In certain cases the papillary reaction may persist even in the absence of the inflammatory response. If the symptoms recur, contact lens wear should be discontinued until patient becomes asymptomatic. At this juncture, it will be beneficial to refit the patient with daily disposable contact lenses and prescribe a topical anti-allergic therapeutic agent to reduce ocular hypersensitivity (Elhers and Donshik 2008). The modalities that are available to decreasing contact lens coating include improving contact lens cleaning, decreasing the wearing time, shortening the replacement interval or modifying the contact lens material or design (Donshik 1994; Elhers and Donshik 2008). Enzymatic cleaning of the lenses on a weekly basis to minimize the accumulation of lens coating is beneficial and should be considered a vital aspect of contact lens hygiene. If a new lens of the same material and design, improved lens hygiene, and regular replacement of lens does not resolve the clinical expression of GPC, the clinician should use a contact lens of different material and design that is more readily tolerated (Allansmith and Ross 1988). Porazinski and Donshik demonstrated that replacing contact lenses at shorter intervals translated into fewer deposits and decreased the antigenic load as well as the mechanical trauma to the ocular surface (Porazinski and Donshik 1999). In another evaluation, Donshik recommended regular cleaning and disinfection of the contact lenses as well as replacing the contact lenses at least every couple of weeks. Moreover, Porazanski and Donshik suggested that patients with a history of allergy may benefit from using a contact lens wear modality that is replaced at 1 day to 2 week intervals. This modality will reduce the coating on the contact lens surface (Porazinski and Donshik 1999).

Patient with trace to mild GPC may benefit from switching from conventional contact lens wear to a frequent replacement plan or daily disposable contact lenses. Additionally, daily lens cleaning and disinfection as well as weekly or biweekly enzymatic treatment may be beneficial (Donshik, Ehlers et al. 2008). Patients with moderate-to severe GPC should discontinue contact lens wear until the inflammatory reaction, corneal staining and apical staining of the tarsal conjunctival papule has completely resolved. These patients may benefit from daily disposable lenses or one-week frequent replacement lenses (Donshik 1994).

Patients with GPC may benefit from either anti-allergic therapy or pulse topical steroidal therapy. The choice of therapy is dependent on the degree of clinical expression of the condition. Palliative therapy, modification of contact lens wear, and anti-allergic pharmaceutical therapy may be sufficient to achieve an adequate therapeutic effect in mild to moderate cases of GPC. Patients with GPC that do not respond to conventional treatment with topical anti-allergic agents will be able to achieve an adequate therapeutic outcome with short-term use of a topical steroid. Patients who have GPC with significant conjunctival papillary hypertrophy or inflammatory component require both a mast cell stabilizer or mast cell stabilizing/antihistamine combination and topical steroid with the intention of tapering the steroid once an adequate clinical response has been achieved (Melton and Thomas 2003).

Bartlett and colleagues demonstrated that Loteprednol etabonate was effective in reducing the size and severity of papillae associated with GPC (Bartlett, Howes et al. 1993). Kymionis et al were able to use topical tacrolimus 0.03% ointment to treat severe GPC that was refractory to conventional therapy with a successful outcome (Kymionis, Goldman et al. 2008).

In managing patients with contact-lens induced giant papillary conjunctivitis, the clinician should evaluate if any of these management modalities, such as changing the edge design, surface properties, fitting characteristics, replacement cycle and modulus of elasticity of the contact lens would provide enhanced benefits (Donshik 2003). If these non-pharmacologic management modalities are ineffective, patients may benefit from a topical mast cell stabilizer or mast cell stabilizing/antihistamine combination, using either once or twice-a-day dosing regimen. The dose for these agents can be administered 5-10 minutes prior to contact lens insertion and if a second dose is needed, it can be administered after the lens is removed at the end of day. It is often beneficial to start anti-allergy medication prior to the allergy season, especially in individuals who are known seasonal allergic sufferers. Once-daily dosed anti-allergic ophthalmic agents, such as Olopatadine 0.2%, may be suitable topical multimodal anti-allergic agents for contact lens wearers who have allergic conjunctivitis.

In cases refractory to anti-allergic or anti-inflammatory agents, surgical intervention may be considered necessary (Kymionis, Goldman et al. 2008).

Complications: The long-term prognosis of a patient with GPC is generally good; however, approximately 5% of the patients develop ocular complications due to chronic inflammation or treatment side effects (Kymionis, Goldman et al. 2008).

Prognosis: Inadequately managed cases have the potential to relapse and chronic cases require ongoing reevaluation. Although the prognosis is typically good for cases that require non-pharmacologic and pharmacologic intervention, prevention is the best strategy.

5.4. Atopic Keratoconjunctivitis

Introduction: In 1952, Hogan introduced the term atopic keratoconjunctivitis (AKC) to describe a bilateral chronic inflammatory disease of the ocular surface and eyelid characterized by chronic conjunctivitis and progressive corneal infiltration often seen in patients with atopic dermatitis (Tuft, Kemeny et al. 1991; Manzouri, Flynn et al. 2006; Uchio, Kimura et al. 2008). AKC is a sight-threatening ocular manifestation of a complex and systemic altered immune response. It is often associated with atopic dermatitis and other allergic conditions (Leonardi, De Dominicis et al. 2007; Nivenius, van der Ploeg et al. 2007; Leonardi, Motterle et al. 2008). It may persist for many years and has the potential to cause ocular surface complications with potentially blinding sequelae (Ozcan, Ersoz et al. 2007; Uchio, Kimura et al. 2008). AKC is the most severe and chronic form of ocular surface allergy-related disorder of the conjunctiva. Calonge and colleagues suggested that AKC is a chronic ocular surface inflammatory condition that atopic dermatitis patients may suffer at any point in the course of their dermatologic disease, independently of its degree of severity (Calonge and Herreras 2007).

AKC is known to occur in 25% – 40% of patients with atopic dermatitis (Casey and Abelson 1997; Manzouri, Flynn et al. 2006). Atopic dermatitis is a pruritic skin condition that affects 3% of the population worldwide (Manzouri, Flynn et al. 2006).

The manifestations of AKC begin in the late teens or early twenties with a peak incidence between the ages of 30 and 50 years. It is more common in males than females. It persists until the fourth or fifth decade of life. AKC has a perennial pattern of occurrence with exacerbations more common in the winter months (Casey and Abelson 1997).

Patients with AKC have an inherited predisposition to atopy. There is a family history of allergic disorders such as asthma. The systemic disorders associated with AKC include hayfever, asthma, atopic dermatitis, food allergies, urticaria and nonhereditary angioedema (Casey and Abelson 1997).

Pathophysiology and Histopathology: The pathogenesis of AKC is multifactorial. Genetic factors, antigen sensitization, neural factors, Th2 type-lymphocytes, cytokines, hormonal factors and conjunctival hyperreactivity all have an influence on the pathogenesis (Leonardi, De Dominicis et al. 2007). The immunopathophysiology of AKC involves chronic IgE-mediated mast cell degranulation and autoimmune Th1- and Th2- type mechanisms with IgE (IgG4) activation (Casey and Abelson 1997; Zhan, Smith et al. 2003; Bonini 2004). The immunopathophysiology of AKC is mediated by T-lymphocytes, eosinophils, mast cells, Th1- and Th2-derived cytokines and other inflammatory cells (Nishida 1999; Butrus and Portela 2005). In AKC, it has been shown that there is an over-expression of mucosal type mast cells and eosinophils in the conjunctiva (Zhan, Smith et al. 2003).

Conjunctival hyperreactivity is a non-specific overreaction to non-specific stimuli, in which ocular symptoms are triggered by non-specific stimuli such as wind, dust and sunlight. This non-specific overreaction may not always be related to allergen levels within the environment (Bonini 2004).

The histopathological and laboratory findings of AKC revealed higher levels of IFN-γ, TNF-α, IL-2, IL-4, IL-5 and IL-10 in the tears, suggesting that both Th1 and Th2 responses may be activated (Leonardi, De Dominicis et al. 2007) as well as significant expression of T-lymphocytes (CD3$^+$, CD5$^+$), T helper-lymphocytes, T suppressor/cytotoxic-lymphocytes (CD8$^+$), macrophages, activated T-lymphocytes (CD25$^+$), B-lymphocytes (CD22$^+$), and dendritic cells (CD1$^+$, HLA-DR+) in substantia propria of the conjunctiva (Foster, Rice et al. 1991).

In AKC, the Helper T-lymphocytes are the primary mediators and effectors of tissue damage. There is recruitment of other cell types, including mast cells, eosinophils, lymphocytes and basophils which produce various allergic and inflammatory mediators. The chronically elevated levels of these cells and other mediators derived from them contribute significantly to the chronic damage seen in AKC (Anzaar, Gallagher et al. 2008).

Clinical Presentation: The most common complaints of patients with AKC are bilateral ocular itching, burning, and tearing. The symptoms are usually perennial (Zhan, Smith et al. 2003). The clinical features of AKC include papillary hypertrophy usually located on the lower tarsal conjunctiva, stringy or ropelike discharge due to the accumulation of cellular debris, fibrin, and mucin, hyperemia of the conjunctiva and episcleral vessels, blepharitis as well as varying degrees of conjunctival and corneal involvement (Casey and Abelson 1997; Bonini 2004; Manzouri, Flynn et al. 2006).

Calonge et al proposed a clinical grading system to help physicians in the diagnosis and management of AKC. Patients with *mild forms of AKC (Grade I)* present with mild/occasional itching, burning and photophobia. The clinical signs include anterior blepharitis, hyperemia/edema/papillae of the tarsal conjunctiva and superficial punctate keratitis. Patients with *mild-to-moderate forms of AKC (Grade II)* present with mildly persistent or moderate/occasional itching, burning and photophobia. In addition to grade I signs, these patients present with meibomian gland dysfunction, hyperemia/edema in the bulbar-limbal conjunctiva region (ciliary injection) and nonpersistent corneal epithelial defects. Patients with *moderate forms of AKC (Grade III)* present with moderately persistent itching, burning and photophobia. In addition to the grade II signs, patients with grade III disease present with meibomitis, conjunctival subepithelial fibrosis, and neovascularization, scarring and thinning of the cornea. Persistent corneal epithelial defects are also present. Patients with *severe forms of AKC (Grade IV)* present with severe itching, burning and photophobia. In addition to the grade III signs, these individuals present with mixed anterior and posterior blepharitis and conjunctival cicatrizing changes such as fornix foreshortening or symblepharon (Calonge and Herreras 2007).

AKC is a chronic disease associated with alterations in the mucin layer of the tear film. This causes increased mucus discharge, corneal epithelial disease and ocular surface desiccation (Leonardi, De Dominicis et al. 2007). Ocular surface mucins are believed to provide a barrier to prevent pathogens and particulate matter from entering the ocular surface epithelium. It has been suggested that mucin may play an important role in increasing the tear film stability and the hydration of the ocular surface (Dogru, Matsumoto et al. 2008). It has been shown that conjunctival squamous metaplasia, tear film instability and goblet cell loss in AKC are associated with a decrease in mucin 5AC and upregulation of mucin 1, 2 and 4 gene expressions. This may explain the lower stability and wettability of the tear film observed in AKC patients (Leonardi, De Dominicis et al. 2007; Dogru, Matsumoto et al. 2008).

The eyelid and periorbital manifestations in AKC include eczema of the periorbital skin and cheeks, maceration, hyperpigmentation of the periocular skin, atopic-related lid dermatitis, atopic-related blepharitis, meibomitis, eyelid margin keratinization, trichiasis/distichiasis, madarosis, rosacea-related blepharitis, ectropion, entropion, profound eyelid edema with Dennie-Morgan folds or Dennie lines, upper eyelid ptosis, fissures in the lateral canthus due to excessive eyelid rubbing and staphylococcal blepharitis (Foster and Calonge 1990; Tuft, Kemeny et al. 1991; Casey and Abelson 1997). Staphylococcus aureus colonization is common in AKC (Leonardi, De Dominicis et al. 2007). Lipases originating from bacteria colonizing the lid margin are believed to degrade some of the lipids as they are secreted, altering the composition of the tear film lipids (Donnenfeld and Pflugfelder 2009).

Conjunctival involvement in AKC include papillary hypertrophy of the tarsal conjunctiva, subepithelial fibrous, hyperemia and chemosis predominantly affecting the inferior forniceal and palpebral conjunctiva, gelatinous perilimbal hyperplasia, cicatrizing conjunctivitis with subepithelial fibrosis and symblepharon, follicles and keratinization involving the lower lid, fornix foreshortening, pseudopterygia and limbal hyperemia (Foster and Calonge 1990; Tuft, Kemeny et al. 1991; Calonge and Herreras 2007).

The ocular inflammatory process and release of allergic mediators onto the ocular surface and tear film are likely to be responsible for the corneal complications (Figure 10). The corneal involvement in AKC includes superficial punctate keratitis, macroerosions, filamentary keratitis, corneal ulceration, plaque formation, sectoral thinning, peripheral micropannus and corneal neovascularization, keratoconus, keratoglobus, pellucid marginal degeneration, pseudogerotoxon and lipid infiltration (Foster and Calonge 1990; Tuft, Kemeny et al. 1991; Casey and Abelson 1997; Zhan, Smith et al. 2003). Limbal scarring and Horner-Trantas dots as well as cataracts do occur in AKC (Tuft, Kemeny et al. 1991).

The perennial nature of the disease distinguishes it from allergic conjunctivitis and vernal keratoconjunctivitis, which usually have a seasonal pattern. Also, AKC tends to have lower lid involvement and to begin in the late teens whereas VKC is characterized by superior tarsal conjunctival papillary hypertrophy and tends to affect mostly children and young adult males (Casey and Abelson 1997). AKC must be considered in the differential diagnosis of chronic cicatrizing conjunctivitis and/or symblepharon (Foster and Calonge 1990).

Diagnosis: The diagnosis of AKC is based on the classic clinical signs and symptoms of the disease. In difficult cases, conjunctival or tear cytological studies can be useful in identifying the inflammatory infiltrate in the conjunctiva. Skin prick testing or the radioallergosorbent (RAST) test can be used to confirm the diagnosis of allergy and identify the offending allergen (Manzouri, Flynn et al. 2006). Although individuals with AKC have high total serum IgE, approximately 45% of patients with AKC are skin test or RAST negative to common allergens (Bonini 2004; Leonardi, De Dominicis et al. 2007). Although IgE antibodies to common allergens are not detectable in all cases of AKC, eosinophils have been found to be present in the tears and conjunctival scrapings of both the skin test/RAST-positive and negative- forms of AKC (Bonini 2004).

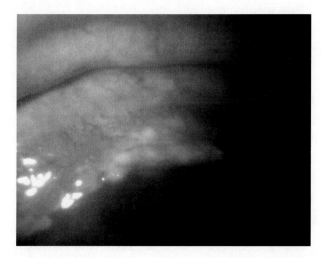

Figure 10. Corneal complications in AKC.

Management: The primary goal in the management of AKC is to prevent recurrences by eliminating or avoiding the trigger factors (Leonardi, Motterle et al. 2008).

The aim of therapy is to control the ocular inflammation, prevent damage to the ocular surface and periocular tissue and preserve vision (Foster and Calonge 1990; Casey and Abelson 1997; Margolis, Thakrar et al. 2007). Educating the patient on the degree of disease activity and the severity of the ocular surface inflammation as well as possible identification of trigger factors is a very important aspect of managing atopic keratoconjunctivitis (Zhan, Smith et al. 2003). Patients should be advised not to rub their eyes since chronic eye rubbing could induce mechanical degranulation of the mast cells, which actually exacerbate the symptoms (Casey and Abelson 1997).

AKC is a chronic ocular allergic disease that requires management with anti-inflammatory and anti-allergic pharmaceutical agents, supportive therapy, prophylactic antibiotics, and other non-pharmacologic management strategies.

The supportive therapy of AKC includes avoiding the trigger factors, applying cool compress, and administering preservative-free ocular lubricants. Cool compresses and preservative-free ocular lubricants provide symptomatic relief when there is intense ocular irritation and burning due to tear film insufficiency. It has been reported that ocular lubrication dilutes and washes away the allergens and inflammatory mediators on the ocular surface (Zhan, Smith et al. 2003).

Patients with the mild form of AKC may benefit from the use of supportive therapy as an adjunct to topical anti-allergic pharmacologic therapy and oral antihistamine. Moderate and severe cases of AKC associated with corneal compromise require topical steroids and prophylactic antibiotics (Berdy 1999). In the absence of corneal compromise, prophylactic antibiotics may not be necessary. It is worth mentioning that patients who present with flare up of their condition no matter how mild, may need a pulsed topical steroidal therapy (Dinowitz, Rescigno et al. 2000; Zhan, Smith et al. 2003). Most cases of AKC will require a topical steroid to control the inflammatory process, since T-lymphocytes and eosinophils play a major role in the immunopathogenesis of the condition (Leonardi and Secchi 2003). Corticosteroid should be used with caution in patients with AKC because of the risk of complications such as infection, cataract, corneal melting, and steroid induced intraocular pressure rise (Casey and Abelson 1997). The chronic blepharitis and meibomianitis associated with AKC requires regular eyelid hygiene, warm compress and long term therapy with systemic antibiotics such as doxycycline that are capable of inhibiting the action of lipase, an enzyme that converts glandular lipids into free fatty acid. The primary objective of this treatment modality is to improve the overall eyelid health and the quality of the tear film (Buckley 1998; McGill, Holgate et al. 1998; Berdy 1999; Dinowitz, Rescigno et al. 2000).

When moderate-to-severe AKC disease is refractory to conventional anti-allergic and anti-inflammatory therapy, the clinician is advised to consider immunosuppressant therapy (Stumpf, Luqmani et al. 2006). Topical immunomodulators such as cyclosporine can be used as a substitute for patients with steroid-dependent AKC. Once an adequate clinical response has been achieved with little or no exacerbations of the inflammatory process, the clinician may consider using topical cyclosporine as a substitute with the intention of weaning the patient off steroid dependency (Zhan, Smith et al. 2003). Clinical studies have shown that topical cyclosporine 2% is a safe and effective steroid-sparing therapeutic agent for AKC. A clinical study has also demonstrated the therapeutic benefits of topical cyclosporine in treating patients with meibomian gland metaplasia and eyelid telangiectasia, a condition that is usually seen in patients with AKC (Donnenfeld and Pflugfelder 2009). Nivenus et al, in their study of eyelid eczema treatment in AKC patients, demonstrated that tacrolimus had the potential to serve as an alternative to steroidal treatment for eczematous eyelid in AKC patients. They also suggested that patients should avoid ultraviolet exposure during treatment with tacrolimus (Nivenius, van der Ploeg et al. 2007).

Concurrent use of oral antihistamines may be necessary to reduce and control the intense itching associated with this condition (Berdy 1999). The eczema and periocular skin inflammation will respond to topical corticosteroid cream or tacrolimus, a non-steroidal alternative with superior efficacy and good safety profile. Preservative-free ocular lubricants and prophylactic antibiotics could be considered as an essential adjunctive therapeutic strategy when therapeutic bandage contact lens are used in managing corneal complications associated with AKC (Lemp and Bielory 2008).

Patients with severe AKC who present with compromised vision due to corneal scar formation, vascularization or corneal ulceration with perforation may benefit from penetrating keratoplasty and other corneal surgical interventions (Casey and Abelson 1997; Zhan, Smith et al. 2003).

The effective management of AKC necessitates a multidisciplinary approach involving the eye care professional, dermatologist, allergist and general medical practitioner. This becomes inevitable when the itching and inflammation extends beyond the ocular and periocular tissue (Casey and Abelson 1997).

Complications: If AKC is left untreated, ocular surface complications can progress to conjunctival scarring with subepithelial fibrosis, fornix foreshortening, symblepharon, corneal neovascularisation and corneal ulceration (Uchio, Kimura et al. 2008). Patients with AKC are predisposed to complications secondary to microbial infection of the eyelids, conjunctiva and cornea (Calonge and Herreras 2007).

The corneal complications seen in AKC are usually associated with tissue thinning of the cornea with consequential induction of refractive changes (Zhan, Smith et al. 2003). Consistent with these observations, reported ocular complications include keratoconus and cataract. Retinal detachment, ocular herpes simplex and general keratitis have also been reported (Foster and Calonge 1990; Anzaar, Gallagher et al. 2008).

AKC is a chronic and potentially blinding immune-mediated ocular surface inflammatory disease that occurs in association with atopic dermatitis (Anzaar, Gallagher et al. 2008). Advanced AKC is characterized by decreased tear production, lid margin keratinization and malposition, conjunctival scarring that result in persistent corneal trauma producing epithelial defects, ectasia, vascularization, and scarring. The ultimate consequence of these ocular sequelae is profound vision loss (Margolis, Thakrar et al. 2007). The key to stopping progressive cicatrization and eventual blinding keratopathy is long-term total control of the conjunctival inflammation (Foster, Rice et al. 1991).

Prognosis: AKC, unlike VKC, does not share the characteristic of spontaneous resolution (Tuft, Kemeny et al. 1991). Without prompt and persistent management, it will progress to potentially sight-threatening sequellae.

5.5. Contact Ocular Allergy

Introduction: Contact ocular allergy (COA) is part toxic-mediated and part immune-mediated hypersensitivity response to haptens, cosmetics, drugs, pollutants or other environmental factors (Leonardi, Motterle et al. 2008). It is predominantly a Th1-lymphocyte-mediated hypersensitivity response that involves the ocular surface, eyelids and periocular skin (Bielory 2007). It is mediated by sensitized T-lymphocytes in which Langerhans' cells process and present environmental allergens such as hapten to T-lymphocytes (Delves 2006; Warwick 2006). It is very common with no gender or racial predilection. It affects individuals of all ages.

Drug-induced allergic conjunctivitis, an ocular adverse reaction, is a delayed hypersensitivity reaction that causes itching and burning of the ocular surface, in response to pharmaceutical agent or their preservatives applied to the eyes or periorbital region (Abelson, Smith et al. 2003; Butrus and Portela 2005; Manzouri, Flynn et al. 2006). *Contact dermatoconjunctivitis,* a delayed cell-mediated hypersensitivity reaction, is characterized by conjunctivitis with dermatitis of the eyelids. It occurs most commonly in individuals using topical ophthalmic pharmaceutical agents (Blondeau 2002). The causative agents include topical pharmaceutical agents such as anesthetics, antibiotics, antivirals, some anti-glaucoma medications; contact lens solutions; and preservatives such as thimerosal or benzalkonium chloride (Schmid and Schmid 2000).

Pathophysiology and Histopathology: In COA, Th1-lymphocytes and their cytokines and, to a limited extent, eosinophils play a role in the immunopathogenesis or disease mechanism. It is related to contact T-lymphocyte-mediated delayed hypersensitivity reaction to haptens (incomplete antigens), which become immunogenic only after they bind to tissue proteins. The antigen is captured by Langerhans cells of the conjunctiva and presented to T-helper-lymphocytes in the regional lymph nodes. The sensitized T-lymphocytes react by secreting cytokines and several chemotactic factors, resulting in recruitment and activation of inflammatory cells and resident cells (Leonardi, De Dominicis et al. 2007). The elicitation phase occurs when memory T-lymphocytes recognize the antigen peptide together with MHC class II molecules on an APC. This interaction between the TCR on the memory CD4[+]T-lymphocytes and MHC on the APC stimulates the memory T-lymphocyte to proliferate and release cytokines that mediate T-lymphocyte mediated hypersensitivity response (Delves 2006). Th1-derived cytokines, such as IFN-γ induces recruitment and activation of macrophages leading to Th1-mediated delayed-type hypersensitivity. Th2-derived cytokines, such as IL-5 stimulate the chemotaxis and activation of eosinophil to the site of inflammation leading to Th2-mediated delayed-type hypersensitivity (Griffiths 2006). The histopathological manifestations reveal dendritic cells, basophils, eosinophils and Th1-lymphocytes (Schmid and Schmid 2000), (Terr 1994).

Clinical Presentation: The clinical manifestation of contact allergy of the eyes include itching, conjunctival hyperemia, chemosis, follicular/papillary reaction involving the inferior palpebral conjunctiva and fornices, punctate keratitis, infiltrative keratitis, as well as dermatitis of the periocular skin and eyelids (Figure 11) (Schmid and Schmid 2000).

Diagnosis: Comprehensive history and clinical presentation of contact ocular allergy is the key to diagnosing the condition. Patch testing is a useful diagnostic tool for contact dermatoconjunctivitis. The differential diagnosis of contact ocular allergy, in particular contact dermatoconjunctivitis, includes keratitis, blepharoconjunctivitis, microbial conjunctivitis and irritant conjunctivitis.

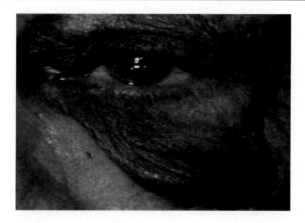

Figure 11. Contact Ocular Allergy.

Management: The management of patients with contact ocular allergy, including drug-induced allergic conjunctivitis and contact dermatoconjunctivitis, involves identifying and removing or avoiding the offending allergen or irritant. Mild forms of these conditions may respond to palliative therapy and antihistamine, as well as, avoiding the offending allergen or irritant. Moderate to severe cases of contact ocular allergy require multimodal anti-allergic agents, oral antihistamine and topical steroids to provide symptomatic relief and control of the inflammatory process (Abelson 1999). A dermatologic immunomodulator or steroidal cream may be necessary in cases presenting with periocular skin inflammation. The downside to long term use of dermatologic steroid cream is the risk of developing infection or skin atrophy. Tacrolimus has a good therapeutic effect with a rapid onset of action. Tacrolimus is a very effective and safe steroid-sparing option for treating the periocular skin inflammation in patients with contact ocular allergy (Kapp 2003; Nakagawa 2006; Paller 2008).

Complications: The complications of contact ocular allergy may arise from persistent exposure to the offending allergen or irritant as well as complications from long-term use of steroids. Contact ocular allergy may cause ocular surface inflammation including keratitis, which can result in visual impairment (Gurwood and Altenderfer 2001).

Prognosis: The prognosis is usually good, but severe cases that are refractory to conventional topical anti-allergic or anti-inflammatory therapy may benefit from using oral therapeutics such as oral corticosteroids.

CONCLUSION

In this chapter we have discussed the basic concepts of immunology, clinical manifestations, disease process and management of allergic disorders of the conjunctiva.

The management of allergic disorders of the conjunctiva presents a challenge to the clinician, calling for adequate knowledge of the immunopathophysiology, clinical features and differential diagnosis of the different types of ocular allergy. A good understanding of the cellular and mediator mechanism that are involved in the disease process of ocular allergy is required to have a successful outcome in the management (Manzouri, Flynn et al. 2006).

On the basis of evidence from several cell and mediator studies, it is therefore suggested that chronic allergic disorders of the conjunctiva are mainly related to a Th2-type allergic inflammation while allergic conjunctivitis is mainly dependent on the classical Type I hypersensitivity immune reaction (Bonini 2004). In chronic forms of allergic disorders of the conjunctiva, such as VKC and AKC, there is a persistent state of mast cell, eosinophil and lymphocyte activation. Chronic allergic disorders of the conjunctiva are associated with a switching from connective-tissue to mucosal-type mast cells, an increased involvement of corneal pathology, tissue remodeling and fibrosis (Leonardi, De Dominicis et al. 2007).

Furthermore, an adequate knowledge of anti-allergic and anti-inflammatory pharmaceutical agents used in the management of allergic disorders of the conjunctiva is necessary. It is important for clinicians to familiarize themselves with the different types of anti-allergic or anti-inflammatory medications, particularly their mode of action, the range of indications, side-effect profile, contra-indications, and relative efficacies. A clinician who has adequate knowledge of these factors will be in a good position to prescribe the type of anti-allergy or anti-inflammatory medications that will be most appropriate for addressing the patient's allergic reaction.

In the management of allergic disorders of the conjunctiva, it is imperative to categorize the severity of the condition into mild, moderate or severe. This will aid in educating the patient and/or their parent on the duration of the treatment, the treatment itself, long-term management plan and prognosis (Collum 1999). The clinician is responsible for educating the patient on the nature of their allergic disease process; the different modalities for managing ocular allergy; the need for long term management; and the correct way of applying topical anti-allergy or anti-inflammatory medication.

The mainstay of the management of allergic disorders of the conjunctiva consists of the use of anti-allergic therapeutic agents such as antihistamine, multiple action anti-allergic agents and mast cell stabilizers. When anti-allergic therapeutic agents are incapable of providing adequate therapeutic effect or do not control the allergic inflammatory process, the clinician should prescribe an anti-inflammatory agent. Topical immunomodulators such as tacrolimus are steroid-free alternatives that could be beneficial when long-term use of topical steroids is not a safe therapeutic option. The once-a-day or twice-a-day dosed multiple action anti-allergic agents have prophylactic and therapeutic properties, and as such, they may be considered the preferred choice for managing allergic conjunctivitis. Mast cell stabilizing drugs are an excellent choice for long-term prophylactic and maintenance therapy in patients with recurrent and perennial ocular allergy (Leonardi 2005). These agents do not have any effect on the histamine already released on the ocular surface. When a clinician decides to use a steroid to control hyperacute or chronic ocular allergic expressions, the topical steroid with an excellent safety profile and suitable for prolonged use such as loteprednol etabonate may be used as the drug of choice. Other suitable topical steroids are rimexolone, prednisolone and fluorometholone (Pavesio and Decory 2008).

Knowledge of the patient's life style is helpful in promoting compliance with recommended treatment protocols. To promote patient compliance, the clinician could prescribe anti-allergic and/or anti-inflammatory therapeutic agents that provide a rapid clinical response and prolonged therapeutic effect. Furthermore, prescribing therapeutic agents that are cost-effective, easy and convenient to use, safe for extended use, and comfortable will also promote compliance. Individuals with busy lifestyles such as students and workers may benefit from using once-a-day or twice-a-day dosed, long-acting topical anti-allergic agents. Agents such as these will improve compliance and also avoid the issue of self-administration in the case of young school-aged children. Once-daily dosed anti-allergic therapeutic agents may be considered the therapeutic agent of choice for school-aged children due to their convenience of use. If a patient complains of stinging or burning effect of the topical anti-allergic medications, in order to ensure compliance, the clinician could advise the patient to keep them in the refrigerator and apply them to the eye in the cold state. This non-pharmacologic management strategy will promote compliance with recommended treatment protocol.

Coated contact lens can have an adverse effect on the ocular surface in patients with GPC, and as such, reducing or eliminating the antigenic load on the contact lens by regular contact lens cleaning and disinfection, weekly enzymatic treatment, decreasing the wearing time, shortening the replacement interval or changing the contact lens material or design should be recommended (Donshik 1994; Donshik, Ehlers et al. 2008).

However, pulse steroidal therapy would become necessary if the allergic expression does not respond to anti-allergic therapy. In acute ocular allergy, the use of anti-allergic medications along with supportive therapy is usually sufficient. In hyperacute cases and chronic ocular allergy, it is preferable to control the inflammatory condition with an anti-inflammatory agent, such as steroids, and a prophylactic anti-allergic agent, such as mast cell stabilizers for long-term maintenance therapy. The correct management of ocular allergy is imperative to avoid an adverse effect on the patient's quality of life, as well as the ocular surface damage that might occur if this condition is under-treated or left untreated.

Allergic conjunctivitis is a benign form of ocular allergy with excellent prognosis whereas chronic ocular allergies are the severe forms with increased potential for developing ocular complications that can adversely affect visual prognosis. The primary aim of treating allergic conjunctivitis is to provide relief from symptoms and to prevent recurrences whereas in chronic ocular allergies, the main objective of treatment and management is to prevent visual complications (Manzouri, Flynn et al. 2006).

The management of allergic disorders of the conjunctiva is aimed at preventing the release of mediators of allergy, controlling the allergic inflammatory cascade and preventing ocular surface damage secondary to the allergic response. To achieve success in the management of ocular allergy, the clinician should have a considerable understanding of the pathophysiology and clinical features of the different types of ocular allergy as well as an adequate knowledge of treatment options and management approaches.

ACKNOWLEDGMENT

The authors wish to thank Dr. Jeffrey S. Nyman for providing the photographs (Figs. 7, 9 and 11) used in this chapter. The authors have no proprietary interest in any of the therapeutic agents mentioned in this chapter.

REFERENCES

Abelson, M. and P. Gomes (2008). "Olopatadine 0.2% ophthalmic solution: the first ophthalmic antiallergy agent with once-daily dosing." Expert Opin Drug Metab Toxicol **4**(4): 453-461.

Abelson, M., P. Gomes, et al. "Efficacy of olopatadine ophthalmic solution 0.2% in reducing signs and symptoms of allergic conjunctivitis." Allergy Asthma Proc **28**(4): 427-433.

Abelson, M. and J. Greiner (2004). "Comparative efficacy of olopatadine 0.1% ophthalmic solution versus levocabastine 0.05% ophthalmic suspension using the conjunctival allergen challenge model." Curr Med Res Opin **20**(12): 1953-1958.

Abelson, M., L. Smith, et al. (2003). "Ocular allergic disease: mechanisms, disease sub-types, treatment." Ocul Surf **1**(3): 127-149.

Abelson, M. B., A. A. Leonardi, et al. (1995). "Histaminase activity in patients with vernal keratoconjunctivitis." Ophthalmology **102**(12): 1958-1963.

Abelson, M. B., L. Smith, et al. (2003). "Ocular allergic disease: mechanisms, disease sub-types, treatment." Ocul Surf **1**(3): 127-149.

Abelson, M. B. L., A.; Smith, L. (2002). "The Mechanisms, Diagnosis and Treatment of Allergy." Review of Ophthalmology **9** (4): 74- 84.

Abelson, M. B. R., S.A. (1999). "How to Handle Drug-induced Allergic Conjunctivitis." Review of Ophthalmology **6**(10): 146-148.

Abu-El-Asrar, A., S. Al-Kharashi, et al. (2001). "Langerhans' cells in vernal keratoconjunctivitis express the costimulatory molecule B7-2 (CD86), but not B7-1 (CD80)." Eye **15**(Pt 5): 648-654.

Abu el-Asrar, A., K. Geboes, et al. (1997). "Adhesion molecules in vernal keratoconjunctivitis." Br J Ophthalmol **81**(12): 1099-1106.

Abu El-Asrar, A., S. Struyf, et al. (2000). "Chemokines in the limbal form of vernal keratoconjunctivitis." Br J Ophthalmol **84**(12): 1360-1366.

Abu El-Asrar, A., S. Struyf, et al. (2001). "Expression of chemokine receptors in vernal keratoconjunctivitis." Br J Ophthalmol **85**(11): 1357-1361.

Abu El-Asrar, A., S. Struyf, et al. (2003). "Role of chemokines in vernal keratoconjunctivitis." Int Ophthalmol Clin **43**(1): 33-39.

Abu El-Asrar, A., I. Van Aelst, et al. (2001). "Gelatinase B in vernal keratoconjunctivitis." Arch Ophthalmol **119**(10): 1505-1511.

Abu El-Asrar, A. M., S. Al-Mansouri, et al. (2006). "Immunopathogenesis of conjunctival remodelling in vernal keratoconjunctivitis." Eye **20**(1): 71-79.

Adkinson, N. F. J. (1990). "The Basic Immunology of Allergic Diseases." Allergy Proc **11**(1): 5-6.

Akbar, A. and J. E. Cook (2006). Regulation of the Immune Response. In: Male D, Brostoff J, Roth DB and Roitt I., editors. Immunology., Mosby Elsevier.

Akinsola, F. B., A. T. Sonuga, et al. (2008). "Vernal keratoconjunctivitis at Guinness Eye Centre, Luth (a five year study)." Nig Q J Hosp Med **18**(1): 1-4.

Alexander, M., S. Allegro, et al. "Efficacy and acceptability of nedocromil sodium 2% and olopatadine hydrochloride 0.1% in perennial allergic conjunctivitis." Adv Ther **17**(3): 140-147.

Allansmith, M. R. and R. N. Ross (1988). "Giant papillary conjunctivitis." Int Ophthalmol Clin **28**(4): 309-316.

Anzaar, F., M. J. Gallagher, et al. (2008). "Use of systemic T-lymphocyte signal transduction inhibitors in the treatment of atopic keratoconjunctivitis." Cornea **27**(8): 884-888.

Asano-Kato, N., K. Fukagawa, et al. (2005). "TGF-beta1, IL-1beta, and Th2 cytokines stimulate vascular endothelial growth factor production from conjunctival fibroblasts." Exp Eye Res **80**(4): 555-560.

Ashrafzadeh, A. and M. Raizman (2003). "New modalities in the treatment of ocular allergy." Int Ophthalmol Clin **43**(1): 105-110.

Askenase, P. (2000). "Proposing Th2 DTH relevant to asthma: cutaneous basophil hypersensitivity then and now." Chem Immunol **78**: 112-123.

Ballow, M., L. Mendelson, et al. (1984). "Pollen-specific IgG antibodies in the tears of patients with allergic-like conjunctivitis." J Allergy Clin Immunol **73**(3): 376-380.

Bandukwala, H., B. Clay, et al. (2007). "Signaling through Fc gamma RIII is required for optimal T helper type (Th)2 responses and Th2-mediated airway inflammation." J Exp Med **204**(8): 1875-1889.

Bartlett, J. D., J. F. Howes, et al. (1993). "Safety and efficacy of loteprednol etabonate for treatment of papillae in contact lens-associated giant papillary conjunctivitis." Curr Eye Res **12**(4): 313-321.

Belfair, N., T. Monos, et al. (2005). "Removal of giant vernal papillae by CO2 laser." Can J Ophthalmol **40**(4): 472-476.

Benjamin, E., R. Coico, et al. (2000). Hypersensitivity reactions: Antibody-Mediated (Type I) reactions. Immunology A Short Course. New York, Wiley-Liss.

Benjamin, E. C., Richard; Sunshine, Geoffrey. (2000). Activation and function of T and B cells. Immunology A Short Course. . New York: , Wiley-Liss.

Berdy, G. (1999). "Atopic keratoconjunctivitis (AKC)." Acta Ophthalmol Scand Suppl(228): 7-9.

Berdy, G., J. Stoppel, et al. (2002). "Comparison of the clinical efficacy and tolerability of olopatadine hydrochloride 0.1% ophthalmic solution and loteprednol etabonate 0.2% ophthalmic suspension in the conjunctival allergen challenge model." Clin Ther **24**(6): 918-929.

Bielory, L. (2007). "Differential diagnoses of conjunctivitis for clinical allergist-immunologists." Ann Allergy Asthma Immunol **98**(2): 105-114; quiz 114-107, 152.

Bielory, L. (2008). "Ocular allergy overview." Immunol Allergy Clin North Am **28**(1): 1-23, v.

Bielory, L. (2008). "Ocular allergy treatment." Immunol Allergy Clin North Am **28**(1): 189-224, vii.

Bielory, L., P. Buddiga, et al. (2004). "Ocular allergy treatment comparisons: azelastine and olopatadine." Curr Allergy Asthma Rep **4**(4): 320-325.

Bielory, L., C. Katelaris, et al. (2007). "Treating the ocular component of allergic rhinoconjunctivitis and related eye disorders." MedGenMed **9**(3): 35.

Blondeau, P. R., J.A. (2002). "Allergic reactions to brimonidine in patients treated for glaucoma." Can J Ophthalmol. **37**(1): 21-26.

Bonini, S. (2004). "Atopic keratoconjunctivitis." Allergy **59 Suppl 78**: 71-73.

Bonini, S. (2006). "Allergic conjunctivitis: the forgotten disease." Chem Immunol Allergy **91**: 110-120.

Bonini, S., M. Coassin, et al. (2004). "Vernal keratoconjunctivitis." Eye **18**(4): 345-351.

Bonini, S., A. Lambiase, et al. (2000). "Vernal keratoconjunctivitis revisited: a case series of 195 patients with long-term followup." Ophthalmology **107**(6): 1157-1163.

Bonini, S., A. Lambiase, et al. (2003). "Cytokines in ocular allergy." Int Ophthalmol Clin **43**(1): 27-32.

Bonini, S., A. Lambiase, et al. (1995). "Estrogen and progesterone receptors in vernal keratoconjunctivitis." Ophthalmology **102**(9): 1374-1379.

Bonini, S., A. Lambiase, et al. (2003). "Allergic chronic inflammation of the ocular surface in vernal keratoconjunctivitis." Curr Opin Allergy Clin Immunol **3**(5): 381-387.

Bonini, S., M. Sacchetti, et al. (2007). "Clinical grading of vernal keratoconjunctivitis." Curr Opin Allergy Clin Immunol **7**(5): 436-441.

Bremond-Gignac, D., J. Donadieu, et al. (2008). "Prevalence of vernal keratoconjunctivitis: a rare disease?" Br J Ophthalmol **92**(8): 1097-1102.

Brody, J. M. F., C. Stephen. (1996). Vernal Conjunctivitis In: Pepose JS, Holland GN, Wilhelmus KR, editors. Ocular Infection and Immunity. . St Louis, Mosby.

Brown, J., T. Wilson, et al. (2008). "The mast cell and allergic diseases: role in pathogenesis and implications for therapy." Clin Exp Allergy **38**(1): 4-18.

Buckley, R. J. (1998). "Allergic eye disease--a clinical challenge." Clin Exp Allergy **28 Suppl 6**: 39-43.

Butrus, S. and R. Portela (2005). "Ocular allergy: diagnosis and treatment." Ophthalmol Clin North Am **18**(4): 485-492, v.

Calder, V. L. and P. M. Lackie (2004). "Basic science and pathophysiology of ocular allergy." Curr Allergy Asthma Rep **4**(4): 326-331.

Calonge, M. and A. Enríquez-de-Salamanca (2005). "The role of the conjunctival epithelium in ocular allergy." Curr Opin Allergy Clin Immunol **5**(5): 441-445.

Calonge, M. and J. Herreras (2007). "Clinical grading of atopic keratoconjunctivitis." Curr Opin Allergy Clin Immunol **7**(5): 442-445.

Calonge, M. and J. M. Herreras (2007). "Clinical grading of atopic keratoconjunctivitis." Curr Opin Allergy Clin Immunol **7**(5): 442-445.

Cameron, J., S. Antonios, et al. "Excimer laser phototherapeutic keratectomy for shield ulcers and corneal plaques in vernal keratoconjunctivitis." J Refract Surg **11**(1): 31-35.

Cameron, J. A. (1995). "Shield ulcers and plaques of the cornea in vernal keratoconjunctivitis." Ophthalmology **102**(6): 985-993.

Cameron, J. A., A. A. Al-Rajhi, et al. (1989). "Corneal ectasia in vernal keratoconjunctivitis." Ophthalmology **96**(11): 1615-1623.

Cameron, J. A. and P. B. Mullaney (1997). "Amblyopia resulting from shield ulcers and plaques of the cornea in vernal keratoconjunctivitis." J Pediatr Ophthalmol Strabismus **34**(4): 261-262.

Casey, R. and M. Abelson (1997). "Atopic keratoconjunctivitis." Int Ophthalmol Clin **37**(2): 111-117.

Chandler, J. W. (1996.). Ocular Surface Immunology In: Pepose JS, Holland GN, Wilhelmus KR, editors. Ocular Infection and Immunity. St Louis, Mosby.

Chang, W. J., D. T. Tse, et al. (2005). "Conjunctival cytology features of giant papillary conjunctivitis associated with ocular prostheses." Ophthal Plast Reconstr Surg **21**(1): 39-45.

Cheer, S. and G. Plosker (2001). "Tacrolimus ointment. A review of its therapeutic potential as a topical therapy in atopic dermatitis." Am J Clin Dermatol **2**(6): 389-406.

Chen, W. (2006). "Dendritic cells and (CD4+)CD25+ T regulatory cells: crosstalk between two professionals in immunity versus tolerance." Front Biosci **11**: 1360-1370.

Chigbu, D. I. (2009). "The management of allergic eye diseases in primary eye care." Cont Lens Anterior Eye **32**(6): 260-272.

Chigbu, D. I. (2009). "The pathophysiology of ocular allergy: a review." Cont Lens Anterior Eye **32**(1): 3-15; quiz 43-14.

Ciprandi, G., S. Buscaglia, et al. (1997). "Azelastine eye drops reduce and prevent allergic conjunctival reaction and exert anti-allergic activity." Clin Exp Allergy **27**(2): 182-191.

Collum, L. M. (1999). "Vernal keratoconjunctivitis." Acta Ophthalmol Scand Suppl(228): 14-16.

Cook, E. B. (2004). "Tear cytokines in acute and chronic ocular allergic inflammation." Curr Opin Allergy Clin Immunol **4**(5): 441-445.

Cook, E. B., J. L. Stahl, et al. (2006). "Allergic tears promote upregulation of eosinophil adhesion to conjunctival epithelial cells in an ex vivo model: inhibition with olopatadine treatment." Invest Ophthalmol Vis Sci **47**(8): 3423-3429.

Corum, I., B. Yeniad, et al. (2005). "Efficiency of olopatadine hydrochloride 0.1% in the treatment of vernal keratoconjunctivitis and goblet cell density." J Ocul Pharmacol Ther **21**(5): 400-405.

Cousins, S. W. and B. T. Rouse (1996). Chemical Mediators of Ocular Inflammation In: Pepose JS, Holland GN, Wilhelmus KR, editors. Ocular Infection and Immunity. St Louis, Mosby.

Coutu, R. B. (1991). "Treatment of vernal keratoconjunctivitis: a retrospective clinical case study. Wallace F. Molinari Ocular Pharmacology Award." Optom Vis Sci **68**(7): 561-564.

Crampton, H. J. (2002). "A comparison of the relative clinical efficacy of a single dose of ketotifen fumarate 0.025% ophthalmic solution versus placebo in inhibiting the signs and symptoms of allergic rhinoconjunctivitis as induced by the conjunctival allergen challenge model." Clin Ther **24**(11): 1800-1808.

D'Arienzo, P., A. Leonardi, et al. (2002). "Randomized, double-masked, placebo-controlled comparison of the efficacy of emedastine difumarate 0.05% ophthalmic solution and ketotifen fumarate 0.025% ophthalmic solution in the human conjunctival allergen challenge model." Clin Ther **24**(3): 409-416.

Del Prete, G., E. Maggi, et al. (1994). "Human Th1 and Th2 cells: functional properties, mechanisms of regulation, and role in disease." Lab Invest **70**(3): 299-306.

Delves, P. J. M., Seamus J.; Burton, Dennis R.; Roitt, Ivan M. (2006). Hypersensitivity. Roitt's Essential Immunology. , Blackwell Publishing.

Delves, P. J. M., Seamus J.; Burton, Dennis R.; Roitt, Ivan M. (2006). Lymphocyte Activation. Roitt's Essential Immunology. , Blackwell Publishing.

Delves, P. J. M., Seamus J.; Burton, Dennis R.; Roitt, Ivan M. (2006). The Production of Effectors. Roitt's Essential Immunology. , Blackwell Publishing.

Deschenes, J., M. Discepola, et al. (1999). "Comparative evaluation of olopatadine ophthalmic solution (0.1%) versus ketorolac ophthalmic solution (0.5%) using the provocative antigen challenge model." Acta Ophthalmol Scand Suppl(228): 47-52.

Dinowitz, M., R. Rescigno, et al. (2000). "Ocular allergic diseases: differential diagnosis, examination techniques, and testing." Clin Allergy Immunol 15: 127-150.

Discepola, M., J. Deschenes, et al. (1999). "Comparison of the topical ocular antiallergic efficacy of emedastine 0.05% ophthalmic solution to ketorolac 0.5% ophthalmic solution in a clinical model of allergic conjunctivitis." Acta Ophthalmol Scand Suppl(228): 43-46.

Dogru, M., Y. Matsumoto, et al. (2008). "Alterations of the ocular surface epithelial MUC16 and goblet cell MUC5AC in patients with atopic keratoconjunctivitis." Allergy 63(10): 1324-1334.

Donnenfeld, E. and S. C. Pflugfelder (2009). "Topical ophthalmic cyclosporine: pharmacology and clinical uses." Surv Ophthalmol 54(3): 321-338.

Donshik, P., W. Ehlers, et al. (2008). "Giant papillary conjunctivitis." Immunol Allergy Clin North Am 28(1): 83-103, vi.

Donshik, P. C. (1994). "Giant papillary conjunctivitis." Trans Am Ophthalmol Soc 92: 687-744.

Donshik, P. C. (2003). "Contact lens chemistry and giant papillary conjunctivitis." Eye Contact Lens 29(1 Suppl): S37-39; discussion S57-39, S192-194.

Donshik, P. C., W. H. Ehlers, et al. (2008). "Giant papillary conjunctivitis." Immunol Allergy Clin North Am 28(1): 83-103, vi.

Durham, S. (1998). "The inflammatory nature of allergic disease." Clin Exp Allergy 28 Suppl 6: 20-24.

Elgebaly, S. A., P. C. Donshik, et al. (1991). "Neutrophil chemotactic factors in the tears of giant papillary conjunctivitis patients." Invest Ophthalmol Vis Sci 32(1): 208-213.

Elhers, W. H. and P. C. Donshik (2008). "Giant papillary conjunctivitis." Curr Opin Allergy Clin Immunol 8(5): 445-449.

Epstein, A. B. (2002). "New Horizons in Ocular Allergy. ." Review of Optometry 139(3): 117-124.

Feldmann, M. and D. Male (1989). Cell Cooperation in the Immune Response. In: Roitt I, Brostoff J & Male D, editors. Immunology. St. Louis, The C.V. Mosby Co.

Foster, C. S. and M. Calonge (1990). "Atopic keratoconjunctivitis." Ophthalmology 97(8): 992-1000.

Foster, C. S., B. A. Rice, et al. (1991). "Immunopathology of atopic keratoconjunctivitis." Ophthalmology 98(8): 1190-1196.

Foulks, G. N., T. Harvey, et al. (2003). "Therapeutic contact lenses: the role of high-Dk lenses." Ophthalmol Clin North Am 16(3): 455-461.

Friedlaender, M. (2006). "Epinastine in the management of ocular allergic disease." Int Ophthalmol Clin 46(4): 85-86.

Fukuda, K. (2005). "[Role of corneal fibroblasts in the pathogenesis of ocular allergic diseases]." Nippon Ganka Gakkai Zasshi 109(11): 717-726.

Fukuda, K., N. Kumagai, et al. (2006). "Fibroblasts as local immune modulators in ocular allergic disease." Allergol Int **55**(2): 121-129.

Galatowicz, G., Y. Ajayi, et al. (2007). "Ocular anti-allergic compounds selectively inhibit human mast cell cytokines in vitro and conjunctival cell infiltration in vivo." Clin Exp Allergy **37**(11): 1648-1656.

Gedik, S., Y. A. Akova, et al. (2006). "Secondary bacterial keratitis associated with shield ulcer caused by vernal conjunctivitis." Cornea **25**(8): 974-976.

Goodman, J. W. (1991). The Immune Response. In: Stites DP, Terr AI, editors. Basic Human Immunology., Appleton and Lange.

Greiner, J., C. Michaelson, et al. "Single dose of ketotifen fumarate .025% vs 2 weeks of cromolyn sodium 4% for allergic conjunctivitis." Adv Ther **19**(4): 185-193.

Griffiths, G. M. (2006). Cell-mediated cytotoxicity. In: Male D, Brostoff J, Roth DB, Roitt I, editors. Immunology. . Mosby Elsevier.

Gupta, A., A. Sharma, et al. (1999). "Mycotic keratitis in non-steroid exposed vernal keratoconjunctivitis." Acta Ophthalmol Scand **77**(2): 229-231.

Gurwood, A. S. and D. S. Altenderfer (2001). "Contact dermatitis." Optometry **72**(1): 36-44.

Hendricks, R. L. and Q. Tang (1996). Cellular Immunity and the Eye In: Pepose JS, Holland GN, Wilhelmus KR, editors. Ocular Infection and Immunity. St Louis, Mosby.

Hingorani, M., V. Calder, et al. (1998). "The role of conjunctival epithelial cells in chronic ocular allergic disease." Exp Eye Res **67**(5): 491-500.

Hjelm, F., F. Carlsson, et al. (2006). "Antibody-mediated regulation of the immune response." Scand J Immunol **64**(3): 177-184.

Holsclaw, D. S., J. P. Whitcher, et al. (1996). "Supratarsal injection of corticosteroid in the treatment of refractory vernal keratoconjunctivitis." Am J Ophthalmol **121**(3): 243-249.

Horak, F., P. Stübner, et al. (2003). "Onset and duration of action of ketotifen 0.025% and emedastine 0.05% in seasonal allergic conjunctivitis : efficacy after repeated pollen challenges in the vienna challenge chamber." Clin Drug Investig **23**(5): 329-337.

Howarth, P. (2002). "Antihistamines in rhinoconjunctivitis." Clin Allergy Immunol **17**: 179-220.

Ilyas, H., C. Slonim, et al. (2004). "Long-term safety of loteprednol etabonate 0.2% in the treatment of seasonal and perennial allergic conjunctivitis." Eye Contact Lens **30**(1): 10-13.

Iovieno, A., A. Lambiase, et al. (2008). "Preliminary evidence of the efficacy of probiotic eye-drop treatment in patients with vernal keratoconjunctivitis." Graefes Arch Clin Exp Ophthalmol **246**(3): 435-441.

Irani, A. M. (2008). "Ocular mast cells and mediators." Immunol Allergy Clin North Am **28**(1): 25-42, v.

Irkeç, M. and B. Bozkurt (2003). "Epithelial cells in ocular allergy." Curr Allergy Asthma Rep **3**(4): 352-357.

Jeng, B. H., J. P. Whitcher, et al. (2004). "Pseudogerontoxon." Clin Experiment Ophthalmol **32**(4): 433-434.

Jones, J. D., V. M. Temino, et al. (2008). "Use of olopatadine ophthalmic solution and reactivity of histamine skin testing." Allergy Asthma Proc **29**(6): 636-639.

Kamani NR, D. S. (1991). Structure and Development of the Immune System. In: Stites DP, Terr AI, editors. Basic Human Immunology. Norwalk, Connecticut., Appleton and Lange; 1991. p. 9-33.

Kapp, A. A., B.R.; Reitamo, S. (2003). "Atopic dermatitis management with tacrolimus ointment (Protopic)." J Dermatolog Treat **14**((Suppl 1)): 5-16.

Katelaris, C., G. Ciprandi, et al. (2002). "A comparison of the efficacy and tolerability of olopatadine hydrochloride 0.1% ophthalmic solution and cromolyn sodium 2% ophthalmic solution in seasonal allergic conjunctivitis." Clin Ther **24**(10): 1561-1575.

Katelaris, C. H. (1999). "Giant papillary conjunctivitis--a review." Acta Ophthalmol Scand Suppl(228): 17-20.

Kato, N., K. Fukagawa, et al. (2006). "Mechanisms of giant papillary formation in vernal keratoconjunctivitis." Cornea **25**(10 Suppl 1): S47-52.

Katsarou, A., M. Armenaka, et al. (2009). "Tacrolimus ointment 0.1% in the treatment of allergic contact eyelid dermatitis." J Eur Acad Dermatol Venereol **23**(4): 382-387.

Keklikci, U., S. Soker, et al. "Efficacy of topical cyclosporin A 0.05% in conjunctival impression cytology specimens and clinical findings of severe vernal keratoconjunctivitis in children." Jpn J Ophthalmol **52**(5): 357-362.

Kirkner, R. (2001). "Lose the CAT...and Other Pearls from Allergists." Review of Optometry **138**(3): 94 - 98.

Kobayashi, A., A. Nagata, et al. (2002). "Surgical treatment of limbal vernal keratoconjunctivitis by resection of a limbal lesion." Jpn J Ophthalmol **46**(6): 679-681.

Kumagai, N., K. Yamamoto, et al. (2002). "Active matrix metalloproteinases in the tear fluid of individuals with vernal keratoconjunctivitis." J Allergy Clin Immunol **110**(3): 489-491.

Kumar, S. (2008). "Combined therapy for vernal shield ulcer." Clin Exp Optom **91**(1): 111-114.

Kumar, S. (2009). "Vernal keratoconjunctivitis: a major review." Acta Ophthalmol **87**(2): 133-147.

Kymionis, G. D., D. Goldman, et al. (2008). "Tacrolimus ointment 0.03% in the eye for treatment of giant papillary conjunctivitis." Cornea **27**(2): 228-229.

Lambiase, A., S. Minchiotti, et al. (2009). "Prospective, multicenter demographic and epidemiological study on vernal keratoconjunctivitis: a glimpse of ocular surface in Italian population." Ophthalmic Epidemiol **16**(1): 38-41.

Lambrecht, B. (2001). "Allergen uptake and presentation by dendritic cells." Curr Opin Allergy Clin Immunol **1**(1): 51-59.

Lanier, L. (1991). Cells of the Immune Response: Lymphocytes and Mononuclear Phagocytes. In: Stites DP, Terr AI, editors. Basic Human Immunology. Norwalk, Connecticut, Appleton and Lange.

Lemanske, R. F. J. K., M.A. (1983). "Late phase allergic reactions." Int J Dermatol **22**(7): 401-409.

Lemp, M. A. and L. Bielory (2008). "Contact lenses and associated anterior segment disorders: dry eye disease, blepharitis, and allergy." Immunol Allergy Clin North Am **28**(1): 105-117, vi-vii.

Leonardi, A. (1999). "Pathophysiology of allergic conjunctivitis." Acta Ophthalmol Scand Suppl(228): 21-23.

Leonardi, A. (2002). "The central role of conjunctival mast cells in the pathogenesis of ocular allergy." Curr Allergy Asthma Rep 2(4): 325-331.

Leonardi, A. (2005). "Emerging drugs for ocular allergy." Expert Opin Emerg Drugs 10(3): 505-520.

Leonardi, A., P. Brun, et al. (2003). "Tear levels and activity of matrix metalloproteinase (MMP)-1 and MMP-9 in vernal keratoconjunctivitis." Invest Ophthalmol Vis Sci 44(7): 3052-3058.

Leonardi, A., P. Brun, et al. (2007). "Matrix metalloproteases in vernal keratoconjunctivitis, nasal polyps and allergic asthma." Clin Exp Allergy 37(6): 872-879.

Leonardi, A., P. Brun, et al. (2005). "Urokinase plasminogen activator, uPa receptor, and its inhibitor in vernal keratoconjunctivitis." Invest Ophthalmol Vis Sci 46(4): 1364-1370.

Leonardi, A., C. De Dominicis, et al. (2007). "Immunopathogenesis of ocular allergy: a schematic approach to different clinical entities." Curr Opin Allergy Clin Immunol 7(5): 429-435.

Leonardi, A., I. A. Fregona, et al. (2006). "Th1- and Th2-type cytokines in chronic ocular allergy." Graefes Arch Clin Exp Ophthalmol 244(10): 1240-1245.

Leonardi, A., L. Motterle, et al. (2008). "Allergy and the eye." Clin Exp Immunol 153 Suppl 1: 17-21.

Leonardi, A. and A. Secchi (2003). "Vernal keratoconjunctivitis." Int Ophthalmol Clin 43(1): 41-58.

Li, J., R. C. Tripathi, et al. (2008). "Drug-induced ocular disorders." Drug Saf 31(2): 127-141.

Luk, F. O., V. W. Wong, et al. (2008). "Perilimbal conjunctival pigmentation in Chinese patients with vernal keratoconjunctivitis." Eye 22(8): 1011-1014.

Lydyard P, G. C. (1989). Cells involved in the Immune Response. In: Roitt I, Brostoff J & Male D, editors. Immunology. St. Louis, The C.V. Mosby Co.

Lydyard, P. G., Carlo E. (2006). Cells, tissue, and organs of the immune system. In: Male D, Brostoff J, Roth DB, Roitt I, editors. Immunology. , Mosby Elsevier.

Mah, F., L. Rosenwasser, et al. (2007). "Efficacy and comfort of olopatadine 0.2% versus epinastine 0.05% ophthalmic solution for treating itching and redness induced by conjunctival allergen challenge." Curr Med Res Opin 23(6): 1445-1452.

Malbec, O. and M. Daëron (2007). "The mast cell IgG receptors and their roles in tissue inflammation." Immunol Rev 217: 206-221.

Male, D. (2006.). Introduction to the Immune System. In: Male D, Brostoff J, Roth DB, Roitt I, editors. Immunology. , Mosby Elsevier.

Male, D. and I. Roitt (1989). Adaptive and Innate Immunity. In: Roitt I, Brostoff J & Male D, editors. Immunology. St. Louis, The C.V. Mosby Co.

Male, D. C., Anne; Owen, Michael; Trowsdale, John; Champion, Brian. (1996). Antigen Processing and Presentation. Advanced Immunology, Mosby Co.

Male, D. C., Anne; Owen, Michael; Trowsdale, John; Champion, Brian. (1996). B cell Activation and Maturation. Advanced Immunology, Mosby Co.

Male, D. C., Anne; Owen, Michael; Trowsdale, John; Champion, Brian. (1996). T lymphocyte Activation and Maturation. Advanced Immunology. , Mosby Co.

Male, D. C., Anne; Owen, Michael; Trowsdale, John; Champion, Brian. (1996). Cytokine and Chemokines. Advanced Immunology. , Mosby Co.

Male, D. R., Ivan. (1989). Adaptive and Innate Immunity. In: Roitt I, Brostoff J, Male D, editors. Immunology. St. Louis, The C.V. Mosby Co.

Manzouri, B., T. Flynn, et al. (2006). "Pharmacotherapy of allergic eye disease." Expert Opin Pharmacother **7**(9): 1191-1200.

Margolis, R., V. Thakrar, et al. (2007). "Role of rigid gas-permeable scleral contact lenses in the management of advanced atopic keratoconjunctivitis." Cornea **26**(9): 1032-1034.

Marini, J. C. (2006). Cell Cooperation in Antibody Response. In: Male D, Brostoff J, Roth DB, Roitt I, editors. Immunology., Mosby Elsevier.

McGill, J., S. Holgate, et al. (1998). "Allergic eye disease mechanisms." Br J Ophthalmol **82**(10): 1203-1214.

Meijer, F., K. Pogany, et al. (1993). "N-acetyl-aspartyl glutamic acid (NAAGA) topical eyedrops in the treatment of giant papillary conjunctivitis (GPC)." Doc Ophthalmol **85**(1): 5-11.

Melton, R. and R. Thomas (2003). "Clinical Guide to Ophthalmic Drugs." Review of Optometry **140**(6): Supplement: 33A -39A.

Metz, D., A. Bacon, et al. (1996). "Phenotypic characterization of T cells infiltrating the conjunctiva in chronic allergic eye disease." J Allergy Clin Immunol **98**(3): 686-696.

Miyazaki, D., T. Tominaga, et al. (2008). "Therapeutic effects of tacrolimus ointment for refractory ocular surface inflammatory diseases." Ophthalmology **115**(6): 988-992.e985.

Moser, M. and K. Murphy (2000). "Dendritic cell regulation of TH1-TH2 development." Nat Immunol **1**(3): 199-205.

Mosman, T. R. (1992). "T lymphocyte subsets, cytokines and effector functions." Annals of the New York Academy of Sciences **664**: 89-92.

Murphy, K. P. T., Paul; Walport, Mark; Janeway, Charles (2008). T-cell mediated immunity. Janeway's immunobiology New York Garland Science

Murphy, K. T., Paul; Walport, Mark; Janeway, Charles (2008). Signaling through immune system receptors. Janeway's Immunobiology. New York, Garland Science.

Nakagawa, H. (2006). "Comparison of the efficacy and safety of 0.1% tacrolimus ointment with topical corticosteroids in adult patients with atopic dermatitis: review of randomised, double-blind clinical studies conducted in Japan." Clin Drug Investig **26**(5): 235-246.

Niederkorn, J. (2008). "Immune regulatory mechanisms in allergic conjunctivitis: insights from mouse models." Curr Opin Allergy Clin Immunol **8**(5): 472-476.

Nishida, T. T., A.W. (1999). "Specific Aqueous Humour Factors induce Activation of Regulatory T cells." Investigative Ophthalmology and Visual Science. **40**(10): 2268-2274.

Nishiwaki-Dantas, M. C., P. E. Dantas, et al. (2000). "Surgical resection of giant papillae and autologous conjunctival graft in patients with severe vernal keratoconjunctivitis and giant papillae." Ophthal Plast Reconstr Surg **16**(6): 438-442.

Nivenius, E., I. van der Ploeg, et al. (2007). "Tacrolimus ointment vs steroid ointment for eyelid dermatitis in patients with atopic keratoconjunctivitis." Eye **21**(7): 968-975.

Noble, S. and D. McTavish (1995). "Levocabastine. An update of its pharmacology, clinical efficacy and tolerability in the topical treatment of allergic rhinitis and conjunctivitis." Drugs **50**(6): 1032-1049.

Oppenheim, J. J., F. W. Ruscetti, et al. (1991). Cytokines. In: Stites DP, Terr AI, editors. Basic Human Immunology. Norwalk, Connecticut, Appleton and Lange.

Owen, M. (1989). Major Histocompatibility Complex. In: Roitt I, Brostoff J & Male D, editors. Immunology. St. Louis, The C.V. Mosby Co.

Ozbek, Z., A. Z. Burakgazi, et al. (2006). "Rapid healing of vernal shield ulcer after surgical debridement: A case report." Cornea **25**(4): 472-473.

Ozcan, A., T. Ersoz, et al. (2007). "Management of severe allergic conjunctivitis with topical cyclosporin a 0.05% eyedrops." Cornea **26**(9): 1035-1038.

Paller, A., L. Eichenfield, et al. (2008). "Three times weekly tacrolimus ointment reduces relapse in stabilized atopic dermatitis: a new paradigm for use." Pediatrics **122**(6): e1210-1218.

Park, A. Y. S., P. (2001). "IL-12: Keeping Cell-Mediated Immunity Alive." Scand. J. Immunol **53**: 529-532.

Pavesio, C. and H. Decory (2008). "Treatment of ocular inflammatory conditions with loteprednol etabonate." Br J Ophthalmol **92**(4): 455-459.

Pawankar, R. (2007). "Inflammatory mechanisms in allergic rhinitis." Curr Opin Allergy Clin Immunol **7**(1): 1-4.

Pelegrin, L., O. Gris, et al. (2008). "Superficial keratectomy and amniotic membrane patch in the treatment of corneal plaque of vernal keratoconjunctivitis." Eur J Ophthalmol **18**(1): 131-133.

Porazinski, A. D. and P. C. Donshik (1999). "Giant papillary conjunctivitis in frequent replacement contact lens wearers: a retrospective study." CLAO J **25**(3): 142-147.

Quah, S. A., C. Hemmerdinger, et al. (2006). "Treatment of refractory vernal ulcers with large-diameter bandage contact lenses." Eye Contact Lens **32**(5): 245-247.

Rao, S. K., S. Meenakshi, et al. (2004). "Perilimbal bulbar conjunctival pigmentation in vernal conjunctivitis: prospective evaluation of a new clinical sign in an Indian population." Cornea **23**(4): 356-359.

Reiss, J., M. B. Abelson, et al. (1996). Allergic conjunctivitis. In: Pepose JS, Holland GN, Wilhelmus KR, editors. Ocular infection and immunity. St. Louis, Mosby.

Reitamo, S., J. Harper, et al. (2004). "0.03% Tacrolimus ointment applied once or twice daily is more efficacious than 1% hydrocortisone acetate in children with moderate to severe atopic dermatitis: results of a randomized double-blind controlled trial." Br J Dermatol **150**(3): 554-562.

Revillard, J. "Innate immunity." Eur J Dermatol **12**(3): 224-227.

Rissoan, M., V. Soumelis, et al. (1999). "Reciprocal control of T helper cell and dendritic cell differentiation." Science **283**(5405): 1183-1186.

Romagnani, S. (1994). "Lymphokine production by human T cells in disease states." Annu Rev Immunol **12**: 227-257.

Rook, G. (1989). Cell-Mediated Immune Responses. In: Roitt I, Brostoff J & Male D, editors. Immunology. St. Louis, The C.V. Mosby Co.

Rosenwasser, L., T. Mahr, et al. "A comparison of olopatadine 0.2% ophthalmic solution versus fluticasone furoate nasal spray for the treatment of allergic conjunctivitis." Allergy Asthma Proc **29**(6): 644-653.

Sanchis-Merino, M., J. Montero, et al. (2008). "Comparative efficacy of topical antihistamines in an animal model of early phase allergic conjunctivitis." Exp Eye Res **86**(5): 791-797.

Sangwan, V. S., S. I. Murthy, et al. (2005). "Cultivated corneal epithelial transplantation for severe ocular surface disease in vernal keratoconjunctivitis." Cornea **24**(4): 426-430.

Schmid, K. L. and L. M. Schmid (2000). "Ocular allergy: causes and therapeutic options." Clin Exp Optom **83**(5): 257-270.

Scoper, S. V., G. J. Berdy, et al. (2007). "Perception and quality of life associated with the use of olopatadine 0.2% (Pataday) in patients with active allergic conjunctivitis." Adv Ther **24**(6): 1221-1232.

Sengor, T., M. Irkec, et al. (1995). "Tear LTC4 levels in patients with subclinical contact lens related giant papillary conjunctivitis." CLAO J **21**(3): 159-162.

Shimmura, S., R. Igarashi, et al. (2003). "Lecithin-bound superoxide dismutase in the treatment of noninfectious corneal ulcers." Am J Ophthalmol **135**(5): 613-619.

Sibéril, S., C. Dutertre, et al. (2006). "Molecular aspects of human FcgammaR interactions with IgG: functional and therapeutic consequences." Immunol Lett **106**(2): 111-118.

Siminovitch, K. (1992). "The new immunology." J Reconstr Microsurg **8**(2): 121-129.

Skotnitsky, C. C., T. J. Naduvilath, et al. (2006). "Two presentations of contact lens-induced papillary conjunctivitis (CLPC) in hydrogel lens wear: local and general." Optom Vis Sci **83**(1): 27-36.

Solomon, A., J. Pe'er, et al. (2001). "Advances in ocular allergy: basic mechanisms, clinical patterns and new therapies." Curr Opin Allergy Clin Immunol **1**(5): 477-482.

Solomon, A., I. Puxeddu, et al. (2003). "Fibrosis in ocular allergic inflammation: recent concepts in the pathogenesis of ocular allergy." Curr Opin Allergy Clin Immunol **3**(5): 389-393.

Solomon, A., E. Zamir, et al. (2004). "Surgical management of corneal plaques in vernal keratoconjunctivitis: a clinicopathologic study." Cornea **23**(6): 608-612.

Spadavecchia, L., P. Fanelli, et al. (2006). "Efficacy of 1.25% and 1% topical cyclosporine in the treatment of severe vernal keratoconjunctivitis in childhood." Pediatr Allergy Immunol **17**(7): 527-532.

Spangler, D., G. Bensch, et al. (2001). "Evaluation of the efficacy of olopatadine hydrochloride 0.1% ophthalmic solution and azelastine hydrochloride 0.05% ophthalmic solution in the conjunctival allergen challenge model." Clin Ther **23**(8): 1272-1280.

Srivastava, A., S. Sur, et al. (2003). "The role of eosinophils in ocular allergy." Int Ophthalmol Clin **43**(1): 9-25.

Stahl, J., E. Cook, et al. (2002). "Pathophysiology of ocular allergy: the roles of conjunctival mast cells and epithelial cells." Curr Allergy Asthma Rep **2**(4): 332-339.

Streilein, J. W. (1996). Regional Immunology of the Eye In: Pepose JS, Holland GN, Wilhelmus KR, editors. Ocular Infection and Immunity. St Louis, Mosby.

Stumpf, T., N. Luqmani, et al. (2006). "Systemic tacrolimus in the treatment of severe atopic keratoconjunctivitis." Cornea **25**(10): 1147-1149.

Suchecki, J. K., P. Donshik, et al. (2003). "Contact lens complications." Ophthalmol Clin North Am **16**(3): 471-484.

Tabbara, K. (2003). "Immunopathogenesis of chronic allergic conjunctivitis." Int Ophthalmol Clin **43**(1): 1-7.

Taylor, A. (2007). "Ocular immunosuppressive microenvironment." Chem Immunol Allergy **92**: 71-85.

Terr, A. I. (1991). Mechanism of Inflammation. In: Stites DP, Terr AI, editors. Basic Human Immunology. Norwalk, Connecticut, Appleton and Lange.

Terr, A. I. (1994). Cell-Mediated Hypersensitivity Disease. In: Stites DP, Terr AI, Parslow TG, editors. Basic & Clinical Immunology. . Norwalk, Connecticut, Appleton & Lange.

Terr, A. I. (1994). Mechanism of Hypersensitivity In: Stites DP, Terr AI, Parslow TG, editors. Basic & Clinical Immunology. . Norwalk, Connecticut:, Appleton & Lange.

Terr, A. I. (1997). Inflammation. In: Stites DP, Terr AI, Parslow TG, editors. Medical Immunology. Stamford, Connecticut, Appleton and Lange.

Tkaczyk, C., Y. Okayama, et al. (2004). "Fcgamma receptors on mast cells: activatory and inhibitory regulation of mediator release." Int Arch Allergy Immunol **133**(3): 305-315.

Tkaczyk, C., Y. Okayama, et al. (2002). "Activation of human mast cells through the high affinity IgG receptor." Mol Immunol **38**(16-18): 1289-1293.

Trattler, W., J. Luchs, et al. (2006). "Elestat (epinastine HCl ophthalmic solution 0.05%) as a therapeutic for allergic conjunctivitis." Int Ophthalmol Clin **46**(4): 87-99.

Trocme, S. D., G. M. Kephart, et al. (1993). "Eosinophil granule major basic protein deposition in corneal ulcers associated with vernal keratoconjunctivitis." Am J Ophthalmol **115**(5): 640-643.

Trowsdale, J. (2006.). Antigen Presentation. In: Male D, Brostoff J, Roth DB, Roitt I., editors. Immunology. , Mosby Elsevier.

Tuft, S. J., I. A. Cree, et al. (1998). "Limbal vernal keratoconjunctivitis in the tropics." Ophthalmology **105**(8): 1489-1493.

Tuft, S. J., D. M. Kemeny, et al. (1991). "Clinical features of atopic keratoconjunctivitis." Ophthalmology **98**(2): 150-158.

Turner, M. (1989). Molecules which recognize Antigen. In: Roitt I, Brostoff J & Male D, editors. Immunology. St. Louis, The C.V. Mosby Co.

Uchio, E., R. Kimura, et al. (2008). "Demographic aspects of allergic ocular diseases and evaluation of new criteria for clinical assessment of ocular allergy." Graefes Arch Clin Exp Ophthalmol **246**(2): 291-296.

Uchio, E., S. Ono, et al. (2000). "Tear levels of interferon-gamma, interleukin (IL) -2, IL-4 and IL-5 in patients with vernal keratoconjunctivitis, atopic keratoconjunctivitis and allergic conjunctivitis." Clin Exp Allergy **30**(1): 103-109.

Verin, P. (1998). "Treating severe eye allergy." Clin Exp Allergy **28 Suppl 6**: 44-48.

Verin, P. H., I. D. Dicker, et al. (1999). "Nedocromil sodium eye drops are more effective than sodium cromoglycate eye drops for the long-term management of vernal keratoconjunctivitis." Clin Exp Allergy **29**(4): 529-536.

Warwick, B. (2006). Hypersensitivity Type IV. In: Male D, Brostoff J, Roth DB, Roitt I, editors. Immunology., Mosby Elsevier. .

Woolhiser, M., K. Brockow, et al. (2004). "Activation of human mast cells by aggregated IgG through FcgammaRI: additive effects of C3a." Clin Immunol **110**(2): 172-180.

Woolhiser, M., Y. Okayama, et al. (2001). "IgG-dependent activation of human mast cells following up-regulation of FcgammaRI by IFN-gamma." Eur J Immunol **31**(11): 3298-3307.

Wraith, D. C. (2006). Immunological Tolerance. In: Male D, Brostoff J, Roth DB and Roitt I., editors. Immunology., Mosby Elsevier.

Zhan, H., L. Smith, et al. (2003). "Clinical and immunological features of atopic keratoconjunctivitis." Int Ophthalmol Clin **43**(1): 59-71.

In: Conjunctivitis: Symptoms, Treatment and Prevention   ISBN: 978-1-61668-321-4
Editor: Anna R. Sallinger, pp. 73-105   © 2010 Nova Science Publishers, Inc.

Chapter II

NOVEL DRUG DELIVERY APPROACHES IN DRY EYE SYNDROME THERAPY

Slavomira Doktorovová[1], Joana R. Araújo[2], Maria A. Egea[2],
Marisa L. Garcia[2] and Eliana B. Souto[1,3,*]

[1]University of Trás-os-Montes and Alto Douro (IBB/CGB-UTAD), Vila Real, Portugal;
[2]University of Barcelona, Barcelona, Spain;
[3]Fernando Pessoa University, Porto, Portugal.

ABSTRACT

Dry eye syndrome or the *keratoconjunctivitis sicca* is a common disease of tear film and ocular surface developed in numerous aetiologies. Tear film instability and ocular surface disturbances that subsequently influence the tear film are among the primarily causes of this disease, but many other factors are involved in tear film disorders. Clinical manifestations commonly include eye discomfort, feeling of a foreign body in the eye, itching or even visual disturbance; inflammation and damage of ocular surface may follow. The therapeutic approaches are based on the dry eye symptoms relief, increasing the patient's comfort and preventing further damage to ocular surface. This can be achieved by renewing the normal function of tear film and ocular surfaces. Although eye surface is easily reached by classical ocular dosage forms, novel drug delivery systems for ocular administration offer advantages in terms of increased residence time on eye surface and/or controlled release of the drug, with enhanced therapeutic effectiveness. Patient's acceptance can also be improved by developing formulations that do not require frequent application, or cause blurred vision, and having a more pleasant appearance. Biodegradable, biocompatible, non-toxic, and mucoadhesive materials are being used for the design of colloidal carriers. Novel polymers for hydrogels suitable for ocular

---

* Correspondence concerning this article should be addressed to: Eliana B. Souto, Faculty of Health Sciences, Fernando Pessoa University, Rua Carlos da Maia, Nr. 296, Office S.1, P-4200-150 Porto, Portugal. Phone: +351-225-074630; Fax: +351-225-074637; Email: eliana@ufp.edu.pt.

administration are reviewed in this chapter, giving overview on their potential benefits and limitations in dry eye syndrome management and reported successful formulations.

Keywords: Dry eye, Keratoconjunctivitis sicca, Sjögren's syndrome, Colloidal carriers, Nanoparticles, Liposomes.

ABBREVIATIONS

AUC	Area Under the Curve
KCS	Keratoconjunctivitis Sicca
NC	Nanocapsules
NE	Nanoemulsion
NLC	Nanostructured Lipid Carriers
NP	Nanoparticles
NS	Nanospheres
NSAIDs	Non Steroidal Anti-Inflammatory Drugs
PECL	Poly-ε-caprolactone
PEG	Polyethylenglycol
PIBCA	Poly-isobutyl-cyanoacrylate
PLGA	Poly(lactic-co-glycolic)acid
PVA	Polyvinyl alcohol
RCE	Rabbit Corneal Epithelium
SLN	Solid Lipid Nanoparticles

1. INTRODUCTION

For many decades, *keratoconjunctivitis sicca* (KCS) or dry eye ocular surface disease, was thought to be limited to dryness of the eyes caused by a reduction of the aqueous phase of the tear film. Now it is understood that this definition does not adequately describe the full clinical picture of dry eye disease, while it is true that the most frequent cause of common dry eye is lachrymal hyposecretion, deviations in tear composition also play a decisive role. As such, the modern definition of dry eye disease is based on the concept of the three layers of the tear film devised by Holly and Lemp [1], which can be directly affected by different stimuli, causing qualitative and quantitative changes. The term "dry eye" is generically used to describe a variety of ocular disorders of diverse pathogenesis that share signs of ocular surface abnormalities and symptoms of discomfort, feeling of dryness, grittiness, and/or foreign body sensation.

Most people experience acute dry eye episodes multiple times during lifetime. Prolonged exposure to dry air (e.g., on a long-haul flight), or to a strong current of air from driving at high speed readily induces transient dry eye even in people with healthy eyes. While these common conditions are harmless and are easily resolve spontaneously, chronic dry eye syndrome can severely impair the patients' quality of life and vocational performance. In severe cases that are left untreated, damage to the cornea may result.

Dry eye syndrome is a superficial eye disorder, meaning that the target site of the drug is the external tissues of the eye. The optimal ocular dosage form suitable for use in dry eye syndrome management should enable the delivery of the actives to the relevant ocular tissue ideally without compromising the irrelevant sites. No systemic uptake of the administered drug should occur. As dry eye syndrome is such a common disease, the use of the final product should at the same time be as convenient as possible for the patient, i.e. should be handled easily, and should not interfere with normal vision, therefore not causing any unpleasant sensation upon administration.

The corneal surface can be easily reached by classical ocular dosage forms like eye drops, aqueous suspensions of drugs, hydrogels, or ophthalmic ointments. Eye drops are the most common ocular dosage forms, ideal for instillation of hydrophilic drugs, offering several advantages including easy manipulation, easy manufacture, and low production costs. The well known limitation is the fast elimination of the aqueous dispersion form the ocular surface by blinking and by tear drainage, not allowing the drug to stay onto the ocular surface for sufficient time. Only a low percentage of the drug will permeate the cornea and reach its site of action within the eye.

Ophthalmic hydrogel formulations are an alternative to eye drops that might provide increased residence time of the drug onto the ocular surface. Despite the transparency, blurring of the vision still may occur. Despite blurred vision is not a serious side effect, the patient's comfort and subsequent compliance may be compromised. Another issue of hydrogel formulations is their higher production costs in comparison to eye drops or ocular ointments.

Many of the actives relevant in dry eye syndrome management are poorly water soluble. The marketed formulations for this kind of drugs include aqueous suspensions of the drug (e.g., Pred Forte™ with 1% prednisolone acetate from Allergan; Alrex™ with 0.2% loteprednol etabonate from Bausch & Lomb) or ophthalmic emulsions (e.g., Restasis™ with 0.05% cyclosporine from Allergan; Durezol™ with 0.05% difluprednate from Sirion Therapeutics). Achieving therapeutic concentrations of the drugs by means of these forms may also be difficult.

Besides practical advantages and well established usage of these classical ocular dosage forms, there is still a space for improvements in terms of bioavailability, targeted delivery of actives to the desired tissues and controlled release. The aims of employing novel dosage forms include: (i) elimination of possible side effects of the drugs or adverse reactions to the formulations constituents; (ii) improvement of drug bioavailability at the required site of action; (iii) provide prolonged therapeutic effect; (iv) assure convenient application of the medicinal product, preferentially in the form of eye drops; (v) to avoid interfering with vision, i.e. be transparent and show a refractive index similar to that of the tears.

As the cornea contains many nerve endings, the size of the carriers that might be used in ophthalmic formulations without causing the sensation of foreign body in the eye and itching is limited to particle diameters below 1 μm [2]. Some authors prefer even smaller particle size for ocular drug delivery e.g. below 500 nm [3] Therefore, any drug carrier intended for ocular administration should have diameter within this size range. Nanoparticle formulations prepared from various materials are being proposed as alternative drug formulation by many research teams. Apart from the suitable size, further reasons for using nanoparticle-based formulation in ocular drug delivery are: (i) the possibility to be applied onto the ocular surface in the same way as eye drops (as aqueous nanoparticle dispersions); (ii) their submicron meter size of the particles avoiding interfering with the vision; and (iii) the possibility to provide a controlled release of the active. Prolonged release of actives is often achieved by encapsulation of the actives into various carriers. The drug must however release from the carrier in such a time that allows its further penetration into the target tissue before the carrier is eliminated from the site.

2. Lachrymal Functional Unit and Dry Eye Syndrome

Tear secretion is controlled and coordinated by the lachrymal functional unit, composed of the main and accessory lachrymal glands, the ocular surface (cornea, conjunctiva and meibomian glands) and the interconnecting innervations. Subconscious stimulation of the free nerve endings populating the cornea, results in the generation of afferent nerve impulses through the ophthalmic branch of the trigeminal nerve on to the mid-brain where they synapse, signal is integrated and sent by efferent branch of the loop through the pterygopalatine ganglion to the lachrymal glands [4].

The eyelids, which serve as a protective device for the eye, moisten the surface of the cornea by producing a tear film of 10 μm thick that prevents desiccation. This tear film consists of three layers: (i) a superficial lipid layer mainly composed of wax and cholesteryl esters and some polar lipids, which plays a major role in maintaining that function; (ii) the aqueous layer, which is important to the maintain the corneal transparency; and a mucous layer sticking to the epithelial cells, responsible for the adherence of the tear film to the cornea. Another essential task of the conjunctiva is the immunological defence provided by Langerhans cells and lymphatic follicles which contain T and B lymphocytes, various subtypes of reticular cells and macrophages.

Tears are also important in wound healing, by providing a pathway by which blood cells make their way from the circulation into central corneal openings, and in the aerobic metabolism of the corneal epithelium, obtaining and dissolving oxygen from the atmosphere. The normal tear quantity, its anti-inflammatory constituents and the secretion of mucin, repair and prevent damage during exposure of the ocular surface in a normal individual to environmental stresses such as wind, low humidity, blinking, or exposure of the surface to bacteria, viruses or particles.

2.1. Causes of the Dry Eye

A number of ocular surface conditions may trigger dry eye disease or be associated with it. Evidence indicates that chronic dry eye results from a T cell-mediated inflammatory pathology [5]. The ocular surface, lachrymal glands, and interconnecting nerves form a homeostatic functional unit that maintains normal tear production and multiple factors, including an age-related drop in systemic androgen levels, autoimmune disorders such as Sjögren's syndrome, or meibomian gland dysfunction, create an environment in which activated T cells are recruited to the ocular surface and lachrymal glands, disrupting the normal nerve traffic and perpetuating a cycle of immune-based inflammation that ultimately results in destruction of the lachrymal glands [6]. Environmental factors such as hot climates, pollution, the use of visual display terminals and contact lenses may also cause chronic ocular surface irritation that can contribute to the onset of dry eye symptoms [7].

Pharmacological and toxic dry eye has been known since the last century. Drugs reported as being relevant for the reduction of lachrymal secretion are atropine, contraceptives, antiestrogen tamoxifen, tranquilizers, acetylsalicylic acid, the antineoplasic busulfan, the antiangina pectoris perhexiline, alpha-adrenergic stimulants and beta-adrenergic blockers. Some toxic chemicals may also desiccate the eye (denaturalized colza oil, botulinum toxin, typhoid fever) [8]. Vitamin A is essential for maintaining the health of epithelial cells throughout the body, affecting cellular regulation and differentiation [9], its deficiency adversely affects epithelial cells. Thus, an absence of this active causes the loss of goblet cells and leads to increased epidermal keratinization and squamous metaplasia of the mucous membranes, generally including the cornea and conjunctiva [10]. This type of avitaminose due to malnutrition in underdeveloped countries and other nutritional conditions such as hyponutrition, alcoholism and dehydration, is also accepted as causes of dry eye.

Sjögren's syndrome, named after the Swedish ophthalmologist Henrik Sjögren, was first described it in 1933, as a chronic autoimmune rheumatic disorder characterized by lymphocytic infiltration of exocrine glands and mucosae [11], leading to destruction of the glandular tissue. Lymphocyte diapedesis and homing to ocular tissues are induced and regulated by multiple signalling pathways. During the initial phase of cell response to injury, immune or inflammatory insults, the corneal and conjunctival epithelial cells can be stimulated to express inflammatory molecules such as cytokines and cell adhesion molecules [12,13]. Chemokines, a family of chemotactic cytokines that signal through G-protein coupled receptors, and Inter Cellular Adhesion Molecule-1 (ICAM-1), one of the most important intercellular adhesion molecules, will in turn promote lymphocyte activation and further recruitment to the ocular tissues and lachrymal glands [14]. As a result, inflammation will occur within the lachrymal functional unit leading towards an alteration in tear quantity and composition, interrupting neuronal reflex signalling and exacerbating inflammation manifestation. The loss of neural function results in sensory isolation of the lachrymal glands and the elimination of requisite neural tone, as a consequence lachrymal glands atrophy, presenting cellular breakdown proteins to the cell surface. Apoptosis (i.e., programmed cell death) of T lymphocytes is a gene-regulated process that functions abnormally in patients with Sjögren's syndrome and appears to contribute to glandular destruction and an altered tear film [15].

Besides the association with Sjögren's syndrome exocrinopathy, dry eye may also be associated with several endocrinopathies, Graves-Basedow's disease, diabetes mellitus, pheochromocytoma, ovariectomy, premature ovarian failure, hypothyroidism and various conditions involving the menstrual cycle, menopause, pregnancy and involution senilis [8].

In patients with atopic dermatitis, which is another skin and mucosae disorder or autoimmune connective tissue disease, KCS is a severe and often chronic ocular surface inflammatory condition, occurring conjunctival scarring and corneal complications, leading to significant visual morbidity. Viral infections, such as infectious mononucleosis, cytomegalovirus, AIDS and viral keratoconjunctivitis (e.g., *Bacillus xerosis*) have also been considered causes of dry eye due to an immune response or to direct involvement of the lachrymal glands. Immunopathological changes include invasion of the epithelium by eosinophils and mast cells and significant infiltration of the stroma by activated T-cells that produce IL-2 and IFN-γ [16, 17].

Changes in the hormonal environment surrounding the ocular surface and lachrymal gland is one of the key factors involved in the etiology of KCS. The common hormonal status in female populations of non-Sjögren's KCS is a decrease in circulating androgens due to decreased function of the ovaries in the post-menopausal woman, and also to secretion of sex hormone binding globulin during pregnancy and birth control pill use [18,19]. Therefore, it is believed that androgens provide trophic support of the lachrymal gland as well as meibomian gland function and its deficiency or inherent insensitivity may lead to meibomian gland disease [20, 21]

Apoptosis is a series of physiological events in the cell which ensure the balance between cell division and loss, therefore contributing for the regulation of tissue development and homeostasis. Pathological apoptosis may also happen, if abnormal increase and/or decrease in the rate of apoptotic cell death in target tissues occurs. Such condition has been demonstrated in various types of diseases including dry eye. Clinically, apoptosis-related markers were found to be upregulated in conjunctival cells from patients with moderate to severe KCS, with or without Sjögren's syndrome [11], indicating an important role in the pathogenesis of KCS.

Other reason for dry eye symptoms includes neurosensorial deprivation of the lachrymal basin caused by an interruption of the trigeminal nerve. Subsidiary corneal damage due to dryness, scarce or incomplete blinking, traumatic aggression or a lack of neurotrophic stimuli results in the release of pro-inflammatory neural transmitters such as substance P. This neuropeptide enhance the activation status of vigilant lymphocytes and the release of cytokines leading to neurogenic inflammation symptoms [22].

Despite the plurality of the underlying causes of dry eye, there are several common histopathologic manifestations of the ocular surface epithelia, namely, the loss of the conjunctival goblet cells, abnormal enlargement of the epithelial cells, increase in cellular stratification, and keratinization [23]. The normal secretory conjunctival mucosa gradually develops into a nonsecretory keratinized epithelium, a process referred to as squamous metaplasia [24].

Obstruction of meibomian gland ducts, whether by epithelial squamous metaplasia, chalazia, or solidified lipids, results in decreased secretion of abnormal tear lipids [25]. Lipases originating from bacteria colonizing the lid margin are believed to degrade some of the lipids as they are secreted, changing lipid composition of the tear film. The partially degraded lipids depict high melting point and, therefore, are more likely to solidify and block meibomian gland orifices at body temperature. Changes in lipid layer of the tear film allows increased evaporation of the aqueous component, leading to many of the signs and symptoms found in chronic dry eye [26].

2.2. Signs and Symptoms of the Dry Eye

The most frequent symptoms of dry eye include irritation, sensation of strange body, existence of filamentous mucosity and transitory blurred vision. Other less frequent symptoms are photophobia, sensation of fatigue and slowness of eyelids. All these symptoms can be exacerbated in those situations where an increase of the evaporation takes place (heat, conditioned air or wind) and can improve closing the eyes. In slight to moderate dry eye, patients can have crisis of intense lachrymation, that does not contradict the existence of dry eye, since these crisis can be due to lachrymation reflects (conjuntival or corneal irritation) or emotional reasons, which usually is normal [8].

Often it is possible to suspect of dry eye, only with observing the signs in pre-corneal tearful film, the marginal tearful layer and the own cornea. For pre-corneal film, the increase of mucous fibers can be detected along with the fact that mucin contaminated with lipids is accumulated in the film and moves with the blinking. In the case of the marginal film, this has a reduced height in dry eye (1 mm for healthy eyes), is concave and contains mucosity, in serious cases it can even lack. Others include punctiform epithelial erosions that can be depicted by the cornea; filaments in the form of comma whose free ends hang on the cornea and move with the blinking; mucous plates that pronounce injuries of varied size and formed by epithelial cells, proteins and lipidic substances. Rare but also possible is the corneal perforation in severe cases.

The evaluation of the breakage time of the pre-corneal tearful film is a simple test to diagnose dry eye and is based on the instillation of fluorescein in the inferior sac. The patient is asked to blink several times and stop, one inspects the film with cobalt blue light. After an interval of time, black spots or lines appear in the tear film which indicates the appearance of dry areas. The time of rupture is measured from the last blinking to the appearance of the first dry spot and is considered abnormal when inferior to 10 seconds. Other possible test is the method of Mengher, which uses corneal reflection, clear when the corneal surface is humidified and distortable by dry spots. Projecting on the cornea a square, the clinician can control the time that takes in distorting the square by the first dry spot.

3. THERAPEUTIC APPROACHES OF THE DRY EYE SYNDROME

Treatment of the dry eye involves the challenges and frustrations associated with the management of a chronic disease. There is generally no cure but, with proper attention and an adequate treatment regimen, it is likely that good vision can be preserved throughout life and a considerable degree of comfort afforded.

General measures to decrease dryness include reviewing the patient's medications to consider replacing one or more drying agents with medications that have fewer anticholinergic effects. Avoiding environmental factors (e.g., wind, dust, smoke, and low humidity), increasing fluid intake (especially water), avoiding use of excessive eye makeup (particularly on the eyelid, because it can soften and enter the eye, creating more concentrated tears), and using moisture-chamber glasses specifically designed to protect the eye from irritants and hold sponges that increase the humidity surrounding the eye, are measures that may help improving eye comfort.

The main objectives of diverse therapeutic options are to alleviate the pain, contribute to a uniform optical surface, prevent corneal injuries and prevent probable causes of dry eye. Traditional therapies, such as punctal occlusion and artificial tears, are palliative measures that attempt to increase the volume of the tear film by either reducing drainage or supplementing the tear film with an aqueous solution [27]. Important factors in the success of dry eye therapy are the full information of patients about the nature of their disease, the goals of the clinician´s choice and the encouragement of compliance with the regimen.

3.1. Current Therapeutic Strategies

Although the definitive cure remains elusive, a number of measures are available for managing various dry eye manifestations. The most appropriate type of treatment modality for each patient must be carefully studied and proceeded, being determined by the severity of the condition. Further research to identify more completely the pathogenetic mechanisms involved in the development of the dry eye is ongoing. It is hoped that the results of such studies will allow the direction of therapy more specifically and even more successfully in the near future.

3.1.1. Tear Substitution: Artificial Tear Substitutes and Lubricants

The eye's primary line of defence is its tear film, a complex isotonic liquid containing a mixture of proteins (including enzymes such as lysozyme, which dissolves gram-negative bacteria) and lipids. Tear replacement by topical artificial tears and lubricants is currently the most widely used therapy for dry eye, with the goal of increasing humidity and improving lubrication at the ocular surface [6].

Tear film substitution by the use of artificial tears has however some limitations. The complex composition of natural tears is difficult to replace and the ability of lachrymal glands to massively increase tear production in response to the introduction of any irritant onto the ocular surface means that eye drops require isotonic, no irritating, and perhaps even astringent formulations. Otherwise, they will be instantly diluted, and even completely flushed out, before they have a chance to diffuse through the cornea - which in itself acts as a barrier for diffusion. Apart from a good tolerance and high surface stability, an ideal tear substitute requires a long retention period, while not being too viscous, as this would have a negative influence on visual acuity, and as far as possible, it should contain no foreign substances, such as irritating preservatives [28].

Lubricants are aqueous solutions of polymers able to meet the requirements of wetting agents, i.e., hydrophilizing the corneal surface and extending adhesion and retention periods in the eye. Available preparations consisting of semi-synthetic cellulose derivates, polyvinyl alcohol, polyvinylpyrrolidone, polyacrylic acid derivates, dextran or hyaluronic acid aqueous solutions reduce the surface tension of the tear fluid, afford improved corneal moistening, thicken and stabilize the pre-corneal tear film, and consequently allow dry eye symptoms relief. However, they all have limited periods of ocular retention. This requirement can be reached by adding to the formulations, ingredients designed to have mucoadhesive properties. Many of these components are formulated as viscous gels [29], which tend to cause irritation, blur vision, make the eyelid sticky and create a sensation of heavy eyelids. Different formulation strategies can simply use less viscous materials [30], biopolymeric systems that allow less viscosity while retaining mucoadhesive properties [31], or the polymer chitosan, which has bioadhesive and lubricating properties [32-34].

Some patients with KCS have particularly viscous, stringy mucus that may be associated with filaments or coarse mucous plaques on the ocular surface, which appear to be major sources of irritation and discomfort [35, 36]. This condition can be ameliorated by daily application of mucolytic solutions, such as 10 to 20% solutions of acetylcysteine 4 to 5 times.

Lipids are usually formulated as ointments which are usually an inconvenience in KCS, since these formulations are not able to mix with the tear film and may damage the pre-corneal film. As a result, these formulations may drastically reduce the breakup time i.e., breaking the tear film within a few seconds when the eye is open. However, there are some preservative-free formulations on the market that can provide relief for patients experiencing symptoms of insufficient moistening action during the night and upon awakening, their application provides a long-lasting means of increasing lubricity between the eyelid and the ocular surface during sleep [35, 36].

To obtain a continuous and adequate treatment, repeated application is required. For this, ophthalmic preparations in multiple-dose containers are necessary and applications from such containers are subject to contamination, being iatrogenic infections with Pseudomonas aeruginosa the most problematic [37]. To ensure a long shelf-life and stability of preparations in multiple-dose containers, in addition to polymers manufacturers commonly employ a variety of stabilizers and preservatives. The most currently used preservatives are quaternary ammonium compounds (benzalkonium chloride, benzododecinium bromide, cetrimide, polyquad), alcohols (chlorobutanol) and other compounds (e.g., chlorhexidine, sorbic acid, potassium sorbate, boric acid, biguanides), acting primarily against the bacterial cell membrane, damaging or destroying it [38-40]. Nevertheless, one must bear in mind that all preservatives have more or less pronounced irritating properties and citotoxicity in the cells of the ocular surface. As such, single-dose preservative-free containers are a suitable alternative to patients having to apply ophthalmic formulations frequently and for extended periods. The drawbacks presented by these single unit-dose tears are the high cost and the induced lack of compliance, because patients must carry numerous vials to maintain adequate dosage over the day.

Other common additives used in artificial tear preparations are buffers, which have the purpose of maintaining the pH of human natural tears as closely as possible when they are applied [38,39]. As a rule, slightly alkaline isotonic or almost isotonic moistening agents are preferred in KCS treatment, as they seem to be more comfortable than neutral or acidic preparations. Accordingly, most commercially available tear substitutes are maintained at a pH value between 7.23 and 7.5 by bicarbonates, phosphates, acetates, citrates, borates and sodium hydroxide.

Another important factor is tear film osmolarity, which is also an irritative factor [41]. In general, its value ranges between 303 and 305 mosm/L and in patients with dry eye this is increased up to 30-40 mosm/L. consequently the attempt is to reduce this increased osmolarity by applying hypotonic electrolyte-based formulations [42, 43]. Bicarbonate seems to be an essential electrolyte in the recovery of the damaged corneal epithelial barrier and in the maintenance of normal ultrastructure [44].

When conditions of dry eye are mild, a tear substitute with low viscosity is recommended, as far as possible no more often than four times per day. In cases of more pronounced dry eye, the frequency of eye drop application must be increased to ten times per day. Besides, the application of commercially available tear substitutes is frequently insufficient for patients with severe forms of KCS, and a too frequent use may result in toxic or allergic reactions due to the cumulative effect of the preservatives. These patients prefer inserts, since these are small, solid, yet soft polymers introduced into the cul-de-sac which, suffer continuous moistening by the natural tear fluid, take several hours to dissolve, and avoid frequent drop applications. The first sustained-release artificial tear inserts becoming available (Lacriserts™) were 5 mg hydroxypropyl cellulose rods that dissolve on contact with the ocular surface, releasing a viscous watery coating that can last 6 to 12 hours [45]. Although being preservative free and used only twice a day, they have the disadvantages of being expensive, difficult to manage, producing the sensation of a foreign body present in the eye and may occasionally cause mild striated vision while being dissolved. Related to this system is a new preservative-free lyophilised drug delivery system with better tolerability, in which hydroxypropylmethyl cellulose detaches from a polymeric carrier upon contact with the tear film [46].

Surgical procedures aiming to substitute tears by fluids from other exocrine glands offers an alternative to the most difficult cases [47]. The parotid salivary gland is a choice being its outward duct transplanted into the conjunctival sac. Besides its higher secretion quantity per time and the different composition of saliva compared to tear fluid, atrophy of the gland often occurs, and because of these disadvantages it is not a usual procedure. Auto-transplantation of areas of normal conjunctiva from one eye to another is a successful surgical modality, particularly in cases of chemical burns.

3.1.2. Tear Preservation

3.1.2.1. Occlusion of the Tear Drainage System

In advanced cases of KCS, occlusion of the puncta leading into the canaliculi and nasolachrymal sac and duct is able to provide an improvement of both objective and subjective complaints. This is currently the most common non-pharmacological therapy for dry eye disease, it prevents the drainage of natural and artificial tears improving the quantity and quality of the aqueous component.

Patients who underwent punctal occlusion may experience diminished ocular surface sensation and a concomitant decrease in tear production [48], being also possible an increase in toxicity of preservatives present in ocular medications. Besides these disadvantages related with a delay in tear clearance and turnover [49], other complications may be reported such as pruritus, discomfort, deviations and rupture of some plugs, supurative canaliculitis and stenosis. Consequently the decision to occlude all the puncta should not be taken lightly and just after the use of unpreserved tears and lubricants have proven to be insufficient and after a positive result to temporary occlusion with absorbable or removable plugs or inserts.

The easier and most commonly performed techniques are tamponade methods, which occlude the drainage system with a foreign body after a previous anesthesia and punctal dilatation [50]. Non-absorbable tamponade can be achieved by inserting plugs made of silicon, HEMA (hydroxyethylmethacrylate) or Teflon (polytetrafluorethylene) into the canaliculus with the head left protruding from the punctum, being easily removed with forceps or by flushing saline [51]. Inserts made of hydroxypropylcellulose or collagen are absorbable, dissolving slowly at body temperature after insertion into the canaliculus, lasting respectively 18 hours and 2 weeks. These are important to assess the patient´s tolerance and avoid future permanent occlusions which may be inadequate in certain cases.

Surgical methods are not usually performed due to the extreme difficulty to reverse them. The exception is the punctum patch, which covers the punctum with autologous conjunctiva and can be easily removed if occlusion results in epiphoria, causing a great deal of discomfort to the patient [52].

When a permanent occlusion is the aim, this usually involves the application of heat, sclerosing or desiccating the lachrymal canaliculi. Thermal methods can be performed by electrically heated probes (cautery), electrodes that coagulate tissues by delivering a high frequency current (diathermy) or argon lasers, being this latter the most flexible method because it can either produce a full or partial occlusion [53].

3.1.2.2. Other Methods of Tear Preservation

Studies have suggested that increased evaporation is one mechanism that produces ocular surface disease associated with dry eyes and some methods of tear preservation act to prevent this evaporation, rather than blocking tear drainage [54]. Moist chambers (watch glass compresses) and tight-fitting goggles (side panels reaching up to the eyebrows) can protect against loss of humidity from the tear film by providing a damp chamber without additional aeration and accumulation of condensation and may, therefore, be useful in more severe cases [55,56]. Swimming goggles should also be mentioned as protective devices from chlorinated water, worn by patients with KCS. Hyperemizing agents, such as hot eye patches, can be applied over the eyelids for a few minutes, increasing the rate of secretion from the meibomian glands.

The attempt to reverse some of the desiccation seen on the corneal surface can also be accomplished with bandage soft contact lenses. These water-filled lenses provide a moist covering and exchange some of the fluid with the epithelium, being particularly useful in the dissolution of filamentary keratitis. Besides constituting an irritable foreign body that can worsen the situation, the use of these lenses is associated with the development of bacterial infections and corneal ulcer with endophthalmitis. They must be used in conjunction with artificial tears as they tend to dry out rapidly and are recommended in only a very small number of patients with intractable filamentary keratitis that cannot be managed by any other treatment modality [57].

If no relief occurs upon occlusion of the outgoing lachrymal canaliculi, and for patients with persistent corneal epithelial defects in severe dry eye disease, tarsorrhaphy (i.e., the suturing together a portion of or the entire upper and lower eyelids) can be undertaken. This procedure decreases the exposed surface of the eye, reducing or avoiding the dry out of the pre-corneal tear film between individual blinks. Although quite simple, it shows however the disadvantage of being cosmetically disfigurating [58].

3.1.3. Pharmacological Stimulation of Natural Tears

Small molecular naturally occurring chemicals and some analogs have been identified that stimulate lachrymal gland secretion. This stimulation is able to act only if a sufficient amount of functioning glandular tissue is still available, since no medication is able to stimulate secretion from an atrophied gland. Some drugs, such as mucolytics (bromhexidine and ambroxol), cholinergic agents (carbachol, bethanecol, pilocarpine), or eledoisin, a natural endekapeptide extracted from the salivary glands of the Mediterranean octopus Eledone moschata, have been adopted into therapy [59].

Although with an unknown mechanism of action, the increase in tear secretion produced is doubtless connected with hyperemia due to vasodilation, and theoretically, drugs that can increase cyclic nucleotide (cAMP or cGMP) levels, increase tear secretion [60].

Apart from the fact that the success of this kind of therapy is often questionable, drugs are expensive and the patient may experience a burning sensation when applying them. It is also possible that the stimulation of previously inflamed ocular surface, as in cases of extreme dryness, could deliver pro-inflammatory tears, worsening the disease.

3.1.4. Treatment of the Underlying Causes of Dry Eye Disease

Although the primary mechanism is a qualitative or quantitative defect in the tear film layers, some types of dry eye are caused by immunological or other primary disorders. Inflammatory mediators liberated by the infiltrating T-cells into the lachrymal gland and conjunctiva, such as IFN-γ, and TNF-α cause lachrymal dysfunction, interfere with normal differentiation, and promote apoptosis of lachrymal gland and ocular surface epithelial cells [61, 62]. Increased levels of inflammatory cytokines have also been demonstrated, especially interleukin-6 (IL-6), in the eyes of patients with or without Sjögren's syndrome [27]. Although the correlation of these findings with the lack of hormonal support, chronic irritation and altered innervational mechanisms in some dry eye states are unknown [4,63], it is predicted that topical anti-inflammatory, immunomodulatory or hormonal agents may be capable of normalizing the disturbed neuro-hormonal reflex between the ocular surface and lachrymal glands. Treatment of any other condition involving conjunctival and corneal surfaces, like a deficit in vitamin A or epidermal growth factor, may complement therapies for dry eye.

3.1.4.1. Cyclosporine A

For the treatment of patients with KCS having primary inflammation of the ocular surface, particularly those who show moderate to severe inflammation, rheumatoid nodules, scleritis and corneal ulcers, immunomodulating agents may be appropriate. Cyclosporine A, largely used to prevent reactions after transplants and in a variety of autoimmune diseases, is an important immunomodulating drug that can also be used in dry eye states.

The efficiency of cyclosporine ophthalmic emulsion for treatment of dry eye was first examined in a randomized, double-masked, placebo-controlled, dose-ranging clinical trial [64]. Although no clear dose-response relationship was seen, cyclosporine 0.05% and 0.1%

emulsions provided significant improvements in symptoms, superficial punctate keratitis, and rose bengal staining from baseline. Cyclosporine 0.05% ophthalmic emulsion was approved by the FDA to increase tear production in patients whose tear production is presumed to be suppressed due to ocular inflammation [65].

Many chronic ocular surface disorders share features with dry eye disease, and their responses to immunomodulation therapy with cyclosporine have been evaluated. Because of this, a number of recent studies have examined topical cyclosporine therapy for various ocular surface disorders. In these trials, cyclosporine 0.05% ophthalmic emulsion showed promise for treatment of posterior blepharitis [66], Laser-assisted in situ keratomileusis associated dry eye [67], contact lens intolerance [68], atopic keratoconjunctivitis [69], and herpetic stromal keratitis [70]. Increasingly evidence demonstrates that topical treatment with cyclosporine A prevents T-cell activation and reverses inflammation, improving symptoms and signs of dry eye disease.

3.1.4.2. Topical Corticosteroids

In recent studies, topical corticosteroids have shown promising results for treating dry eye, as they may help increasing goblet cell density and reduce the accumulation of inflammatory cells within ocular surface tissues [71,72]. Lee et al. reported that ocular surface nerve growth factor (NGF) may play an important role in ocular surface inflammation processes associated with dry eye, since KCS patients showed elevated levels of tear NGF, which decreased by treatment with 0.1% prednisolone [73].

The inflammatory factors are decreased and the integrity of ocular surface is improved after the application of corticosteroid, the nerves of cornea and conjunctiva can be stimulated by blinking more effectively. The reflective secretion becomes normal, then the quality and quantity of tears are also improved. Although corticosteroid can ameliorate the symptoms and signs rapidly, its chronic use for dry eye and for almost any other ocular disease must be restricted, because of severe side effects (e.g., increased infection, ocular hypertension, and cataract formation), being therefore more suitable for acute treatment of dry eye exacerbations.

3.1.4.3. Non-steroidal Anti-inflammatory Drugs (NSAIDs)

Topical non-steriodal anti-inflammatory drugs (NSAIDs) are nowadays widely used for the treatment of several ocular conditions, including corneal traumatic and inflammatory diseases and could be considered a good alternative to steroids to avoid the well known complications of corticotherapy in the treatment of patients with chronic diseases.

NSAIDs can be useful in resolving symptoms of ocular discomfort in Sjögren's syndrome patients [74]. A more complete study about the role of these agents in dry eye disease should be therefore undertaken. However, these drugs should be used with caution and under close monitoring, and the treatment should be promptly discontinued if corneal epithelial defects develop or worsen during treatment. The most commonly reported adverse effects are symptoms of stinging and irritation, superficial punctate keratitis, corneal infiltrates and melting [75,76].

3.1.4.4. Systemic Tetracyclines

Typical bacterial conjunctivitis is caused by the common staphylococcus and diplococcus pneumoniae to the less common organisms of the haemophilus group. Infection is generally in both eyes with the patients experiencing discomfort in the form of grittiness, moderate photophobia and minimal pain. Discharge from the infection causes symptoms of eyelids stuck together on wakening and a "crusty" appearance. Bacterial conjunctivitis responds well to lid hygiene and topical ointments of antibiotics alone or in combination with steroids [77]. In severe cases oral tetracycline and its derivates (e.g., doxycycline) is the treatment of choice, especially in rosacea-associated meibomitis [78].

3.1.4.5. Sexual Hormones

As noted earlier, evidence has strengthened the link between hormonal dysfunction and ocular surface disease, and as androgen and estrogen receptors are widely distributed on the ocular surface and lachrymal gland tissues [79], they represent potential targets for topical application of these hormones as an effective therapy for aqueous-deficient and evaporative dry eye. A topical estradiol-ointment was tested in a clinical trial, proving great potential to improve KCS symptoms [80].

3.1.4.6. Topical Vitamin A

Vitamin A is provided to the corneal epithelium by tears and can exist in three forms, namely, retinol, retinal and retinoic acid, being this latter the most abundant. This nutrient is known to regulate the proliferation and differentiation of corneal epithelial cells and to preserve conjunctival goblet cells. Thus, a lack of vitamin A in the eye may be responsible for xerophthalmia, a keratinisation or formation of a horny layer and drying out of the conjunctiva and cornea, which may produce blindness.

There are serious ocular complications derived from the systemic use of retinoid acid derivates (mainly 13-cis-retinoic acid and isotretinoin), including dry eye signs and symptoms, blepharoconjunctivitis and contact lens intolerance. Bearing this in mind, the indication for therapy with vitamin A is limited to those patients with a loss of goblet cells in very severe dry eye conditions. Usually, vitamin A has been used in the form of a 0.01% ophthalmic ointment, as an adjunct therapy with artificial lubricants in the treatment of eye diseases, such as dry eye and superior limbic keratoconjunctivitis [81, 82]. In 1985 Tseng demonstrated that topical all-trans retinoic acid ointment was effective in the treatment of severe cases of KCS, Stevens-Johnson syndrome, drug-induced pseudopemphigoid, and surgery-induced dry eye, being useful in reversing cellular changes noted in the conjunctiva [83].

3.1.4.7. Topical Autologous Serum

Autologous serum eyedrops have been proposed as a way to deliver essential tear components, e.g., epidermal growth factor, hepatocyte growth factor, fibronectin, neurotrophic growth factor and vitamin A. All of these have shown to play an important role in maintaining ocular surface epithelial milieu and are not included in commercially available artificial tear preparations. Although this kind of treatment is beneficial in cases of persistent epithelial defects [84], superior limbic keratoconjunctivitis [85] and neurotrophic keratopathy

[86], because of the nature of study designs and presence of punctum plug occlusion in the patients, its solitary effects were not assessed till recently. A randomized case-control prospective study found significant improvements in tear stability, ocular surface vital staining scores, and pain symptom scores in patients treated with autologous serum eye drops compared with other assigned to non-preserved artificial tears, none of which had punctal occlusion [87]. Autologous serum provides growth factors and vitamins that are useful for an altered ocular surface. However, there are some problems preventing its widespread use in ocular disorders, including risk of contamination, arbitrary dilution, and a current lack of regulations.

3.1.4.8. Omega-6

Recent studies have shown the beneficial effect of oral omega-6 supplementation (γ-linolenic acid and its precursor linoleic acid) in **Sjögren's** syndrome and dry eye with an inflammatory component [88, 89]. Reduced symptoms of dry eye were reported, as well as an improvement in objective signs such as corneal staining and reduced conjunctival expression of HLA-DR (human leukocyte antigens involved in several autoimmune conditions, disease susceptibility and disease resistance) [90]. Supplementation with linoleic and γ-linoleic acids was shown to increase tear production and reduce dry eye symptoms after photorefractive keratectomy [49].

3.1.4.9. Botulinum Toxin A

Botulinum toxin A, a dichain protein, is one of seven neurotoxins produced by *Clostridium botulinum*. When injected locally, it causes paralysis of the orbicularis oculi muscle by interfering with the release of acetylcholine at neuromuscular junctions. This paralysis acts on the canaliculi inducing a decreased pump function during blink. Because of the reduction of lachrymal drainage after botulinum toxin A injections, this treatment has been suggested for dry eyes [91]. Studies confirmed increased tearing after injections in the eyes of **Sjögren's** syndrome patients with severe xerophthalmia and blepharospasm [92], and decreased lachrymal drainage after injections in dry eye patients [93]. However, when applied to patients with pathologic hyperlachrymation, a significant reduction of this lachrymation is observed [94]. Further studies are required to assess the clinical value of these injections as an additional treatment for dry eye patients.

3.1.4.10. Acupuncture

Acupuncture is an ancient technique that has shown some benefit in the treatment of **Sjögren's** syndrome related xerostomia [95] and of KCS [96]. Although acupuncture is not in the common clinical practice of ophthalmologists, their positive effects are attributed to parasympathetic activation not producing any adverse effects. Thus longer observations in a significant number of patients to optimize the technique and further prospective objective measurements of both the tear film and its components should be the subjects of further research.

3.1.4.11. Antiviral Agents

Adenoviral infections are some of the most common external eye infections, causing inflammation of the membrane on the back of the eyelid. Evidence has been accumulated about the associations of viruses with **Sjögren's** syndrome, such as Epstein-Barr, Human Herpes and Human T lymphotropic virus [97,98]. Antiretrovirals such as zidovudine, must be tested to assess the tolerance and efficacy in improving dry eye symptoms and signs since they may be beneficial in primary **Sjögren's** syndrome [99-101]. As new information about novel therapeutic molecules becomes available, designs for clinical trials undoubtedly will undergo further evolution. This is critical to surmount the regulatory barriers to successful development of new, more efficient treatments for patients with dry eye disease.

3.2. Novel Therapeutic Strategies

3.2.1. Polymeric Nanoparticles

Various types of natural and synthetic polymers were used for preparation of nanoparticulate carriers of drugs relevant in dry eye syndrome therapy. The materials and production methods are being extensively reviewed [3,102]. By selection or further chemical modification of the polymer structure, the characteristics necessary for drug loading and increase of bioavailability in target tissues may be accomplished.

The selection of the material used for production of nanoparticles for ocular delivery should consider the ocular tolerance of the material, and its stability in the tear film i.e. in presence of lysozyme and mucin. Likewise, the material should not interact with mucin of ocular surface to large extent, no significant increase of mucin viscosity should be observed, as increased mucin viscosity may lead to further eye structure damage [103].

Polymers such as poly (D,L-lactic-co-glycolic)acid (PLGA) or poly-ε-caprolactone (PECL) attracted much attention for nanoparticle preparation since these materials are biodegradable [104] and generally biocompatible [102]. Their suitability for ocular delivery has also been shown for several formulations. In fact, no mucosa damage [105] or irritation [106] were observed after PLGA nanoparticles administration in rabbit eyes up to 24 hours by corneal hydration test. With respect to improvement of bioavailability of the drugs in ocular tissues, mucoadhesive polymers are interesting to improve residence time in the eye.

PLGA nanoparticles were proposed for delivery of NSAIDs such as diclofenac sodium salt [106] and flurbiprofen [105]. In this latter case, the drug is available from the nanoparticles in non-dissociated form, in contrast to marketed formulations containing sodium salt. Corneal permeation of flurbiprofen from this system was shown to be superior to aqueous solution or even to a marketed formulation containing a penetration enhancer (e.g., polyvinyl alcohol).

Other NSAIDs have been encapsulated in Eudragit RL and RS, which are copolymers of polyethylacrylate, methyl-methacrylate, and chlorotrimethyl-ammonioethylmethacrylate. Although not showing mucoadhesive properties themselves, these polymers provide a positively charged surface of nanoparticles with a very small diameter, which could enable them to remain onto the ocular surface for the required time to assure efficient drug release [107]. Suspensions of nanoparticles prepared from Eudragit RS and RL were shown non toxic and well tolerated upon administration onto the eye surface [107-109]. Encapsulation of flurbiprofen and ibuprofen led to increased drug concentration in the aqueous humor of the eye despite applying lower concentrations than those in commercially available eye drops. Therefore, these systems were proposed to help maintain miosis during cataract surgery [108,109]. These systems could also be useful in dry eye syndrome therapy. Nevertheless, formulations aiming to target the anterior eye segments are already reported in the literature.

Cyclosporine A is typically studied as a model drug in various colloidal drug delivery systems. Nanoparticles prepared from e.g. PECL [110] or poly-isobutyl-cyanoacrylate (PIBCA) [111] were examined for the possibility to increase the drug concentration that would permeate the cornea and increase the availability of this peptide for further ocular tissues. Despite various methodologies used to evaluate the drug concentration in the eye, the colloidal carrier systems were clearly more efficient than any oil solution of cyclosporine A. For example, nanocapsules composed of PECL as polymeric shell and medium chain triglycerides as oil core could assure 5 times higher concentration, in comparison to the oily solution, that could be remained within 3 days after administration [110]. An interesting comparison of cyclosporine A nanocapsules, carbopol hydrogel and nanocapsules-loaded hydrogel formulations was assessed by an *ex vivo* study [111]. All of these formulations being superior in effectively of corneal absorption than olive oil solution, the achieved concentrations increased from nanocapsules followed by hydrogel and reaching nanocapsules-loaded hydrogel the highest values. In addition, a slight ocular surface damage was seen for carbopol hydrogel or nanocapsules formulation but not for nanocapsules-loaded hydrogel formulation.

The highest cyclosporine A concentrations were reported from PECL nanoparticles with mucoadhesive coating (hyaluronic acid) and cationic surfactant/preservative (benzalkonium chloride) [112]. The concentrations of cyclosporine A in cornea and conjunctiva were found 6-8 times higher when compared to cyclosporine A administered dissolved in castor oil. Administration of cyclosporine A in hyaluronic acid coated nanoparticles lead to significantly increased uptake of the drug by cornea, especially during the first 4 hours after administration.

In case of treatment of inflammation of the exterior parts of the eye, which is the case of KCS, the increase of drug concentration needs to be carefully considered. It is of high importance to achieve therapeutic concentration of administered drugs in cornea and conjunctiva while not reaching irrelevant tissues and avoiding systemic absorption of the drug. This requires a careful selection of the materials and dosage forms used in dry eye syndrome treatment, so that only the target tissues are exposed to the drug. The nanoparticles not always penetrate the cornea but they rather stay adsorbed on its surface or in the cul-de-sac and act as drug reservoir. Together with the fact the drug release from the carrier is quite slow and continuous; the bioavailability of the drug can be improved.

3.2.1.1. Natural Polymers

Among the polymeric material with the highest relative mucoadhesive properties, hyaluronic acid, sodium alginate and mostly chitosan are investigated for ocular delivery improvement.

Chitosan is a modified (deacetylated) naturally occurring polysaccharide with positive charge. Depending on degree of deacetylation and molecular weight, slight differences in its characteristics are present. Chitosan draw much attention in ocular drug delivery systems design as it shows excellent mucoadhesive properties [113]. These are ascribed to the ability of its amonium groups to bind with sialic acid residues of mucin. Non-modified chitosan is water insoluble at physiological pH, but is capable of swelling [33], which makes it a suitable material for hydrogel and nanoparticle preparation chitosan properties can be further modified by derivatisation of its amino groups. This offers possibility to synthesise wide spectra of chitosan derivates with different solubility conditions and subsequently varying penetration rate. For example, a quaternized derivative N-trimethylchitosan chloride is water-soluble irrespectively of pH, which makes this material a useful transmucosal penetration enhancer [114]. On the other hand, an amphiphilic cholesterol-3-hemisuccinate-chitosan derivate insoluble in neutral pH and self-assembling into particles with size well below 1 μm could be maintained in cornea (78.3%) and conjunctiva (20.1% as measured by γ-scintigraphy of ^{99m}Tc-labeled nanoparticles) without permeating into the posterior segment of the eye [115]. This clearly shows the suitability of Chitosan to design tailor-made systems for reaching the desired part of the eye.

Chitosan nanoparticles can be obtained by simple preparation method – ionic gelation, based on the interaction of the cationic polymer with pentasodium tripolyphosphate [116]. Despite using mild conditions in terms of temperature or pressure, the use of organic solvents is not avoided. Chitosan nanoparticles were intensively tested for their biocompatibility with ocular tissues, with an optimized performance. Almost 100% viability on relevant cell lines was observed (IOBA NHC [117], Chang cells [103]), no irritation or damage in the outer ocular tissues after in vivo testing. De Campos et al. evaluated the stability of chitosan nanoparticles in conditions similar to those physiological of eye surface [103]. Again, the suitability of these systems was confirmed, as the nanoparticles did not suffer any degradation in presence of lysozyme or mucin. Also, mucin viscosity was not affected by the presence of such polysaccharide-based systems. The potential of chitosan in ocular drug delivery, illustrated by many nanoparticle or nanocapsules formulations or colloidal carriers coatings, was recently reviewed by Paolicelli et al. [33].

Cyclosporine A-loaded chitosan nanoparticles were instilled in eye rabbits following bioavailability assessment in conjunctiva and cornea, in comparison to a cyclosporine solution in chitosan or water [118]. Peptide concentration was significantly higher after administration of nanoparticles than of the solutions. The therapeutic dose could be maintained in conjunctiva and cornea up to 48 hours. These chitosan nanoparticles were shown to accumulate in the external ocular tissues, and to remain on the ocular surface. It was therefore anticipated that chitosan nanoparticles have higher affinity to conjunctiva than cornea [103]. In case of cyclosporine A, small quantities of drug were detected in systemic circulation, however, in such a concentration that is not expected to cause any side effects [118]. With regard to concentrations reached within the eye (i.e., iris/ciliary body and aqueous humour), blood and plasma, clearly highest concentration could be found in external ocular tissues, intraocular concentrations of the drug was not enhanced. Considering ocular surface diseases, such as the KCS, this characteristic make non-modified chitosan a very promising material for drug delivery systems design.

Indomethacin-loaded chitosan nanoparticles were also tested for ocular wound healing purposes [34]. Upon application on healthy eye, normal histological image of cornea was obtained. For this purpose, a chitosan nanoemulsion was favoured over chitosan nanoparticles.

3.2.1.2. Polymeric Coating of Various Carrier Systems

The effectiveness of colloidal carriers on the eye strongly depends on their surface characteristics. As shown by various research groups, presence and type of the coating of the colloidal carriers are governing its ability to permeate through cornea. A comparison between polyethylene glycol (PEG)-coated and chitosan-coated PECL nanocapsules clearly showed that the surface characteristics influence the fate of the nanoparticles in the eye. While PEG-coated nanocapsules could proceed through the cornea by transcellular pathway, chitosan coated particles could enter the corneal cells, but were maintain within them [119]. By selecting the surface characteristics of the colloidal carrier, it can be targeted to the particular part of the eye. Chitosan has been used as coating of various colloidal carriers intended for ocular drug delivery. These include nanoparticles prepared from various polymers [120], lipid nanoparticles [121] or liposomes [122,123]. The combination of chitosan with phospholipids seems to be in particular useful in ocular drug delivery. The complexes prepared from these materials, either chitosan-coated liposomes [124] or chitosan nanoparticles with a phospholipid shell [122], could penetrate through corneal tissues easily. Depending on composition, the extent of the permeation could be controlled. A hyaluronic acid coating may also be used to enhance cyclosporine A concentration in corneal tissues reported after administration of nanoparticles [112].

3.2.2. Solid Lipid Nanoparticles

Colloidal carriers based on lipids offer the advantage of use of naturally occurring or very similar material, which is presumed to be well tolerated and non toxic. These characteristics need however to be shown for every type of material and stabilizing agent used for the manufacture. Since ophthalmic emulsions have already reached the market, one might antecipate that other lipid-based drug delivery systems applications will be seen in near future.

Lipid nanoparticles were developed after polymeric nanoparticles on the concept of replacing the oil phase of an emulsion by a solid lipid and thus obtaining particles with small size (50-1000 nm) that are solid at room temperature. Lipid nanoparticles already tested for ocular delivery include solid lipid nanoparticles (SLN), nanostructured lipid carriers (NLC). The production methods and drug incorporation models are reviewed elsewhere [125].

Suitability of lipid nanoparticles for ocular drug delivery was first shown by Cavalli *et al.* who reported a tobramycin-loaded SLN formulation [126]. Already in this study, prolonged pre-corneal residence times were observed when compared to an aqueous solution of fluorescamine, and higher bioavailability of the incorporated drug than from a marketed aqueous solution was achieved. With regards to KCS, NSAIDs and cyclosporine A formulations were also reported.

Ibuprofen-loaded NLC could be used to improve ocular bioavailability, which could be further enhanced by stearylamine incorporation to obtain a positive surface charge. Thus the pre-corneal retention times could be prolonged [127]. Diclofenac sodium salt was encapsulated SLN composed of a mixture of lipid from goat fat plated with a phospholipid [128]. The coating was found to be important factor influencing both the release of diclofenac from the particles, as well as its penetration through cornea construct. The phospholipid coating was the prerequisite of controlled release and higher permeation rate through the cornea [129].

Several research groups developed SLN formulations to deliver cyclosporine A. As this peptide is poorly soluble in water, a lipid based system may be a successful solution for its formulation. Formulations with particle size less than 500 nm and stability over 6 months were reported [130], and, as expected, typically high loading capacities (over 90%) were achieved [131,132]. Both blank and cyclosporine-loaded SLN were biocompatible with rabbit corneal epithelium (RCE) cells, maintaining the percentage of living cells comparable with those cultivated with growth medium [131].

Penetration or permeation of cyclosporine A suspension into RCE cells or excised corneal tissues could not be observed in several reports [121,131], but cyclosporine could be detected within the cells [121] and found to permeate the corneal tissues [121,131] after being delivered by SLN. However, Gokce *et al.* did not find the differences between the permeation of cyclosporine A suspension and protein-loaded SLN significantly [131]. An *in vivo* study showed that cyclosporine administered in SLN could eventually reach the vitreous body of the eye and could be detected 48 hours after administration [133].

The pre-corneal residence time of SLN or NLC formulations could be further improved by inducing positive surface charge e.g. by stearylamine [130,134], or by mucoadhesive coating cysteine-PEG stearate coating [135]. To improve the ability to permeate the corneal tissue, nanoparticles prepared from solid lipid and chitosan mixtures were proposed [121]. Indeed, in cell culture these formulations have proven to be more efficient to enhance cyclosporine A penetration into epithelial cells. All of these reports show the potential of lipid nanoparticles to be used in ocular therapy for cyclosporine.

Considering the practical point of view, the lipid nanoparticle formulations could be sterilized either by autoclaving [130,131] or by freeze-drying [136] without compromising the colloidal nature of the formulations. The methods used in preparation of the referred formulations are generally simple and do should be applicable in large scale production as well. If low wt% of lipid is used in the formulation, it remains liquid and slightly opalescent, which should not cause much inconvenience upon ocular administration. Despite these promising results, there are still only a few reports on SLN or NLC for ocular drug delivery. Practical use of these formulations can be considered only after conveying more detailed studies.

3.2.3. Liposomes

Liposomes are drug delivery systems suitable for delivery of both hydrophilic and lipophilic drugs, feasible for various administration routes [137]. Extensive testing of liposomes application in ophthalmology revealed their suitability in terms of sufficient bioavailability improvement of drugs relevant in ocular diseases treatment and acceptable toxicological profile [138]. The mechanisms of bioavailability improvement of drugs administered in liposomes may include their adherence to the ocular surface, as well as the optimal rate of drug release. Prolonged residence times on corneal surface where observed with liposomes with positive surface charge.

Examples of ocular bioavailability improvements by liposome encapsulation include NSAIDs [139], and immunosupressives, such as the sirolimus or rapamycin, which was found in therapeutic concentrations throughout the eye when administered in liposomes [140]. Immunosuppressive peptides, antibiotics, and NSAIDs, are often formulated in different colloidal carriers, which may be superior to liposomes in terms of stability upon administration, also long term storage stability and manufacture costs. What makes liposomes in particular relevant in KCS therapy is the composition of natural (or similar to natural) amphiphilic phospholipids. There are strong evidences that evaporative dry eye needs treatment focused on the lipid layer of the tear film. Aqueous tear supplements are not sufficient in these cases, as well as there might be no need for administration of immunosuppressives. Although artificial tears and ophthalmic gels with triglyceride content are commercially available and do bring relief in this type of KCS, liposomal formulations were proposed. Currently, there are two liposome-containing over-the-counter products available on the market (TearsAgain Liposome Spray™, Optima Pharmaceutical GmbH and Clarymist™). Both are administered on closed eyelids. A few reports from clinical studies of these formulations indicate their significantly superior clinical benefits over triglyceride containing eye gel [141], or aqueous artificial tears eye drops [142], or sprays [143] presented in some controlled parameters. Improvements were reported in particular in eyelid edge inflammation. These data hint that phospholipids administered in form of colloidal carriers might be more beneficial than in form of solution or gel. However, a direct proof of the proposed mechanism of action (improvement of tear film stability) is still missing. Also, the price of these products is considerably higher than that of any conventional ophthalmic formulation.

4. CONCLUSIONS AND FUTURE TRENDS

The research and development of advanced drug delivery systems may bring additional advantages in the management of KCS. The materials and formulations summarized here show potential of improving the bioavailability of the drugs relevant in KCS management. Since only a few of these systems reached the pharmaceutical market in any administration route (Liposomes in i.v., dermal and ocular; NLC in dermal), the prior concern of these systems would be their actual safety upon administration in human eye. Various methods were used to assess the safety of the proposed systems making the comparison of the different types of colloidal carrier unclear; however, the most of these results are positive in terms of sufficient safety.

Table 1 gives an overview of the drug incorporated in different colloidal carriers and the advantages reported from their testing. The formulations of NSAIDs group generally achieved longer residence time onto the ocular surface, and can deliver also water insoluble drugs such as flurbiprofen or diclofenac in their non-dissociated form. Except from chitosan-coated formulations, the NSAIDs were loaded into material which does not show much pronounced mucoadhesive properties. The improved pre-corneal residence times could be attributed to the positive charge the nanoparticles had, and simply to the colloidal size of these particles, assuring slightly adhesive properties.

Also cyclosporine A concentration improvements could be achieved using different materials. The highest concentrations reported in the research literature were obtained when using colloidal carriers with mucoadhesive coatings, however, non-adhesive material based carriers could also produce promising results. Cyclosporine A was shown to have the ability to accumulate in cornea and conjunctiva which may act as drug reservoir and release it over extended period of time [144], therefore a high residence time onto the ocular surface, maintained for sufficient time seem to be the most important factor for a successful formulation. Again, the small size gives advantage itself, associated with a positive surface charge might ensure the contact with the ocular surface. As the mucin content may vary drastically in KCS conditions, mucoadhesiveness of the material itself may not be sufficient to enable the drug to stay on the ocular surface for a sufficient time. Therefore, the advantages that colloidal carriers may bring is their bioavailability improvement by enhanced drug permeation into the eye and improved residence time on the ocular surface, which can be assured by adhesiveness, a feature that colloidal carriers typically have, stressed by positive surface charge of the carriers.

Table 1. Examples of drugs entrapped into colloidal carriers based on polymeric, polyssacharide or lipid materials, for ocular administration

Drug	Formulation	Improvements	Reference
Cyclosporine -A	PIBCA NS PIBCA NS incorporated in Carbopol hydrogel	Higher effectiveness in corneal absorption of drug as compared to olive oil solution; limited damage of corneal tissue (NS hydrogel)	[111]
	PECL NP	Increase in AUC, therapeutic concentrations maintained during 3 days	[110]
	Hyaluronic acid coated PECL NS	6-8 times higher corneal levels than from castor oil emulsion, higher corneal uptake of the drug in first 4 hours after administration	[145]
	Chitosan NP	Therapeutic dose maintained for 24 hours in conjunctiva; 48 hours in cornea	[118]
	SLN	Enhanced permeation and penetration through RCE cells and corneal construct, no ocular irritation nor corneal damage	[130-132, 135, 146]
	Thiolated PEG-coated NLC	Enhanced pre-corneal retention time, controlled release over 12 hours	[135]
Diclofenac	PLGA NP	No irritation up to 24 hours post-administration (Draize test)	[106]
	Eudragit RS NP		[147]
	SLN	Enhanced corneal permeation, non-dissociated drug available	[128, 148]
Ibuprofen	Eudragit RS 100 NP	Therapeutic effect achieved with lower administered concentration	[108, 149]

	Eudragit RL 100 NP		[150]
	NLC	Enhanced pre-corneal retention time	[127]
Flurbiprofen	Eudragit RS RL NP	Higher drug concentration in the aqueous humour achieved in comparison with eye drops, non-dissociated drug available, no corneal damage	[109]
	PLGA NP	Corneal penetration superior to drug buffer solution or drug solution containing PVA	[105, 151]
Indomethacin	Chitosan-coated emulsion		[152]
	Chitosan NE, NPs	NE: significantly higher concentrations in aqueous humour first hour post-administration	[34]
	Chitosan NC	Increased corneal transport	[153]
Piroxicam	Eudragit RS 100	Anti-inflammatory effect observed up to 24 hours	[154]

PIBCA, poly-isobutyl-cyanoacrylate; PLGA, poly(lactic-co-glycolic)acid; PVA, polyvinyl alcohol; RCE, Rabbit corneal epithelium.AUC, area under the curve; NS, nanospheres; NC, nanocapsules; NP, nanoparticles; SLN, solid lipid nanoparticles; NLC, nanostructured lipid carriers, PECL, poly-ε-caprolactone; PEG, polyethylenglycol;

REFERENCES

[1]   Holly FJ, Lemp MA: Tear physiology and dry eyes. *Surv Ophthalmol* 1977, 22:69-87.
[2]   Ali Y, Lehmussaari K: Industrial perspective in ocular drug delivery. *Adv Drug Deliv Rev* 2006, 58:1258-1268.
[3]   Nagarwal RC, Kant S, Singh PN, Maiti P, Pandit JK: Polymeric nanoparticulate system: A potential approach for ocular drug delivery. *Journal of Controlled Release* 2009, 136:2-13.
[4]   Stern ME, Beuerman RW, Fox RI, Gao J, Mircheff AK, Pflugfelder SC: A unified theory of the role of the ocular surface in dry eye. *Adv Exp Med Biol* 1998, 438:643-651.
[5]   Niederkorn JY, Stern ME, Pflugfelder SC, De Paiva CS, Corrales RM, Gao J, Siemasko K: Desiccating stress induces T cell-mediated Sjogren's Syndrome-like lacrimal keratoconjunctivitis. *J Immunol* 2006, 176:3950-3957.
[6]   Stern ME, Gao J, Siemasko KF, Beuerman RW, Pflugfelder SC: The role of the lacrimal functional unit in the pathophysiology of dry eye. *Exp Eye Res* 2004, 78:409-416.
[7]   Nakamori K, Odawara M, Nakajima T, Mizutani T, Tsubota K: Blinking is controlled primarily by ocular surface conditions. *Am J Ophthalmol* 1997, 124:24-30.
[8]   Lemp MA, Marquardt R: *The dry eye: A comprehensive guide.* Springer-Verlag (Berlin, New York); 1992.

[9]   Kobayashi TK, Tsubota K, Takamura E, Sawa M, Ohashi Y, Usui M: Effect of retinol palmitate as a treatment for dry eye: a cytological evaluation. *Ophthalmologica* 1997, 211:358-361.

[10]   Hatchell DL, Sommer A: Detection of Ocular Surface Abnormalities in Experimental Vitamin A Deficiency. *Arch Ophthalmol* 1984, 102:1389-1393.

[11]   Brignole F, Pisella PJ, Goldschild M, De Saint Jean M, Goguel A, Baudouin C: Flow cytometric analysis of inflammatory markers in conjunctival epithelial cells of patients with dry eyes. *Invest Ophthalmol Vis Sci* 2000, 41:1356-1363.

[12]   Jones D, Monroy D, Ji Z, Atherton S, Pflugfelder S: Sjogren's syndrome: cytokine and Epstein-Barr viral gene expression within the conjunctival epithelium. *Invest Ophthalmol Vis Sci* 1994, 35:3493-3504.

[13]   Pflugfelder SC, Solomon A, Dursun D: Dry eye and delayed tear clearance: 'a call to arms'. *Adv Exp Med Biol* 2002, 506:739-743.

[14]   Tsubota K, Goto E, Fujita H, Ono M, Inoue H, Saito I, Shimmura S: Treatment of dry eye by autologous serum application in Sjogren's syndrome. *Br J Ophthalmol* 1999, 83:390-395.

[15]   Vivino FB, Katz WA: jögren's syndrome: Clinical picture and diagnostic tests. *Journal of Musculoskeletal Medicine* 1995, 12:40-52.

[16]   Foster CS, Rice BA, Dutt JE: Immunopathology of atopic keratoconjunctivitis. *Ophthalmology* 1991, 98:1190-1196.

[17]   Metz D, P., Hingorani M, Calder V, L., Buckley R, J., Lightman S, L.: T-cell cytokines in chronic allergic eye disease. *J Allergy Clin Immunol* 1997, 100:817-824.

[18]   Vermeulen A, D. M, D. P: Commentary to the Article--Low Levels of Sex Hormone-Binding Globulin and Testosterone Are Associated with Smaller, Denser Low Density Lipoproteins in Normoglycemic Menc. *J Clin Endocrinol Metab* 1998, 83:1822a-.

[19]   Warren DW: Hormonal Influences on the Lacrimal Gland. *Int Ophthalmol Clin* 1994, 34:19-25.

[20]   Sullivan DA, Schaumberg DA, Suzuki T, Schirra F, Liu M, Richards S, Sullivan RM, Dana MR, Sullivan BD: Sex steroids, meibomian gland dysfunction and evaporative dry eye in Sj ogren's syndrome. *Lupus* 2002, 11:667-.

[21]   Sullivan DA, Sullivan BD, Evans JE, Schirra F, Yamagami H, Liu M, Richards SM, Suzuki T, Schaumberg DA, Sullivan RM, Dana MR: Androgen deficiency, meibomian gland dysfunction, and evaporative dry eye. *Am NY Acad Sci* 2002, 966.

[22]   Richardson JD, Vasko MR: Cellular Mechanisms of Neurogenic Inflammation. *J Pharmacol Exp Ther* 2002, 302:839-845.

[23]   Nelson JD, Havener VR, Cameron JD: Cellulose Acetate Impressions of the Ocular Surface: Dry Eye States. *Arch Ophthalmol* 1983, 101:1869-1872.

[24]   Tseng SC, Hirst LW, Maumenee AE, Kenyon KR, Sun TT, Green WR: Possible mechanisms for the loss of goblet cells in mucin-deficient disorders. *Ophthalmology* 1984, 91:545-552.

[25]   Driver P, J., Lemp M, A.: Meibomian gland dysfunction. *Surv Ophthalmol* 1996, 40:343-367.

[26]   Shimazaki J, Sakata M, K. T: Ocular surface changes and discomfort in patients with meibomian gland dysfunction. *Arch Ophthalmol* 1995, 113:1266-1270.

[27]   Pflugfelder SC, Tseng SC, Sanabria O, Kell HOD, Garcia CG, Felix C, Feuer W, Reis BL: Evaluation of subjective assessments and objective diagnostic tests for diagnosing tear-film disorders known to cause ocular irritation. *Cornea* 1998, 17:38 -56.

[28]   Asbell PA: Increasing importance of dry eye syndrome and the ideal artificial tear: consensus views from a roundtable discussion*. *Current Medical Research and Opinion* 2006, 22:2149-2157.

[29]   Bron AJ, Daubas P, Siou-Mermet R, Trinquand C: Comparison of the efficacy and safety of two eye gels in the treatment of dry eyes: Lacrinorm and Viscotears. *Eye* 1998, 12 (Pt 5):839-847.

[30]   Bron AJ, Tiffany JM, Embleton J: Topical delivery of microvolumes using a forced-flow system (Optidyne). In *Lacrimal Gland, Tear Film and Dry Eye Syndromes*. Volume Vol. 2. Edited by (Ed.) SDA. New York: Plenum; 1998

[31]   Oechsner M, Keipert S: Polyacrylic acid/polyvinylpyrrolidone bipolymeric systems. I. Rheological and mucoadhesive properties of formulations potentially useful for the treatment of dry-eye-syndrome. *Eur J Pharm Biopharm* 1999, 47:113-118.

[32]   Barbu E, Verestiuc L, Iancu M, Jatariu A, Lungu A, Tsibouklis J: Hybrid polymeric hydrogels for ocular drug delivery: nanoparticulate systems from copolymers of acrylic acid-functionalized   chitosan   and   N-isopropylacrylamide   or   2-hydroxyethyl methacrylate. *Nanotechnology* 2009, 20:225108.

[33]   Paolicelli P, de la Fuente M, Sanchez A, Seijo B, Alonso MJ: Chitosan nanoparticles for drug delivery to the eye. *Expert Opin Drug Deliv* 2009, 6:239-253.

[34]   Badawi AA, El-Laithy HM, El Qidra RK, El Mofty H, El dally M: Chitosan based nanocarriers for indomethacin ocular delivery. *Arch Pharm Res* 2008, 31:1040-1049.

[35]   Lemp MA: Dry eye syndromes: treatment and clinical trials. Adv Exp Med Biol 1994, 350:553-559.

[36]   Lemp MA: Management of the dry-eye patient. *Int Ophthalmol Clin* 1994, 34:101-113.

[37]   Marchese A, Bozzolasco M, Gualco L, Schito GC, Debbia EA: Evaluation of spontaneous contamination of ocular medications. *Chemotherapy* 2001, 47:304-308.

[38]   Murube J, Murube A, Zhuo C: Classification of artificial tears. II: Additives and commercial formulas. *Adv Exp Med Biol* 1998, 438:705-715.

[39]   Murube J, Paterson A, Murube E: Classification of artificial tears. I: Composition and properties. *Adv Exp Med Biol* 1998, 438:693-704.

[40]   Tripathi BJ, Tripathi RC: Cytotoxic effects of benzalkonium chloride and chlorobutanol on human corneal epithelial cells in vitro. *Lens Eye Toxic Res* 1989, 6:395-403.

[41]   Murube J: Tear osmolarity. *Ocul Surf* 2006, 4:62-73.

[42]   Gilbard JP: Human tear film electrolyte concentrations in health and dry-eye disease. *Int Ophthalmol Clin* 1994, 34:27-36.

[43]   Gilbard JP, Rossi SR: Changes in tear ion concentrations in dry-eye disorders. *Adv Exp Med Biol* 1994, 350:529-533.

[44]   Ubels JL, McCartney MD, Lantz WK, Beaird J, Dayalan A, Edelhauser HF: Effects of preservative-free artificial tear solutions on corneal epithelial structure and function. *Arch Ophthalmol* 1995, 113:371-378.

[45] Wander AH, Koffler BH: Extending the duration of tear film protection in dry eye syndrome: review and retrospective case series study of the hydroxypropyl cellulose ophthalmic insert. *Ocul Surf* 2009, 7:154-162.

[46] Diestelhorst M, Grunthal S, Suverkrup R: Dry Drops: a new preservative-free drug delivery system. *Graefes Arch Clin Exp Ophthalmol* 1999, 237:394-398.

[47] Geerling G, Sieg P, Bastian GO, Laqua H: Transplantation of the autologous submandibular gland for most severe cases of keratoconjunctivitis sicca. *Ophthalmology* 1998, 105:327-335.

[48] Yen MT, Pflugfelder SC, Feuer WJ: The effect of punctal occlusion on tear production, tear clearance, and ocular surface sensation in normal subjects. *Am J Ophthalmol* 2001, 131:314-323.

[49] Macrì A, Giuffrida S, Amico V, Iester M, Traverso CE: Effect of linoleic acid and gamma-linolenic acid on tear production, tear clearance and on the ocular surface after photorefractive keratectomy. *Greafes Arch Clin Exp Ophthalmol* 2003, 241:561-566.

[50] Redmond JW: Punctal occlusion with collagen implants. Ophthalmic Surg 1992, 23:642.

[51] Willis RM, Folberg R, Krachmer JH, Holland EJ: The treatment of aqueous-deficient dry eye with removable punctal plugs. A clinical and impression-cytologic study. *Ophthalmology* 1987, 94:514-518.

[52] Murube J: Surgical treatment of dry eye. *Orbit* 2003, 22:203-232.

[53] Benson DR, Hemmady PB, Snyder RW: Efficacy of laser punctal occlusion. *Ophthalmology* 1992, 99:618-621.

[54] Rolando M, Refojo MF: Tear evaporimeter for measuring water evaporation rate from the tear film under controlled conditions in humans. *Exp Eye Res* 1983, 36:25-33.

[55] Tsubota K, Yamada M, Urayama K: Spectacle side panels and moist inserts for the treatment of dry-eye patients. *Cornea* 1994, 13:197-201.

[56] Tsubota K: New approaches to dry-eye therapy. *Int Ophthalmol Clin* 1994, 34:115-128.

[57] Farris RL: Contact lenses and the dry eye. *Int Ophthalmol Clin* 1994, 34:129-136.

[58] Stamler JF, Tse DT: A simple and reliable technique for permanent lateral tarsorrhaphy. *Arch Ophthalmol* 1990, 108:125-127.

[59] Calonge M: The treatment of dry eye. *Surv Ophthalmol* 2001, 45 Suppl 2:S227-239.

[60] Gilbard JP, Rossi SR, Heyda KG, Dartt DA: Stimulation of tear secretion by topical agents that increase cyclic nucleotide levels. *Invest Ophthalmol Vis Sci* 1990, 31:1381-1388.

[61] Pflugfelder SC, Solomon A, Stern ME: The Diagnosis and Management of Dry Eye: A Twenty-five-Year Review. *Cornea* 2000, 19:644-649.

[62] Smith RE: The Tear Film Complex: Pathogenesis and Emerging Therapies for Dry Eyes. *Cornea* 2005, 24:1-7.

[63] Stern ME, Beuerman RW, Fox RI, Gao J, Mircheff AK, Pflugfelder SC: The pathology of dry eye: the interaction between the ocular surface and lacrimal glands. *Cornea* 1998, 17:584-589.

[64] Stevenson D, Tauber J, Reis BL: Efficacy and safety of cyclosporin a ophthalmic emulsion in the treatment of moderate-to-severe dry eye disease - A dose-ranging, randomized trial. *Ophthalmology* 2000, 107:967-974.

[65] Sall K, Stevenson OD, Mundorf T, K., Reis B, L.: Two multicenter, randomized studies of the efficacy and safety of cyclosporine ophthalmic emulsion in moderate to severe dry eye disease. *Ophthalmology* 2000, 107:631-639.

[66] Perry HD, Doshi-Carnevale S, Donnenfeld ED, Solomon Re, Biser SA, Bloom AH: Efficacy of Commercially Available Topical Cyclosporine A 0.05% in the Treatment of Meibomian Gland Dysfunction. *Cornea* 2006, 25:171-175.

[67] Salib G, M., McDonald M, B., Smolek M: Safety and efficacy of cyclosporine 0.05% drops versus unpreserved artificial tears in dry-eye patients having laser in situ keratomileusis. *J Cataract Refract Surg* 2006, 32:772-778.

[68] Hom MM: Use of Cyclosporine 0.05% Ophthalmic Emulsion for Contact Lens-Intolerant Patients. *Eye Contact Lens* 2006, 32:109-111.

[69] Akpek EK, Dart JK, Watson S, Christen W, Dursun D, Yoo S, P. T, Schein OD, Gottsch JD: A randomized trial of topical cyclosporin 0.05% in topical steroid-resistant atopic keratoconjunctivitis. *Ophthalmology* 2004, 111:476-482.

[70] Rao S, N.: Treatment of Herpes Simplex Virus Stromal Keratitis Unresponsive to Topical Prednisolone 1% With Topical Cyclosporine 0.05%. *Am J Ophthalmol* 2006, 141:771-772.

[71] Avunduk AM, Avunduk MC, Varnell ED, Kaufman HE: The comparison of efficacies of topical corticosteroids and nonsteroidal anti-inflammatory drops on dry eye patients: a clinical and immunocytochemical study. *Am J Ophthalmol* 2003, 136:593-602.

[72] Pflugfelder SC, Maskin SL, Anderson B, Chodosh J, Holland EJ, d, e Palva CS, Bartels SP, Micuda T, Proskin HE, Vogel R: A randomized, double-masked, placebo-controlled, multicenter comparison of loteprednol etabonate ophthalmic suspension, 0.5%, and placebo for treatment of keratoconjunctivitis sicca in patients with delayed tear clearance. *Am J Ophthalmol* 2004, 138:444-457.

[73] Lee HK, Ryu IH, Seo KY, Hong S, Kim HC, Kim EK: Topical 0.1% Prednisolone Lowers Nerve Growth Factor Expression in Keratoconjunctivitis Sicca Patients. *Ophthalmology* 2006, 113:198-205.

[74] Avisar R, Robinson A, Appel I, Yassur Y, Weinberger D: Diclofenac sodium, 0.1% (Voltaren Ophtha), versus sodium chloride, 5%, in the treatment of filamentary keratitis. *Cornea* 2000, 19:145-147.

[75] Guidera A, C., Luchs J, I., Udell I, J.: Keratitis, ulceration, and perforation associated with topical nonsteroidal anti-inflammatory drugs. *Ophthalmology* 2001, 108:936-944.

[76] Hsu J, K. W., Johnston WT, Read R, W., McDonnell P, J., Pangalinan R, Rao N, Smith R, E.: Histopathology of corneal melting associated with diclofenac use after refractive surgery. *J Cataract Refract* Surg 2003, 29:250-256.

[77] Dougherty JM, McCulley JP, Silvany RE, Meyer DR: The role of tetracycline in chronic blepharitis. Inhibition of lipase production in staphylococci. *Invest Ophthalmol Vis Sci* 1991, 32:2970-2975.

[78] Cetinkaya A, Akova YA: Pediatric ocular acne rosacea: long-term treatment with systemic antibiotics. *Am J Ophthalmol* 2006, 142:816-821.

[79] Esmaeli B, Harvey JT, Hewlett B: Immunohistochemical evidence for estrogen receptors in meibomian glands. *Ophthalmology* 2000, 107:180-184.

[80]   Akramian J, Wedrich A, Nepp J, Sator M: Estrogen therapy in keratoconjunctivitis sicca. *Adv Exp Med Biol* 1998, 438:1005-1009.

[81]   Ohashi Y, Watanabe H, Kinoshita S, Hosotani H, Umemoto M, R. M: Vitamin A eye drops for superior limbic keratoconjunctivitis. *Am J Ophthalmol* 1988, 105:523-527.

[82]   Selek H, Unlü N, Orhan M, M. I: Evaluation of retinoic acid ophthalmic emulsion in dry eye. *Eur J Ophthalmol* 2000, 10:121-127.

[83]   Tseng S: Topical retinoid treatment for dry eye disorders. *Trans Ophthalmol Soc U K* 1985, 104:489-495.

[84]   Tsubota K, Shimazaki J: Surgical treatment of children blinded by Stevens-Johnson syndrome. *Am J Ophthalmol* 1999, 128:573-581.

[85]   Goto E, Shimmura S, Shimazaki J, Tsubota K: Treatment of Superior Limbic Keratoconjunctivitis by Application of Autologous Serum. *Cornea* 2001, 20:807-810.

[86]   Matsumoto Y, Dogru M, Goto E, Ohashi Y, Kojima T, Ishida R, Tsubota K: Autologous serum application in the treatment of neurotrophic keratopathy. *Ophthalmology* 2004, 111:1115-1120.

[87]   Kojima T, Ishida R, Dogru M, Goto E., Matsumoto Y, Kaido M, Tsubota K: The effect of autologous serum eyedrops in the treatment of severe dry eye disease: A prospective randomized case-control study. *Am J Ophthalmol* 2005, 139:242-246.

[88]   Aragona P, Bucolo C, Spinella R, Giuffrida S, Ferreri G: Systemic Omega-6 Essential Fatty Acid Treatment and PGE1 Tear Content in Sjogren's Syndrome Patients. *Invest Ophthalmol Vis Sci* 2005, 46:4474-4479.

[89]   Barabino S, Rolando M, Camicione P, Ravera G, Zanardi S, Giuffrida S, Calabria G: Systemic Linoleic and [gamma]-Linolenic Acid Therapy in Dry Eye Syndrome With an Inflammatory Component. *Cornea* 2003, 22:97-101.

[90]   Tsubota K, Fujihara T, Saito K, Takeuchi T: Conjunctival epithelium expression of HLA-DR in dry eye patients. *Ophthalmologica* 1999, 213:16-19.

[91]   Sahlin S, Chen E: Evaluation of the lacrimal drainage function by the drop test. *Am J Ophthalmol* 1996, 122:701-708.

[92]   Spiera H, Asbell PA, Simpson DM: Botulinum toxin increases tearing in patients with Sjogren's syndrome: a preliminary report. *J Rheumatol* 1997, 24:1842-1843.

[93]   Sahlin S, Chen E, Kaugesaar T, Almqvist H, Kjellberg K, Lennerstrand G: Effect of eyelid botulinum toxin injection on lacrimal drainage. *Am J Ophthalmol* 2000, 129:481-486.

[94]   Riemann R, Pfennigsdorf S, Riemann E, Naumann M: Successful treatment of crocodile tears by injection of botulinum toxin into the lacrimal gland: a case report. *Ophthalmology* 1999, 106:2322-2324.

[95]   Blom M, Kopp S, Lundeberg T: Prognostic value of the pilocarpine test to identify patients who may obtain long-term relief from xerostomia by acupuncture treatment. *Arch Otolaryngol Head Neck Surg* 1999, 125:561-566.

[96]   Nepp J, Derbolav A, Haslinger-Akramian J, Mudrich C, Schauersberger J, Wedrich A: [Effect of acupuncture in keratoconjunctivitis sicca]. *Klin Monatsbl Augenheilkd* 1999, 215:228-232.

[97] Tsubota K, Fujishima H, Toda I, Katagiri S, Kawashima Y, Saito I: Increased levels of Epstein-Barr virus DNA in lacrimal glands of Sjogren's syndrome patients. *Acta Ophthalmol Scand* 1995, 73:425-430.

[98] Willoughby CE, Baker K, Kaye SB, Carey P, O'Donnell N, Field A, Longman L, Bucknall R, Hart CA: Epstein-Barr virus (types 1 and 2) in the tear film in Sjogren's syndrome and HIV infection. *J Med Virol* 2002, 68:378-383.

[99] Pot C, Chizzolini C, Vokatch N, Tiercy JM, Ribi C, Landis T, Perren F: Combined antiviral-immunosuppressive treatment in human T-lymphotrophic virus 1-Sjogren-associated myelopathy. *Arch Neurol* 2006, 63:1318-1320.

[100] Steinfeld S, Simonart T: New approaches to the treatment of Sjogren's syndrome: soon beyond symptomatic relief? *Dermatology* 2003, 207:6-9.

[101] Steinfeld SD, Demols P, Van Vooren JP, Cogan E, Appelboom T: Zidovudine in primary Sjogren's syndrome. *Rheumatology (Oxford)* 1999, 38:814-817.

[102] Moghimi SM, Vega E, Garcia ML, Al-Hanbali OAR, Rutt KJ: Polymeric nanoparticles as drug carriers and controlled release implant devices. In *Nanoparticulates as drug carriers*. Edited by Torchilin VP. London: Imperial College Press; 2006: 29-42

[103] de Campos A, Diebold Y, Carvalho E, Sánchez A, José Alonso M: Chitosan Nanoparticles as New Ocular Drug Delivery Systems: in Vitro Stability, in Vivo Fate, and Cellular Toxicity. *Pharm Res* 2004, 21:803-810.

[104] Deshpande A, Heller J, Gurny R: Bioerodible polymers for ocular delivery. *Crit Rev Ther Drug Carrier Syst* 1998, 15:381-420.

[105] Vega E, Gamisans F, Garcia ML, Chauvet A, Lacoulonche F, Egea MA: PLGA Nanospheres for the Ocular Delivery of Flurbiprofen: Drug Release and Interactions. *Journal of Pharmaceutical Sciences* 2008, 97:5306-5317.

[106] Agnihotri SM, Vavia PR: Diclofenac-loaded biopolymeric nanosuspensions for ophthalmic application. *Nanomedicine-Nanotechnology Biology and Medicine* 2009, 5:90-95.

[107] Pignatello R, Bucolo C, Puglisi G: Ocular tolerability of Eudragit RS100 (R) and RL1009 (R) nanosuspensions as carriers for ophthalmic controlled drug delivery. *Journal of Pharmaceutical Sciences* 2002, 91:2636-2641.

[108] Pignatello R, Bucolo C, Ferrara P, Maltese A, Puleo A, Puglisi G: Eudragit RS100 (R) nanosuspensions for the ophthalmic controlled delivery of ibuprofen. *European Journal of Pharmaceutical Sciences* 2002, 16:53-61.

[109] Pignatello R, Bucolo C, Spedalieri G, Maltese A, Puglisi G: Flurbiprofen-loaded acrylate polymer nanosuspensions for ophthalmic application. *Biomaterials* 2002, 23:3247-3255.

[110] Calvo P, SĂˇnchez A, MartĂ-nez J, LĂłpez MI, Calonge M, Pastor JC, Alonso MJ: Polyester nanocapsules as new topical ocular delivery systems for cyclosporin A. *Pharmaceutical Research* 1996, 13:311-315.

[111] Le Bourlais CA, Chevanne F, Turlin B, Acar L, Zia H, Sado PA, Needham TE, Leverge R: Effect of cyclosporine A formulations on bovine corneal absorption: ex-vivo study. *J Microencapsul* 1997, 14: 457-467

[112] Yenice I, Mocan M, Palaska E, Bochot A, Bilensoy E, Vural I, Irkeç M, Hincal A: Hyaluronic acid coated poly-epsilon-caprolactone nanospheres deliver high concentrations of cyclosporine A into the cornea. *Exp Eye Res* 2008, 87:162-167.

[113] Lehr C-M, Bouwstra JA, Schacht EH, Junginger HE: In vitro evaluation of mucoadhesive properties of chitosan and some other natural polymers. *International Journal of Pharmaceutics* 1992, 78:43-48.

[114] Zambito Y, Zaino C, Di Colo G: Effects of N-trimethylchitosan on transcellular and paracellular transcorneal drug transport. *European Journal of Pharmaceutics and Biopharmaceutics* 2006, 64:16-25.

[115] Yuan XB, Li H, Yuan YB: Preparation of cholesterol-modified chitosan self-aggregated nanoparticles for delivery of drugs to ocular surface. *Carbohydrate Polymers* 2006, 65:337-345.

[116] Calvo P, Remunán-López C, Vila-Jato JL, Alonso MJ: Novel hydrophilic chitosan-polyethylene oxide nanoparticles as protein carriers. *Journal of Applied Polymer Science* 1997, 63:125-132.

[117] de Salamanca A, Diebold Y, Calonge M, Garcia-Vazquez C, Callejo S, Vila A, Alonso MJ: Chitosan nanoparticles as a potential drug delivery system for the ocular surface: toxicity, uptake mechanism and in vivo tolerance. *Invest Ophthalmol Vis Sci* 2006, 47:1416-1425.

[118] De Campos AM, Sanchez A, Alonso MJ: Chitosan nanoparticles: a new vehicle for the improvement of the delivery of drugs to the ocular surface. Application to cyclosporin A. *Int J Pharm* 2001, 224:159-168.

[119] De Campos AM, Sanchez A, Gref R, Calvo P, Alonso MJ: The effect of a PEG versus a chitosan coating on the interaction of drug colloidal carriers with the ocular mucosa. *Eur J Pharm Sci* 2003, 20:73-81.

[120] Yuan XB, Yuan YB, Jiang W, Liu J, Tian EJ, Shun HM, Huang DH, Yuan XY, Li H, Sheng J: Preparation of rapamycin-loaded chitosan/PLA nanoparticles for immunosuppression in corneal transplantation. *International Journal of Pharmaceutics* 2008, 349:241-248.

[121] Sandri G, Bonferoni MC, Gökçe EH, Ferrari F, Rossi S, Caramella C: Chitosan Associated Solid Lipid Nanoparticles: Assessement of Penetration Enhancement Properties Using RCE cell line. *In 37th Controlled Release Society Annual Meeting & Exposition*; 18-23 July 2009; Copenhagen, Denmark. 2009

[122] Diebold Y, Jarrin M, Saez V, Carvalho EL, Orea M, Calonge M, Seijo B, Alonso MJ: Ocular drug delivery by liposome-chitosan nanoparticle complexes (LCS-NP). *Biomaterials* 2007, 28:1553-1564.

[123] Mehanna MM, Elmaradny HA, Samaha MW: Mucoadhesive liposomes as ocular delivery system: physical, microbiological, and in vivo assessment. *Drug Dev Ind Pharm* 2009.

[124] Li N, Zhuang C, Wang M, Sun X, Nie S, Pan W: Liposome coated with low molecular weight chitosan and its potential use in ocular drug delivery. *Int J Pharm* 2009.

[125] Souto EB, Müller RH: Lipid nanoparticles (SLN and NLC) for drug delivery. In *Nanoparticles for Pharmaceutical Applications*. Volume 01-2007. Edited by Domb AJ,

Tabata Y, Ravi Kumar MNV, Farber S. Los Angeles, California: American Scientific Publishers; 2007: 103-122

[126] Cavalli R, Gasco MR, Chetoni P, Burgalassi S, Saettone MF: Solid lipid nanoparticles (SLN) as ocular delivery system for tobramycin. *Int J Pharm* 2002, 238:241-245.

[127] Li X, Nie SF, Kong J, Li N, Ju CY, Pan WS: A controlled-release ocular delivery system for ibuprofen based on nanostructured lipid carriers. *International Journal of Pharmaceutics* 2008, 363:177-182.

[128] Attama AA, Reichl S, Muller-Goymann CC: Diclofenac sodium delivery to the eye: In vitro evaluation of novel solid lipid nanoparticle formulation using human cornea construct. *International Journal of Pharmaceutics* 2008, 355:307-313.

[129] Attama AA, Muller-Goymann CC: Investigation of surface-modified solid lipid nanocontainers formulated with a heterolipid-templated homolipid. *Int J Pharm* 2007, 334:179-189.

[130] Cengiz E, Demirel M, Yazan Y: Ocular Fate of Cyclosporine-A with Solid Lipid Nanoparticles. *In 6th World Meeting on Pharmaceutics, Biopharmaceutics and Pharmaceutical Technology*; 7-10 April 2008; Barcelona, Spain. 2008

[131] Gökçe EH, Sandri G, Bonferoni MC, Rossi S, Ferrari F, Güneri T, Caramella C: Cyclosporine A loaded SLNs: Evaluation of cellular uptake and corneal cytotoxicity. *International Journal of Pharmaceutics* 2008, 364:76-86.

[132] Niu M, Shi K, Sun Y, Wang J, Cui F: Preparation of CyA-loaded solid lipid nanoparticles and application on ocular preparations. *Journal of Drug Delivery Science and Technology* 2008, 18:293-297.

[133] Başaran E, Demirel M, Sırmagül B, Yazan Y: Cyclosporine-A incorporated cationic solid lipid nanoparticles for ocular delivery. *J Microencapsul* 2009, doi:10.1080/02652040902846883.

[134] Niu M-m, Yu Y-w, Shi K, Zhang L-q, Lin W-h, Cui F-d: A novel solid lipid nanoparticles loaded in situ gel for CyA delivery and its lacrimal pharmacokinetics in rabbit tears. *Journal of Shengyang Pharmaceutical university* 2009, 26:507-511

[135] Shen J, Wang Y, Ping Q, Xiao Y, Huang X: Mucoadhesive effect of thiolated PEG stearate and its modified NLC for ocular drug delivery. *Journal of Controlled Release* 2009, 137:217-223.

[136] Gökçe EH, Sandri G, Bonferoni MC, Güneri T, Caramella C: Freeze-drying of Cyclosporine A Loaded Solid Lipid Nanoparticles *In 37th Controlled Release Society Annual Meeting & Exposition*; 18-23th July 2009; Copenhagen, Denmark. 2009

[137] Samad A, Sultana Y, Aqil M: Liposomal Drug Delivery Systems: An Update Review. *Curr Drug Deliv* 2007, 4:297-305.

[138] Ebrahim S, Peyman GA, Lee PJ: Applications of liposomes in ophthalmology. *Survey of Ophthalmology* 2005, 50:167-182.

[139] Sun KX, Wang AP, Huang LJ, Liang RC, Liu K: Preparation of diclofenac sodium liposomes and its ocular pharmacokinetics. *Yao Xue Xue Bao* 2006, 41:1094-1098.

[140] Pleyer U, Lutz S, Jusko W, Nguyen K, Narawane M, Ruckert D, Mondino B, Lee V, K N: Ocular absorption of topically applied FK506 from liposomal and oil formulations in the rabbit eye [published erratum appears in Invest Ophthalmol Vis Sci 1993 Nov;34(12):3481]. *Invest Ophthalmol Vis Sci* 1993, 34:2737-2742.

[141] Dausch D, Lee S, Dausch S, Kim JC, Schwert G, Michelson W: Vergleichende Studie zur Therapie des Trockenen Auges bedingt durch Lipidphasenstörungen mit lipidhaltigen Tränenpräparaten [Comparative Study of Treatment of the Dry Eye Syndrome due to Disturbances of the Tear Film Lipid Layer with Lipid-Containing Tear Substitutes]. *Klin Monatsbl Augenheilkd* 2006, 223:974-983.

[142] Khaireddin R, Schmidt KG: Vergleichende Untersuchung zur Therapie des evaporativen trockenen Auges [Comparative Investigation of Treatments for Evaporative Dry Eye]. *Klin Monatsbl Augenheilkd* 2009.

[143] Craig JP, Purslow C, Murphy PJ, Wolffsohn JS: Effect Of A Liposomal Spray On The Preocular Tear Film. *In 5th International Conference on the Tear Film & Ocular Surface: Basic Science and Clinical Relevance*; Taormina, Sicily, Italy. 2007

[144] Oh C, Saville BA, Cheng Y-L, Rootman DS: A Compartmental Model for the Ocular Pharmacokinetics of Cyclosporine in Rabbits. *Pharm Res* 1995, 12:433-437.

[145] Yenice I, Mocan MC, Palaska E, Bochot A, Bilensoy E, Vural I, Irkec M, Hincal AA: Hyaluronic acid coated poly-epsilon-caprolactone nanospheres deliver high concentrations of cyclosporine A into the cornea. *Experimental Eye Research* 2008, 87:162-167.

[146] Varia J, Dodiya S, Sawant K: Cyclosporine a loaded solid lipid nanoparticles: optimization of formulation, process variable and characterization. *Curr Drug Deliv* 2008, 5:64-69.

[147] Castelli F, Messina C, Pignatello R, Puglisi G: Effect of pH on diclofenac release from Eudragit RS100 (R) microparticles. A kinetic study by DSC. *Drug Delivery* 2001, 8:173-177.

[148] Attama AA, Schicke BC, Paepenmuller T, Muller-Goymann CC: Solid lipid nanodispersions containing mixed lipid core and a polar heterolipid: Characterization. *European Journal of Pharmaceutics and Biopharmaceutics* 2007, 67:48-57.

[149] Bucolo C, Maltese A, Puglisi G, Pignatello R: Enhanced ocular anti-inflammatory activity of Ibuprofen carried by an Eudragit RS100((R)) nanoparticle suspension. *Ophthalmic Research* 2002, 34:319-323.

[150] Castelli F, Messina C, Sarpietro MG, Pignatello R, Puglisi G: Eudragit as controlled release system for anti-inflammatory drugs - A comparison between DSC and dialysis experiments. *Thermochimica Acta* 2003, 400:227-234.

[151] Vega E, Egea MA, Valls O, Espina M, Garcia ML: Flurbiprofen loaded biodegradable nanoparticles for ophtalmic administration. *Journal of Pharmaceutical Sciences* 2006, 95:2393-2405.

[152] Yamaguchi M, Ueda K, Isowaki A, Ohtori A, Takeuchi H, Ohguro N, Tojo K: Mucoadhesive Properties of Chitosan-Coated Ophthalmic Lipid Emulsion Containing Indomethacin in Tear Fluid. *Biological & Pharmaceutical Bulletin* 2009, 32:1266-1271.

[153] Calvo P, Alonso MJ, Vila-Jato JL, Robinson JR: Improved Ocular Bioavailability of Indomethacin by Novel Ocular Drug Carriers. *Journal of Pharmacy and Pharmacology* 1996, 48:1147-1152.

[154] Adibkia K, Shadbad MRS, Nokhodchi A, Javadzedeh A, Barzegar-Jalali M, Barar J, Mohammadi G, Omidi Y: Piroxicam nanoparticles for ocular delivery:

Physicochemical characterization and implementation in endotoxin-induced uveitis. *Journal of Drug Targeting* 2007, 15:407-416.

In: Conjunctivitis: Symptoms, Treatment and Prevention   ISBN: 978-1-61668-321-4
Editor: Anna R. Sallinger, pp. 107-139   © 2010 Nova Science Publishers, Inc.

Chapter III

PHARMACOLOGICAL TREATMENT OF OCULAR INFLAMMATORY DISEASES WITH NOVEL LIPID BASED DRUG DELIVERY SYSTEMS

Tais Gratieri[1], Elisabet Gonzalez-Mira[2], Renata F. V. Lopez[1], Maria A. Egea[2], Marisa L. Garcia[2] and Eliana B. Souto[3,4,*

[1]Universidade de São Paulo, São Paulo, Brazil;
[2]University of Barcelona, Barcelona, Spain;
[3]University of Trás-os-Montes and Alto Douro (IBB/CGB-UTAD), Vila Real, Portugal;
[4]Fernando Pessoa University, Porto, Portugal.

ABSTRACT

Novel strategies for ocular anti-inflammatory therapies are extensively being investigated to increase drug bioavailability and decrease adverse side effects of common treatments. Colloidal carriers based on lipid materials are becoming a suitable alternative due to several advantages, including solubilization of hydrophobic/lipophilic anti-inflammatory drugs followed by bioavailability enhancement, modification of pharmacokinetic parameters, and protection of sensitive drugs from physical, chemical or biological degradation. Furthermore, by modulating the surface properties e.g. with viscosity-enhancing agents or mucoadhesive polymers may also improve drug bioavailability since the carriers are maintained in the target area for longer time. Likewise, submicron meter particles allow efficient crossing of biological barriers protecting the eye and transport enabling efficient drug delivery to the target tissues and fluids of the anterior segment (cornea, conjunctiva, sclera, anterior uvea) or posterior segment (uveal region, vitreous fluid, choroids and retina). Lipid-based colloidal carriers broadly comprise micro and nanoemulsions, liposomes and lipid nanoparticles (Solid

---

* Correspondence concerning this article should be addressed to: Eliana B. Souto, Faculty of Health Sciences, Fernando Pessoa University, Rua Carlos da Maia, Nr. 296, Office S.1, P-4200-150 Porto, Portugal. Phone: +351-225-074630; Fax: +351-225-074637; Email: eliana@ufp.edu.pt.

Lipid Nanoparticles and Nanostructured Lipid Carriers). These have been already tested for ocular delivery of several anti-inflammatory drugs including corticosteroids and non-steroidal anti-inflammatory drugs, revealing a great potential discussed herein. Novel drug delivery systems are being improved on a daily basis since they are considered a promising strategy to enhance the ocular bioavailability of topically administered drugs.

Keywords: Liposomes, Microemulsions, Nanoemulsions, Solid Lipid Nanoparticles, Nanostructured Lipid Carriers, Ocular Inflammation, Corticosteroids, Non-Steroidal Anti-Inflammatory Drugs.

ABBREVIATIONS

COX	Cyclooxygenase
FDA	Food and Drug Administration
HLB	Hydrophilic-Lipophilic Balance
IOP	Intraocular Pressure
LUV	Large Unilamellar Vesicles
NLC	Nanostructured Lipid Carriers
NSAIDs	Non Steroidal Anti-Inflammatory Drugs
MLV	Multilamellar Vesicles
OLV	Oligolamellar Vesicles
pI	Isoelectric Point
o/w	Oil-in-water
SLN	Solid Lipid Nanoparticles
SUV	Small Unilamellar Vesicles.

1. INTRODUCTION

Inflammation is the manifestation of vascular and cellular response of the host tissue to injury. Injury to the tissue may be inflicted by physical or chemical agents, invasion of pathogens, ischemia, and excessive (hypersensitivity) or inappropriate (autoimmunity) operation of immune mechanisms [1]. Regardless whether an inflammatory insult is the inciting agent or a result of another pathogenic mechanism, ocular inflammation may occur on a large and diverse group of conditions that could compromise human health. The classic signs and symptoms of inflammation, including itching, pain, redness, heat and swelling, often result from ocular inflammatory conditions such as giant papillary conjunctivitis [2], seasonal (intermittent) allergic conjunctivitis [3,4], uveitis [5], dry eye [6], as well as inflammation following injury and/or surgery [7,8]. Such clinical conditions are associated with local changes in blood flow and the invasion of immune cells and inflammatory mediators. If left untreated, ocular inflammation may lead to temporary or permanent vision loss [9].

The pharmacological approach to manage inflammation involves administration of anti-inflammatory agents, i.e., corticosteroids, non-steroidal anti-inflammatory drugs (NSAIDs), and other pharmacologically active compounds.

Corticosteroids are normally used to treat severe inflammation of external eye tissues, which includes inflammation following injury and/or surgery [7,8], uveitis [10] and severe cases of keratoconjuntivitis [11]. These drugs are very potent and effective, however, can produce a plethora of adverse ocular and systemic events, such as induction or exacerbation of glaucoma [12], tear-film instability, epithelial toxicity, progression of cataracts and increased risk of opportunistic infections [13,14].

NSAIDs have proven to be relatively safe in the topical management of ocular inflammations and can be used in less severe cases including for the surgically induced miosis [15,16], management of post-operative inflammation [17], treatment of allergic conjunctivitis [18], prevention and treatment of cystoid macular oedema [19,20] for in the control of pain associated with corneal abrasions [21,22]. There are, however, some reported adverse side effects include impaired corneal sensation [23], persistent epithelial defects [24], superficial punctate keratitis [25].

Despite the several effective anti-inflammatory agents available nowadays, the main challenge remains in the treatment of most ocular diseases by means of achieving local therapeutic concentrations of the drug, limiting its adverse side effects.

The eye is characterized by physiological barriers that limit drug entrance from blood circulation to its inner structures. These are the blood aqueous and the blood-retinal barriers [26]. As a consequence, systemic or oral drug therapy requires large drug dosages to reach the site of action in proper amounts, which may cause significant systemic side-effects [27].

Intravitreal, periocular and subconjunctival injections could minimize systemic exposure of the drug, but the use of these systems is followed by a series of disadvantages. The intravitreally injected drug is rapidly eliminated by the eye's natural circulatory process and therefore frequent injections may be required. Likewise, large dosages are often needed, giving rise to toxicological problems. Besides, there are also relevant side effects, e.g. pain, discomfort, increased intra ocular pressure, intraocular bleeding, increased chances for infection, and the possibility of retinal detachment. The major complication for intravitreal injection is endophtalmitis which can result in severe vision loss [28-30]. In addition, ocular injections are not well accepted by patients.

Ocular implants could represent and alternative to repeated injections as they are able to sustain drug release [31,32], however the insertion of these devices is invasive and can be followed by serious complications, such as retinal detachment, local haemorrhage (in case of intravitreal implants), cataract and increased intra ocular pressure [33]. The need of challenging surgical techniques has hampered the further development of these systems for routine clinical use.

The topical administration would be the preferred route for management of ocular inflammations, especially for inflammations affecting the anterior chamber structures. Nevertheless, unfortunately in several cases, the topical treatment is not effective enough due to protection mechanisms of the human eye, as lachrymal secretion and blinking reflex, which cause rapid drainage of the formulation [34]. Only 5% of the applied drug in conventional eye drops penetrates the cornea and reaches the intraocular tissues with the rest of the dose undergoing transconjunctival absorption or drainage via the nasolachrymal duct before transnasal absorption. This results in loss of drug into the systemic circulation and provides also undesirable systemic side effects [35]. Besides that, tight junctions between cells of the corneal epithelium provide an effective barrier against the penetration of most compounds. The short precorneal residence time allied with cornea impermeability results in low bioavailability and frequent dosing is usually needed to compensate the rapid precorneal drug loss.

Regardless the administration route many anti-inflammatory drugs do not possess the required physicochemical properties to be absorbed, and reach or enter target tissues. Most of the NSAIDs are weakly acidic drugs, which ionize at the pH of the lachrymal fluid and therefore have limited permeability through the anionic cornea which has an isoelectric point (pI) of 3.2. Reducing the pH of the formulation increases the unionized fraction of the drug which enhances permeation. However, being acidic, NSAIDs are inherently irritant [36], and reducing the pH of formulation further increases their irritation potential, and decrease their aqueous solubility [1]. Also the ocular administration of corticosteroids often results in insufficient drug concentration due to poor absorption, rapid metabolism and elimination, being the permeation through the cornea dependent on the drug partition coefficient and molecular-weight [37].

A promising strategy to overcome these problems involves the development of suitable drug carriers systems. The in vivo fate of the drug is no longer mainly dependent on by the properties of the drug, but on the carrier itself, which should allow a controlled and localized release of the active drug according to the specific needs of the therapy, whilst maintaining the simplicity and convenience of the dosage form. Various approaches, e.g. viscosity enhancement [38], use of mucoadhesive [39] or particulate [40] drug delivery systems, vesicular systems [41] and prodrugs [42,43], are being explored. Among these, lipid based drug delivery systems has received much attention due to the many advantages they can provide. Major advantages include: (i) prolonged and controlled action at the corneal surface; (ii) controlled ocular delivery by preventing the metabolism of the drug from the enzymes present at the tear/corneal epithelial surface; (iii) good biocompatibility due to the use of physiological and biodegradable lipids of low systemic toxicity; and (iv) for some formulations, the possibility of production on large industrial scale.

Considering this, the aim of the present chapter is to discuss the anti-inflammatory therapies available and describe the novel lipid based drug delivery systems such as microemulsions, nanoemulsions, liposomes and lipid nanoparticles, used for controlled release and drug targeting.

2. MECHANISM OF INFLAMMATION

Intraocular inflammation is a clinical ocular disorder developed after eye injury by several biological, chemical or physical agents. Ischemia, hypersensitivity or autoimmunity causes may be involved. The ocular inflammation is involved in many pathological clinical conditions and other diseases affecting the anterior or posterior segment of the eye. Ocular structures, such as eyelids, conjunctiva, cornea (keratitis), and anterior or middle uvea (iritis, ciclitis) can be affected. The inflammatory response consists of miosis, lachrymation, conjunctival hyperaemia and breakdown of the blood aqueous barrier followed by protein leakage into the aqueous humour [44]. Inflammation in the back of the eye can be choroiditis (if affecting the uvea posterior), or retinitis (if affecting the retina). Vasculitis may also occur if the retinal vessels are inflamed.

Postoperative inflammation is also common after tissue injury upon surgical incision in cataract or other ophthalmic surgery. This incision triggers the inflammatory cascade, which begins with activation of phospholipase A2. The degree of postoperative inflammation following cataract surgery is linked to several surgery-dependent factors (e.g. surgical technique, intraocular lens type) and patient-dependent factors (e.g. history of inflammatory disease and degree of iris pigmentation). Extracapsular cataract extraction with posterior chamber lens implantation has become a safe procedure. However, during the surgery or postoperative period, specific complications related to prostaglandins and other inflammatory mediators may occure.g. acute pain and discomfort, intraoperative miosis, decrease in visual acuity, posterior capsule fibrosis, keratopathy, fibrin reaction, chronic uveitis, raised intraocular pressure (IOP), synechiae or secondary membrane.

Inflammation is regulated by a complicated mechanism responsible for the rupture of the blood ocular barrier and the attraction of leukocytes towards the eye. This cellular trafficking is regulated by the release of inflammatory mediators and cytokines. As a result of the injury, the phospholipids existing in the cell membranes are broken down into arachidonic acid, which is then converted to prostaglandins by cyclooxygenase (COX) or converted to hydroxy acids and leukotrienes by 5-lipoxygenase. The produced arachidonic acid enters either the COX or lipoxygenase pathway. Activation of COX pathway results in formation of prostaglandins and thromboxanes, whereas the lipoxygenase pathway yields eicosanoids (hydroxyeicosatetraenoic acid and leukotrienes).

Prostaglandins play an important role in the initiation and maintenance of ocular inflammation, being the mediators within the cellular and humoral inflammation cascade, including allergic reactions and pain response. These inflammatory mediators, which show chemokinetic activity, are present in the most tissues of the eye, being the conjunctiva and the anterior uvea the ocular structures which exhibit the most ability of synthesize prostaglandins. In the sclera, cornea, lens, choroid and retina this ability is weaker. Ocular prostaglandins released in the inflammatory process may act at different levels: prostaglandins E1 and E2 increase the IOP by local vasodilatation and increased permeability of blood aqueous barrier but prostaglandin F2 lowers the IOP by increasing uveoscleral outflow. At iris level, they act on the smooth muscle to cause miosis [1]. On the other hand, PGs cause vasodilatation and increase the vascular permeability resulting in increased aqueous humour protein concentration [45].

Corneal nociceptor terminals are excited by exogenous noxious stimuli and also by inflammatory substances released by damaged cells (arachidonic acid, metabolites, neuropeptides, biogenic amines, and kinins). Inflammatory mediators, such prostaglandins may directly activate corneal nociceptive terminals or induce sensitization, and contribute to the sustained ocular pain that follow corneal damage [45]. Accordingly, anti-inflammatory agents are also prescribed as analgesic drugs to reduce postoperative pain after photorefractive surgery [46]. Moreover, the anti-inflammatory agents elicit their action at different levels of arachidonic acid cascade. Corticosteroids act by blocking the enzyme phospholipase A2 to inhibit arachidonic acid production, thereby preventing the synthesis of all the PGs, thromboxanes and eicosanoids. On the other hand, NSAIDs exert their anti-inflammatory action by inhibiting the enzymes COX-1 and COX-2.

Ocular inflammation of the anterior segment of the eye is generally managed by topical administration of drugs, which are also approved by FDA for postoperative use. To provide a better control of the inflammatory condition and to prevent undesired side effects (as miosis) during the surgical procedure itself, their clinical use may be both in pre and post operative approaches [36]. Anti-inflammatory agents have also been used in preoperative prophylaxis [47].

2.1. Corticosteroids

Corticosteroids are anti-inflammatory agents since they inhibit phospholipase A2 and subsequently inhibit both the COX and lipoxigenase pathways [48]. Steroids interact with specific DNA sequences of cellular nucleus, changing the production of inhibitory proteins, and inhibiting the production of additional inflammatory mediators. Steroids also reduce the macrophages and neutrophils migration to the inflamed area, decreasing vascular permeability and suppressing the action of various lymphokines [49]. They also inhibit oedema, capillary dilatation, cellular infiltration, fibroblastic proliferation and deposition of collagen. Cortocisteroids are therefore the most current option to treat the inflammation associated with cataract surgery. They are recommended for preventing and/or treating postoperative ocular inflammation.

Since the corneal epithelium is lipophilic and the stroma is hydrophilic, molecules comprising both lipophilic and hydrophilic moieties (e.g., acetates or alcohols) penetrate the cornea to a greater degree rather than totally hydrophilic compounds (e.g., phosphate solutions) [50]. Prednisolone (acetate, phosphate) is most common topical corticosteroid, but others (e.g. fluocinolone acetonide [51], dexamethasone [52], fluorometholone [53], medrysone [54], and rimexolone [13]), have been used to treat inflammation, reducing adverse effects after surgical procedures [55]. These steroids can be used in ocular disorders that involve some inflammatory surface reaction such as dry eye, based on immune response and induced by many cytokines [6,56].

Corticosteroids offer the most potent efficacy in treating inflammation; however, they can induce significant side effects. Their short-term use helps minimizing the risk while still reaping significant benefits. Some of the most serious side effects of prolonged topical steroid application include ocular hypertension, glaucoma, cataracts, mydriasis, ptosis, inhibition of corneal epithelial or stoma healing, punctate staining, corneal-sclera melting, damage to the optic nerve, and defects in visual acuity and visual fields [57].

2.2. Non-steroidal Anti-inflamatory Drugs (NSAIDs)

NSAIDs comprise several chemically heterogeneous compounds which inhibit prostaglandins and thromboxane formation from arachidonic acid through the inhibition of the enzymes COX-1 and COX-2. Endogenous prostaglandins increase the permeability of the blood ocular barriers affect intraocular pressure and produce miosis and conjunctival hyperemia.

NSAIDs may be an effective alternative to costicosteroids in the topical management of ocular inflammations, being nowadays used in postoperative inflammation [58,59], inhibition of intra-operative miosis [60], treatment of seasonal allergic conjunctivitis [61], prevention and treatment of cystoid macular oedema [62], in pain relief [63], to decrease bacterial colonization of contact lenses and prevent bacterial adhesion to corneal cells [64].

NSAIDs for ocular inflammation include water soluble indoleacetic acid, aryl acetic acid, aryl propionic acid and enolic acid derivatives. The majority of the molecules are weak acids, which ionize at the pH of the lachrymal fluid and thus have limited permeability through the anionic cornea. Reducing the pH of the formulation increases the non-ionized fraction, enhancing drug permeation but increases the risk of irritation. There are some NSAIDs approved by the FDA for the treatment of post-operative inflammation after cataract surgery (kerotolac, flurbiprofen, bromfenac, diclofenac and nepafenac (a prodrug that is converted in its active form amfenac by intraocular enzymatic hydrolysis) [65]. These drugs are also prescribed for postoperative pain relief after photo-refractive surgery, being the analgesic action partially attributed to reduction of prostaglandins production [45].

The main advantage of using topical NSAIDs is the avoidance of undesirable effects of steroids, in particular for patients susceptible to corticosteroid-responsive IOP elevations, or with recurrent herpes simplex infection or delayed wound healing. Although NSAIDs are widely recognized as providing most of the clinical benefits of steroids while avoiding major adverse side effects, they also have limitations. These include ocular irritation and discomfort following application, conjunctival injection, mild punctate keratopathy, mydriasis, allergic and hypersensitivity reactions [36].

3. NOVEL LIPID-BASED DRUG DELIVERY SYSTEMS FOR OCULAR INFLAMMATORY DISEASES

Enhanced ocular retention of oily vehicles has been reported for more than 30 years [66], being attributed to their interaction with the superficial oily layer of the tear film. As a consequence, initial attempts to overcome the poor bioavailability of topically instilled drugs typically involved the use of ointments and emulsions. Ointments and emulsions ensured superior drug bioavailability by increasing the contact time with the eye, minimizing the dilution by tears, and resisting nasolachrymal drainage [67]. However, these vehicles have the major disadvantage of being uncomfortable and providing blurred vision. They still can be found for a series of anti-inflammatory drugs but are mainly used for either administration overnight or for treatment on the outside and edges of the eyelids [68]. Since only a limited percentage of the administered drug reaches the target tissue, patient compliance is an important aspect to consider when developing an ophthalmic delivery system. As such, attention should be paid to the facility of administration and to the sensorial feeling after the administration, since discomfort after administration (e.g., burning sensation), could induce tear production, followed by drug dilution and drainage through nasolachrymal duct.

Other important aspect to consider is the retention time, drug loading capacity and drug protection from metabolic degradation. In fact, if the system is able to prolong the retention, while loading a sufficient amount of drug in a protected manner, the interval between administrations can be lengthened. For instance, in case of intravitreal injections, the reduction on the number of injections would also reduce the potential side-effects. Apart from these, all the factors that would influence the overall costs should also be considered, as possibility of scaling up of production, sterilizing and the physical and chemical storage stability of the product.

The novel lipid based delivery systems as microemulsions, nanoemulsions, liposomes, SLN and NLC are now being used in attempt to attend all these requirements. The advantages and limitations of each system, and their suitability for the treatment of ocular inflammatory diseases will be reviewed in the following sections.

3.1. Microemulsions

The concept of microemulsions was first described in 1943 by Hoar and Schulman who generated a clear single-phase solution by titrating a milky emulsion with hexanol [69]. Microemulsions are defined as a system composed of water, oil and an amphiphile molecule which is a single optically isotropic and thermodynamically stable liquid solution' [70].

They are formulated using high concentration of surfactants, to decrease the interfacial tension at the oil/water interface and usually also co-surfactants (e.g., alcohol, amides and sulphoxides), to keep the interfacial layer highly flexible and fluid. In this way, a clear or translucent system composed of very small droplets (~100 nm) of oil or water is obtained stabilized by an interfacial film (Figure 1). These systems are called "Ternary systems" if only surfactants are used, or "Pseudoternary systems" if surfactants and co-surfactants are used together taken as a single-phase [71]. The ionic surfactants are generally too toxic to be used at high concentrations in ocular preparations, therefore, non-ionic surfactants are preferred [72].

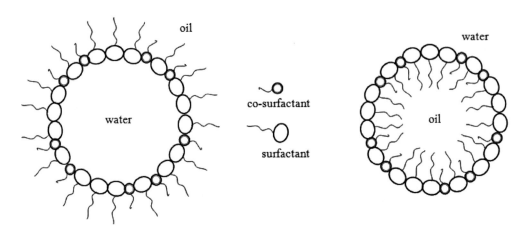

Figure 1. Schematic representation of microemulsions (adapted from Bonacucina et al. [73]).

The intrinsic properties of microemulsions confer special advantages to its use as ophthalmic drug delivery systems. Firstly, as they are thermodynamicaly stable they can be easily prepared and easily sterilized. Secondly, they have a high solubilizing capacity [74]. Besides, the surfactants and co-surfactants can act as penetration enhancers to facilitate corneal penetration of drugs [70] what could be further potentialized by the good spreadability on the cornea and mixing with the precorneal film constituents, due to the low surface tension of microemulsions [75]. Most likely due to their oily nature, microemulsions have demonstrated prolonged retention in comparison with aqueous solutions [72], which could reduce frequency of drug administration and contribute to patient compliance. Moreover, as they are transparent systems, it is possible to obtain formulations with refractive index close to the water, corneal and lachrymal fluid values (from 1.33 to 1.36) [76], avoiding, in this way, impairment of vision and discomfort, which are frequent after administration of macroemulsions, ointments and some gels. In addition, the low viscosity allows normal blinking and is preferred by users, as it facilitates administration.

Microemulsions have been designed to increase bioavailability of corticosteroids in the aqueous humor after topical administration. It was possible to achieve improved pharmacokinetic parameters of dexamethasone (0.1% w/v) in rabbits using a microemulsion. This specific system was composed of 15.0% w/w of non-ionic surfactant (polyoxyethyleneglycerol triricinoleate), 5.0% w/w of isopropyl myristate as the oil phase, ultrafiltrated water with benzalkonium chloride (0.01% w/w) as the aqueous phase, and 15.0% w/w of propyleneglycol as the cosurfactant. Furthermore, the greater drug penetration in the eye was observed allowing the possibility of decreasing the number of application of eye drops per day [76].

Though microemulsions have excellent advantages and seem to be promising ophthalmic drug delivery systems, limitations in selection of surfactant/co-surfactant system and potential toxicity associated with higher concentration of surfactant/co-surfactant often restricts its use [77]. In this way, a more feasible approach is the use of nanoemulsions, which are emulsions with extremely small droplet size, which also possess a series of advantages concerning ocular delivery but, most importantly, are formulated with small percentage of surfactants and co-surfactants.

3.2. Nanoemulsions

Emulsions with droplet size in the nanometric range (typically from 20–200 nm) are often referred to in the literature as miniemulsions [78], submicron emulsions [79], nanoemulsions [80-83], fine emulsions [84]. Due to small droplet size, in the same way as microemulsions, nanoemulsions can appear transparent or translucent to the naked eye. Although some authors decide to use the terms microemulsions and nanoemulsions interchangeably, there is a fundamental difference between these systems, which is that microemulsions are systems under thermodynamically stable equilibrium, while nanoemulsions are non-equilibrium systems with a spontaneous tendency to separate into the constituent phases [85], even though nanoemulsions may possess a relatively high kinetic stability, even for several years [86].

In comparison to microemulsions the major advantage is the use of less percentage of surfactants and co-surfactants, making them safer in terms of toxicity. Oil-in-water (o/w) nanoemulsions physically resemble a simple aqueous-based eye drops dosage form since more than 90% of the external phase is aqueous and oil concentrations are normally below 5% to prevent blurred vision [82,83]. Following topical administration, these systems suffer the protection mechanisms of the eye, and, can be drained by the tears. Therefore, nanoemulsions are likely to be destabilized by the tear fluid electrolytic and dynamic action. When it happens, the water phase of the emulsion is drained off while the oil phase of the emulsion remains in the cul-de-sac for a long period of time and functions as a drug reservoir [82,83]. Such hypothesis has been proven adding a fluorescent marker to nanoemulsions formulations. In this experiment 39.9 ±10.2% of the fluorescence was measured one minute after topical instillation of a nanoemulsion in the eye, while only 6.8 ± 1.8% of fluorescence was still present after a regular eye drop instillation [87].

Nanoemulsions present a series of advantages to conventional eye drops, ointments and gels. They are naturally biodegradable, easily sterilized, can improve ocular bioavailability, both by prolonging formulation residence time and by increasing corneal permeability and providing substantial drug solubilization either at the innermost oil phase or at the o/w interface. Nanoemulsion strongly improved the solubilization of indomethacin and sodium diclofenac [74]. However, one limitation of this system is the low possibility of controlling drug release due to the small size and the liquid state of the carrier [88].

The earlier attempts on applying nanoemulsions for ocular delivery of anti-inflammatory drugs were made using anionic formulations. The in vitro corneal penetration of indomethacin from anionic nanoemulsions composed of lecithin and Miglyol 840 oil has demonstrated to be more than 3-fold that of the commercial eye drops. In addition, this property was comparable between nanoparticles and nanocapsules made of poly-ε-caprolactone with similar particle size of the nanoemulsions (200-250 nm), which therefore excludes the influence of the inner structure or chemical composition of the colloidal systems on the corneal penetration of indomethacin [89]. As further animal studies showed that microparticles containing indomethacin hardly increased drug penetration, the authors concluded that the main factor responsible for the favourable corneal transport of indomethacin was the colloidal nature of these carriers rather than their inner structure or composition [90]. Similar results (i.e., a 3.8-fold indomethacin permeation increase in comparison to commercially available eye drops), were obtained using an anionic nanoemulsion composed of 20% oily phase, 0.2-1% phospholipids and 0.2-0.5% amphoteric agents. In this formulation, the pH value was adjusted to 3.8 in order to maintain the indomethacin in the oily phase, preventing its ionization (pKa = 4.5). In this case, the increase of indomethacin permeation can be also attributed to the low ionization of the drug at emulsion pH. This resulted in a higher partition to the lipophilic epithelium layer compared to the indomethacin aqueous solution that was adjusted to pH 6.8, where the drug is markedly ionized [79]. On the other hand, in vivo the lower pH of the external phase would result in pH-induced lachrymation and loss of drug from the conjunctival sac resulting in reduced bioavailability and return of the pH of lachrymal fluid back to physiological range would reduce ocular penetration of drug due to ionization [1].

Another preparation made of 4.0% (w/v) of polysorbate 80, a non ionic surfactant and 5.0% (w/v) was capable of a 5.7-fold increase in the ocular penetration of difluprednate, a synthetic glucorticoid, in comparison with the drug ophthalmic suspension [81].

The scientific literature reports the occurrence of electrostatic interactions between the cationic emulsified droplets and anionic cellular moieties of the ocular surface [91]. In addition to the intrinsic corneal cells membrane negative charge, a layer of the glycoprotein mucin (a mixture of neutral and acidic mucopolysaccharides) secreted by goblet cells at the conjunctival surface is adjacent to the corneal epithelium, what makes it negatively charged with an isoelectric point of 3.2 [92]. The hypothesis of electrostatic interaction between positively charged emulsions and the cornea surface has been supported by various studies demonstrating that positive charge may prolong the residence time of the drop on the epithelial layer of the cornea and thus enable better drug penetration through the cornea to the internal tissues of the eye. Animal studies have demonstrated that the contact angle of one droplet of the different dosage forms on the cornea is found to be 70° for saline, 38° for an anionic nanoemulsion and 21.2° for a cationic nanoemulsion. The values of the spreading coefficient were found to be -47, -8.6 and -2.4 mN/m, respectively. It can be clearly deduced that both nanoemulsions had better wettability properties on the cornea compared to saline, being the positively charged superior than the negatively one. In these systems, it is likely that the drug is not released from the oil droplet in a hydrophilic tear compartment but rather partitioned directly from the oil droplets to the cell membranes on the corneal epithelium [82,83].

A positively charged nanoemulsion containing piroxicam demonstrated to be effective in lowering the ulcerative cornea score, following alkali burn of rabbit corneas [93]. Likewise, the comparison of indomethacin corneal penetration from the positively charged nanoemulsion Indocollyre® (a marketed hydro-PEG ocular solution) and a negatively charged nanoemulsion revealed better performance of the positively charged formulation, as its spreading coefficient on cornea was four times higher than that of the negatively charged emulsion [94].

A study evaluating the residence time of indomethacin after instillation in rabbit eyes compared the performance of chitosan-coated emulsion with a non-coated emulsion. The coated emulsion had a mean particle size of 117.6 nm and positively charged (zeta potential of 27.7 mV), whereas the non-coated emulsion was of smaller mean size (94.8 nm) and slightly negatively charged (-6.2 mV). Coated emulsion provided mean concentrations 3.6-fold and 3.8-fold higher than the non-coated at 0.5 hr and 0.75 hr after instillation, respectively. The drug levels in cornea, conjunctiva, and aqueous humour 1 hr after instillation were also higher than those obtained after administration of the non-coated emulsion. After in vitro mucoadhesive tests the authors concluded that the residence time of the emulsion in tear fluid was attributed to the mucoadhesive properties of chitosan [95].

Chitosan nanoparticles were also compared to positively charged chitosan nanoemulsions for ocular indomethacin delivery. In vivo studies and histopathological examination revealed that rabbit eyes treated with nanoemulsion showed clearer healing of corneal chemical ulcer with moderate effective inhibition of polymorph nuclear leuckocytic infiltration, compared with nanoparticles preparation. Using nanoemulsions, therapeutic concentrations of indomethacin were achieved in the cornea and were significantly higher than those obtained following instillation of indomethacin solution [80].

3.3. Liposomes

Liposomes are phospholipid vesicles formed by one or several lipid bilayers. In each bilayer the nonpolar fatty acid tails are placed in the interior, whereas the polar heads are turned outside containing an aqueous phase both inside and between the bilayers (Figure 2). As such, appearance and permeability of phospholipid layers are similar to those of biological membranes [96].

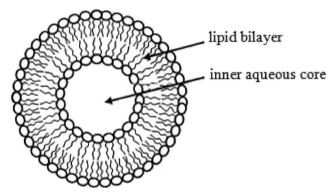

Figure 2. Schematic representation of a liposome (adapted from Bonacucina et al. [73]).

Liposomes were first introduced by Bangham et al. in the 1960s [97]. Studying the behaviour of lecithin and other phospholipids, the authors found that they are able to form spheres in dilute aqueous solutions. They defined liposomes as the smallest artificial vesicles of spherical shape that can be produced from natural nontoxic phospholipids and cholesterol. Bangham et al. were the first to study the physicochemical properties of these colloidal mesophases, such as their particle size distribution, osmotic behaviour, and surface charge [73].

Liposomes are formed spontaneously when phospholipids are hydrated in aqueous media. The mean size can vary from 20 to above 1000 nm, depending on composition, preparation method and number of bilayers. According to the number of bilayers they are distinguished as small unilamellar vesicles (SUV) (25-50 nm), large unilamellar vesicles (LUV) (100-200 nm), oligolamellar vesicles (OLV) and multilamellar vesicles (MLV) (1-2 μm) (Figure 3).

Since liposomes are composed of similar substances as cell membranes it is expected that they are biocompatible and biodegradable preparations. Most liposomes are prepared by using lecithin of egg or vegetable (soy bean) origin. Furthermore, a common component used in liposomes preparations is cholesterol, which is applied to improve characteristics (e.g., fluidity), to reduce the permeability of water-soluble molecules through the membrane in order to control release and to increase the stability of the bilayer membrane in the presence of biological fluids (e.g., blood/plasma) [96].

Several factors can influence the fate of drugs in liposome ocular delivery, namely: (i) the chemical composition of the liposomal product (lipids, surfactants, and other molecules); (ii) mean size of the vesicle; (iii) surface charge; (iv) drug-liposome interaction; and (v) the production process. Because of their amphiphilic character, liposomes are able to entrap both hydrophilic and hydrophobic compounds in the aqueous compartments or within the lipid bilayers, respectively [98,99]. Nevertheless, the encapsulation efficiency is generally higher for lipophilic rather than for hydrophilic molecules [96]. Liposomes can provide controlled release of incorporated drugs since the spherical lipid shield formed by bilayer membranes provides a permeability barrier to drug release. In this way, the drug is protected from degradation and clearance, and toxicity resultant from high peak concentrations is avoided. This property can be especially useful for posterior segment applications [100].

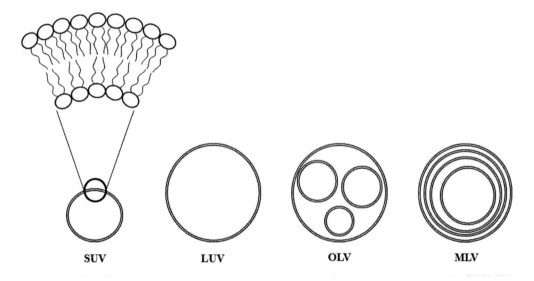

| SUV | LUV | OLV | MLV |

Figure 3. Schematic representations of different types of liposomes, depending on the shape, size and number of bilayers: small unilamellar vesicles (SUV), large unilamellar vesicles (LUV), oligolamellar vesicles (OLV) and multilamellar vesicles (MLV) (adapted from Bonacucina et al. [73]).

The increased residence time of drugs, and maintenance of their therapeutic concentrations for longer time intervals, could reduce the number of subconjunctival and intravitreal injections usually required in some treatments [101-104], while allowing higher doses without toxicity from initial concentration [84]. In this way, liposomes can minimize some of the adverse side effects encountered by these administration routes, increasing therapeutic effectiveness when no other options are available. Intravitreal injection of liposomes containing antibiotics [105-109], antifungal agents [110], antiviral agents [111-114], immunosuppressives [115], oligonucleotides [116,117] and other pharmaceutically active compounds, have been evaluated, but unfortunately not the same effort has been found for liposomes containing anti-inflammatory drugs.

In a recent study, the potential of target-delivering corticosteroids to inflamed eye was suggested using intravenous injection of a sugar chain modified liposome containing dexamethasone in experimental autoimmune uveoretinitis mice. The authors verified that while intravenous administration of the drug alone provided a wide distribution in all tissues (eye, brain, heart, lung, liver, kidney, spleen and intestine), the intravenous injection of the modified liposome was almost concentrated to the eye, even though drug concentration in liposome formulation was the double of the formulation containing drug alone [118].

For the anterior segment, topical ocular administration of drugs incorporated into liposomes also showed several advantages, as increased corneal adherence [119], therefore, prolonged residence time [120], and improved bioavailability. Moreover, the controlled release allows prolonged effect [121], therefore time between administrations can be lengthened. In addition, liposomes offer the convenience of an ophthalmic drop and confinement of the action at the site of administration [122].

The use of liposomes for the topical delivery of anti-inflammatory agents has been investigated since 1983, when Singh et al. encapsulated triamcinolone acetonide in large MLV composed of phosphatidylcholine and cholesterol. These liposomes produced higher drug levels in ocular tissues of rabbits in compared to a standard suspension of the steroid. A more than two-fold drug concentration was obtained and maintained in the aqueous humour for up to 5 h when using the liposome formulation [123].

Probably due to fact that topical steroids poorly penetrate the cornea with intact epithelium, first studies on liposomes for topical delivery focused on the application of these compounds. The efficacy of liposomes containing dexamethasone and its ester was investigated and compared to similar aqueous suspensions of each drug. The authors verified that the liposome containing dexamethasone valerate provided the highest ocular drug levels. In the case of dexamethasone or dexamethasone palmitate, the liposomes provided a lower drug level in comparison with the suspension. In this study, a high esterase activity was observed in the corneal homogenate supernatant, and most of the steroid taken up after instillation of dexamethasone valerate was metabolized to free alcohol [124].

Radiolabeled cationic liposomes were used for dexamethasone delivery [125,126]. This corticosteroid achieved high concentrations in the rabbit cornea, aqueous humour, iris, ciliary body, and sclera for up to 4 hours. Drug levels remained high for 6 hr in the conjunctiva. The authors anticipated that the saturated phospholipids in liposomes may protect them from tear lysozyme and esterase activity, resulting in greater bioavailability.

Diclofenac sodium was also loaded in cationic liposomes prepared by reverse phase evaporation [127]. They were shown to provide a 211% increase in aqueous humour concentration of drug compared with conventional aqueous eye drop formulation. In another study, notable advantages for ocular drug delivery were achieved by coating liposomes containing sodium diclofenac with chitosan. The authors reported that this procedure conferred a positive charge and slightly increased liposomes particle size, while the drug encapsulation was not affected. The coating procedure also prolonged in vitro drug release profile, improved physicochemical stability, and increased bioadhesion. This resulted in a prolonged retention compared to the non-coated liposome or drug solution, and displayed a potential penetration enhancing effect for transcorneal delivery. In the ocular tolerance study, no irritation or toxicity was caused by continual administration of low molecular weight chitosan-coated liposome in a total period of 7 days [128].

Significant progress has been made in demonstrating the advantages of liposome-mediated drug delivery in ophthalmology. In some cases, liposomes have shown to improve efficacy, reduce toxicity, prolong activity and provide site specific delivery. Despite those reasons, which make liposomes a potentially useful system for ocular delivery, until nowadays there were very few attempts on applying them for the treatment of ocular inflammatory diseases. Problems normally encountered were short shelf life, limited drug loading capacity, use of aggressive conditions for preparation, and problems in sterilization [129]. Temperatures required for autoclaving can cause irreversible damage to vesicles while filtration reduces the vesicle to an average of 200 nm limiting its use to small vesicles.

Several anti-inflammatory drugs have been successfully incorporated in liposomes, particularly in the last decade, e.g., aceclofenac [130], piroxicam [131,132], salicylic acid [133], indomethacin [134], ibuprofen [135], flurbiprofen [136], ketoprofen [137], dexamethasone [138], and betamethasone [139,140]. In some cases high encapsulation efficiency and long-term stability during storage were achieved [136,141]. Therefore, as these main formulation problems are being solved it is expected that in the next years studies applying liposomes containing anti-inflammatory agents for ocular drug delivery will increase massively and therefore more therapeutic options will become available.

3.4. Lipid Nanoparticles (SLN and NLC)

Solid lipid nanoparticles (SLN) are the first generation of nanoparticles composed of lipids that are solid at room and body temperatures, stabilized with an emulsifying layer in an aqueous dispersion, i.e.,, they resemble the nanoemulsions by replacing the inner liquid lipid with a solid lipid. They were developed in the beginning of the 90s. The main advantage of SLN over nanoemulsions is the possibility of a controlled drug delivery, since drug mobility in a solid lipid is lower compared with an oily phase. Other advantages of such carriers include the use of physiological compounds in the composition, the fast and effective production process, including the possibility of large scale production, the avoidance of organic solvents in the production procedures, and the possibility to produce high concentrated lipid suspensions [142]. The main disadvantage, however, is the low drug loading capacity [143], which is mainly related to the possibility of drug expulsion during storage [144].

Drug localization within SLN, as well as the capacity of these particles to retain the drug, will depend on the composition of the formulation (lipid, active compound, surfactant), as well as on the production conditions (hot vs. cold homogenization). The drug may be placed in between the chains of the fatty acids or in between the lipid layers and also in imperfections (e.g., amorphous clusters). After heating the melted lipids crystallize in higher energy conformations. These conformations are not very organized, allowing drugs to be loaded. During shelf life polymorphic transitions occur and low energy conformations are adopted, reducing the number of imperfections in the crystal lattice and expulsing the drug (Figure 4) [145,146]. Perfect lipid crystals are usually formed when the lipid molecules are chemically similar, e.g., pure triglycerides [147].

Nanostructured lipid carriers (NLC) are another type of lipid nanoparticles being developed to overcome some limitations of SLN. NLC are prepared not only from solid lipids but from a blend of a solid lipid with a certain amount of oil, to maintain a melting point above 40°C. Mixing especially very different molecules, such as long chain glycerides of the solid lipid with short chain glycerides of the liquid lipid, creates crystals with many imperfections [148]. Apart from localizing drug in between fatty acid chains or lipid lamellae, these imperfections provide a space for additional loading of active molecules. These latter can be incorporated in the particle matrix in a molecular dispersed form, or be arranged in amorphous clusters. There is also more flexibility for modulation of drug release, increasing the drug loading and preventing its leakage.

There are three models describing the NLC structure [148], namely, the imperfect type, the amorphous type, and the multiple type (Figure 4). Several comprehensive reviews have been devoted to this topic [144,148-152].

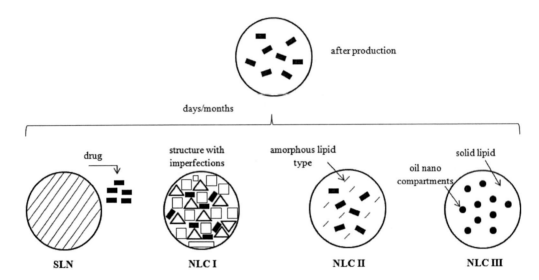

Figure 4. Crystallization process during storage to perfect crystal in SLN (left) and schematic model showing the NLC different structures: imperfect type (NLC I); amorphous type (NLCII) and multiple type (NLC III) (adapted from Müller et al. [148]).

Distribution of the drug depends on its physicochemical characteristics and on the composition of the particles, but it is influenced by the partition coefficient of the drug [153]. Lipid nanoparticles (SLN and NLC) are an interesting system for the ocular delivery of drugs. Similar to emulsions they are composed of accepted excipients, and can be produced on large industrial scale, using an established and low cost homogenization process. The lipid nanoparticles show additionally the advantages of a solid matrix similar to polymeric nanoparticles, having the ability to protect chemically labile ingredients and to modulate release (from very fast to extremely prolonged release). The possibility of surface modifications can be used to prolong pre-corneal residence time. Similarly to liposomes, several SLN and NLC have been successfully prepared for the incorporation of anti-inflammatory drugs but aimed for different administration routes, as intravenous, oral, pulmonary and transdermal. Examples of anti-inflammatory drug used include flurbiprofen [154-156], indomethacin [157-159], ketoprofen [158,160], naproxen [160], ketorolac [161], valdecoxib [162], sodium diclofenac [163], dexamethasone [164], hydrocortisone [163,165], betamethasone [166], triamcinolone acetonide [167,168], and methotrexate [169,170]. Therefore, it is expected that in the recent future lipid nanoparticles will become available for the treatment of ocular inflammatory diseases. Apart from the drug loading difficulties, several compounds commonly used in the treatment of ocular diseases have been incorporated in lipid nanoparticles, such as tobramycin [171], gatifloxacin [172], cyclosporine [173], and timolol maleate [174]. Lipid nanoparticles have shown sustained release and enhancement of drug bioavailability [171]. In the last years, SLN have attempted also a big development as non-viral systems for DNA delivery, but there are still few papers about their use in gene therapy. An example of this development is the work by del Pozo-Rodríguez et al. who evaluated the transfection capacity of SLN in the human retinal pigment epithelial established cell line in order to elucidate the potential application of this vector in the treatment of retinal diseases [175].

Lipid nanoparticles can be attractive systems for the ocular delivery of poorly water soluble drugs. For instance, hydrocortisone was loaded into SLN in a high extent (97% of total 0.5%, w/w). In vitro drug permeation studies through human cornea construct revealed that the permeation coefficients of hydrocortisone-loaded SLN were reduced in comparison to aqueous and oily solutions of the drug. However, the permeated amount was higher from the SLN due to a much higher hydrocortisone concentration achieved. The authors also observed that the high drug load of the nanoparticles provides prolonged drug release [176]. Sustained release and high permeation through bio-engineered cornea was also observed for SLN containing diclofenac sodium. Using phospholipids together with homolipid from goat, the authors obtained high loading efficiencies (94%), which has been attributed it to complex formation between phospholipids and the drug, and also to drug association in the structures formed at the particle surface [177].

Ibuprofen has been widely used for the treatments of ocular inflammations. However, it is limited by a short biological half-life time (1.5–2 h) that leads to a short duration of action [178]. In order to overcome the shortcoming, multiple intakes of ibuprofen are required to maintain the effective concentration in human bodies which potentially lead to the occurrences of some side effects [179]. Due to its poor solubility in water, ibuprofen is an ideal candidate to be incorporated in lipid carriers. Since 2006 it has been successfully incorporate in SLN and NLC for diverse routes of delivery [178,180-184]. However, the first paper reporting a NLC intended for ocular drug delivery was published by Li et al. in 2008 [185]. They investigated four different compositions of NLC for the ocular delivery of ibuprofen. The effect of Gelucire 44/14 (as solid lipid material), Transcutol P (as permeability enhancer) and stearylamine (as charge-inducing reagent) on particle size, zeta potential, ocular irritation and corneal permeability were studied. The result showed that both Gelucire 44/14 and Transcutol P could enhance the drug corneal permeability to some extent; and stearylamine could prolong the pre-corneal retention of drug. Ibuprofen-loaded NLC displayed controlled-release profile. By optimizing the NLC composition, a suitable formulation was developed showing higher drug bioavailability in comparison to eye drops [185]. This prolonged pre-corneal retention has been attributed to the positively charged NLC.

The surface composition of the colloidal carriers may affect their affinity towards the ocular mucosa. The positive surface charge was found to have a positive effect in prolong the residence time of nanoemulsion droplet containing indomethacin on the epithelial layer of the cornea [94]. Nanoparticles coated with a bioadhesive polymer, such as hyaluronic acid or chitosan, indicated that the nature of the coating layers affect the interaction of the carriers with the corneal epithelial cells [186,187]. Based on these facts, a promising tool for ocular drug delivery is the use of NLC with surface modifications that could increase mucoadhesive properties, and leading to prolonged precorneal retention and, as a consequence, increased bioavailability. Such particles have recently been obtained by surface modification of cyclosporine loaded NLC with cysteine-polyethylene glycol stearate [188].

Surfactants applied in SLN for the treatment of ophthalmic diseases are selected from the group comprising: (i) lecithins, as they are, (e.g., Lipoids, phospholipids and hydrogenated forms thereof and synthetic and semi-synthetic derivates thereof); (ii) bile salts (e.g., sodium glycocholate, sodium taurocholate and taurodeoxycholate); (iii) polysorbates and sorbitans (e.g., Tween 20, Tween 40, Tween 80, Span 20, Span 40, and Span 60); and (iv) viscosity enhancers, particularly gelatin. The co-surfactants are selected from the group comprising: (i) low molecular weight alcohols or glycols (e.g., butanol, hexanol and hexadiol); (ii) low molecular weight fatty acids (e.g., butyric acid and octanoic acid); (iii) phosphoric acid esters, (iv) benzylic alcohol and (v) bile salts [189].

Table 1. Aspects to be considered on choosing an ophthalmic delivery system and the performance of novel lipid-based systems

Aspects to consider	Novel lipid-based systems				
	Microemulsion	Nanoemulsion	Liposome	SLN	NLC
Facility of administration	+ + +	+ + +	+ +	+ +	+ +
Sensorial after administration – (avoidance of blurred vision, burning sensation)	+ + +	+ + +	+ +	+ +	+ +
Drug loading capacity	+ + +	+ + +	+ +	-	+ +
Possibility of drug targeting	-	-	+ + +	+ +	+ +
Pre-corneal retention time	+ +	+ +	+ +	+ +	+ +
In vitreous residence time	-	-	+ +	-*	-*
Controlled drug release	-	-	++	++	++
Avoidance of toxicity	-	++	+++	++	++
Scaling up of production	+++	+++	-	+++	+++
Easy to sterilize	+++	+++	-	+++	+++
Storage stability	+++	++	-	++	++

+ + + excellent, + + very good, + good, - poor, -*not reported.

Several factors should be considered when choosing surfactants for lipid nanoparticles in general, namely, hydrophilic-lipophilic balance (HLB) value, route of administration, toxicity, and the effect on lipid modification and particle size. Surfactants with HLB values in the range of 8-18 are suitable for the preparation of o/w dispersion. Non-ionic surfactants are preferred over the ionic ones for ocular formulations because of their lower toxicity and irritancy. In general, the order of the toxicity of surfactants is from cationic to anionic, non-ionic, and ultimately amphoteric.

Table 2. Advantages and disadvantages of novel lipid-based drug delivery systems and anti-inflammatory drugs incorporated for ophthalmic delivery

Lipid based delivery system	Advantages	Disadvantages	Anti-inflammatory drugs used for ocular delivery
Microemulsion	High solubility of both hydrophilic and hydrophobic drugs Easy preparation and sterilization Prolonged pre-corneal residence time Enhanced drug penetration Transparent systems	Large amounts of surfactants and co-surfactants needed Potential toxicity	Dexamethasone [194]
Nanoemulsions	Small amount of surfactant – toxicological safety High solubility of both hydrophilic and hydrophobic drugs Easy preparation – large scale production Easy sterilization May be transparent Prolonged pre-corneal residence time	Difficult to control drug release Thermodynamically instable systems	Indomethacin [80, 89, 90, 94, 95] Piroxicam [93] Difluprednate [81] Predinisolone [84]
Liposomes	Biocompatible and biodegradable Able to entrap both hydrophilic and hydrophobic drugs Controlled release Provide drug protection from metabolic degradation Prolonged residence time – pre-corneal and in vitreous	Poor stability Difficult to prepare and sterilize High cost	Diclofenac sodium [127, 128] Dexamethasone [124-126, 195]
SLN	Easy preparation – large scale production Easy sterilization Improved ocular bioavailability Prolonged pre-corneal residence time Controlled release	Limited drug loading	Hydrocortisone [176] Diclofenac sodium[177]
NLC	Easy preparation – large scale production Easy sterilization Drug loading of lipophilic and possibly hydrophilic Improved ocular bioavailability Prolonged pre-corneal residence time Controlled release	Hydrophilic drugs can show burst effects	Ibuprofen [185]

Table 3. List of surfactants, co-surfactants commonly used in SLN and NLC

Amphoteric surfactants	Non-ionic surfactants	Ionic surfactants	Co-surfactants
Egg phosphatidylcholine Egg lecithin Soy phosphatidylcholine (Epikuron 200, 95% SP) (Lipoid S100) (Lipoid S75, 68% SP) (Lipoid S75, 68% SP) (Phospholipon 90G, 90%)	Poloxamer 188 Poloxamer 207 Poloxamine 908 Polyglycerol methyl glucose distearate Solutol HS15 Span 20, 40, 60 Trehalose Tween 20, 40, 60 Tyloxapol	Sodium cholate Sodium dodecyl sulfate Sodium glycocholate Sodium oleate Sodium taurocholate Sodium taurodeoxycholate	Butanol Butyric acid

One important factor in the choice of a surfactant for lipid nanoparticles should be considered: different surfactants have variable influences on the in vivo biodegradation of the lipid matrix. For instance, non-ionic surfactants are more effective for inhibiting the degradation of lipid matrix in vivo. Finally, the choice of surfactants and co-surfactants also affects the particle size. Lipid nanoparticles made of the same lipids may have different sizes because of the use of different surfactants [190].

The development of lipid nanoparticles for ocular drug delivery has not received as much attention as other administration routes. However, some interesting properties highlighting their potential for ocular administration are their adhesiveness [191] and the longer retention time on the corneal surface and in the cul-de-sac, probably related to their relatively small size [171]. The nanoparticles are presumed to be entrapped and retained in the mucus layer [192].

Table 4. Comparison between SLN/NLC and polymeric nanoparticles
(adapted from Date et al. [193])

	SLN/NLC	Polymeric nanoparticles
Ocular delivery	Possible	Possible
Ability to deliver hydrophobic and hydrophilic drugs	Yes	Yes
Physical stability	+++	+++
Biological stability	++	+++
Biocompatibility	+++	++
Ease of sterilization	++	++
Drug targeting	++	++
Drug loading	Low to moderate (SLN), moderate to high (NLC)	Moderate
Ease of commercialization	++	+
Ability to deliver biotechnological therapeutics	++	++

4. CONCLUSIONS AND FUTURE TRENDS

For the treatment of ocular inflammatory diseases, one should keep in mind that there are not ideal anti-inflammatory agents or administration regimens. As such, the pharmacological treatment should be chosen considering drug mechanism of action, disease specific conditions, possible side effects and the drug ability on reaching the site of infection in therapeutic concentrations. Although microemulsions present excellent advantages over conventional systems, as high drug solubilization, long stability and enhanced corneal penetration, they suffer from limitations in selection of surfactants/co-surfactants due to its potential toxicity. On the contrary, nanoemulsions can be easily prepared with less amount of surfactants, being in this way well tolerated. They can be used to increase pre-corneal residence time as well as penetration of drugs, though its major drawback is the limited ability on sustaining the drug release. Liposomes and SLN could be therefore a suitable alternative. However, the former represents a challenge when considering large scale production, whereas the latter depicts a low drug loading capacity. NLC have emerged as a novel delivery system that could incorporate the advantages of the lipid based delivery systems and overcome their limitations. In the last few years, several NLC formulations have been successfully prepared for the incorporation of anti-inflammatory drugs but have not yet been fully employed in the treatment of ocular diseases. It is expected that in the next years more studies will be performed using lipid based systems for the ocular route, resulting, in this way, in more efficient therapeutic options for the treatment of inflammatory diseases.

REFERENCES

[1]   Ahuja, M.; Dhake, A.; Sharma, S.; Majumdar, D., Topical ocular delivery of NSAIDs. *AAPS J* 2008, 10, (2), 229-241.

[2]   Elhers, W. H.; Donshik, P. C., Giant papillary conjunctivitis. *Curr Opin Allergy Clin Immunol* 2008, 8, (5), 445-9.

[3]   Leonardi, A.; Motterle, L.; Bortolotti, M., Allergy and the eye. *Clin Exp Immunol* 2008, 153 Suppl 1, 17-21.

[4]   Bielory, L.; Friedlaender, M. H., Allergic conjunctivitis. *Immunol Allergy Clin North Am* 2008, 28, (1), 43-58.

[5]   Yeh, S.; Faia, L. J.; Nussenblatt, R. B., Advances in the diagnosis and immunotherapy for ocular inflammatory disease. *Semin Immunopathol* 2008, 30, (2), 145-64.

[6]   Pflugfelder, S. C., Antiinflammatory therapy for dry eye. *Am J Ophthalmol* 2004, 137, (2), 337-42.

[7]   Struck, H. G.; Bariszlovich, A., Comparison of 0.1% dexamethasone phosphate eye gel (Dexagel) and 1% prednisolone acetate eye suspension in the treatment of post-operative inflammation after cataract surgery. *Graefes Archive for Clinical and Experimental Ophthalmology* 2001, 239, (10), 737-742.

[8]   Hoang-Xuan, T.; Hannouche, D., Medical treatment of ocular burns. *Journal Francais D Ophtalmologie* 2004, 27, (10), 1175-1178.

[9]   Pavesio, C. E.; Decory, H. H., Treatment of ocular inflammatory conditions with loteprednol etabonate. *Br J Ophthalmol* 2008, 92, (4), 455-459.

[10] Abad, S.; Seve, P.; Dhote, R.; Brezin, A. P., Guidelines for the management of uveitis in Internal Medicine. *Revue de Medecine Interne* 2009, 30, (6), 492-500.

[11] Messmer, E. M., Therapeutic options in vernal keratoconjunctivitis. *Ophthalmologe* 2009, 106, (6), 557-561.

[12] Group, L. E. U. U. S., Controlled evaluation of loteprednol etabonate and prednisolone acetate in the treatment of acute anterior uveitis. Loteprednol Etabonate US Uveitis Study Group. *Am J Ophthalmol* 1999, 127, (5), 537-544.

[13] Raizman, M., Corticosteroid therapy of eye disease. Fifty years later. *Arch Ophthalmol* 1996, 114, (8), 1000-1001.

[14] McGhee, C. N.; Dean, S.; Danesh-Meyer, H., Locally administered ocular corticosteroids: benefits and risks. *Drug Saf* 2002, 25, (1), 33-55.

[15] Psilas, K.; Kalogeropoulos, C.; Loucatzicos, E.; Asproudis, I.; Petroutsos, G., The Effect of Indomethacin, Diclofenac and Flurbiprofen on the Maintenance of Mydriasis During Extracapsular Cataract-Extraction. *Documenta Ophthalmologica* 1992, 81, (3), 293-300.

[16] Stewart, R.; Grosserode, R.; Cheetham, J. K.; Rosenthal, A., Efficacy and safety profile of ketorolac 0.5% ophthalmic solution in the prevention of surgically induced miosis during cataract surgery. *Clin Ther* 1999, 21, (4), 723-732.

[17] Russo, P.; Papa, V.; Russo, S.; Di Bella, A.; Pabst, G.; Milazzo, G.; Balestrazzi, A.; Caporossi, A., Topical nonsteroidal anti-inflammatory drugs in uncomplicated cataract surgery: Effect of sodium naproxen. *Eur J Ophthalmol* 2005, 15, (5), 598-606.

[18] Swamy, B. N.; Chilov, M.; McClellan, K.; Petsoglou, C., Topical non-steroidal anti-inflammatory drugs in allergic conjunctivitis: Meta-analysis of randomized trial data. *Ophthalmic Epidemiol* 2007, 14, (5), 311-319.

[19] Yavas, G. F.; Ozturk, F.; Kusbeci, T., Preoperative topical indomethacin to prevent pseudophakic cystoid macular edema. *J Cataract Refract Surg* 2007, 33, (5), 804-807.

[20] Warren, K. A.; Fox, J. E., Topical Nepafenac As An Alternate Treatment for Cystoid Macular Edema in Steroid Responsive Patients. *Retina-the Journal of Retinal and Vitreous Diseases* 2008, 28, (10), 1427-1434.

[21] Aslam, S. A.; Sheth, H. G.; Vaughan, A. J., Emergency management of corneal injuries. *Injury-International Journal of the Care of the Injured* 2007, 38, (5), 594-597.

[22] Wilson, S. A.; Last, A., Management of corneal abrasions. *Am Fam Physician* 2004, 70, (1), 123-128.

[23] Sun, R.; Gimbel, H. V., Effects of topical ketorolac and diclofenac on normal corneal sensation. *J Refract Surg* 1997, 13, (2), 158-161.

[24] Shimazaki, J.; Saito, H.; Yang, H. Y.; Toda, I.; Fujishima, H.; Tsubota, K., Persistent epithelial defect following penetrating keratoplasty: an adverse effect of diclofenac eyedrops. *Cornea* 1995, 14, (6), 623-627.

[25] Gills, J. P., Voltaren associated with medication keratitis. *J Cataract Refract Surg* 1994, 20, (1), 110.

[26] Barar, J.; Javadzadeh, A. R.; Omidi, Y., Ocular novel drug delivery: impacts of membranes and barriers. *Expert Opin Drug Deliv* 2008, 5, (5), 567-581.

[27] Schalenbourg, A.; Leys, A.; de, C.; Coutteel, C.; Herbort, C. P., Corticosteroid-induced central serous chorioretinopathy in patients with ocular inflammatory disorders. *Klinische Monatsblatter fur Augenheilkunde* 2002, 219, (4), 264-267.

[28] Cunningham, M. A.; Edelman, J. L.; Kaushal, S., Intravitreal steroids for macular edema: The past, the present, and the future. *Surv Ophthalmol* 2008, 53, (2), 139-149.

[29] Del Amo, E. M.; Urtti, A., Current and future ophthalmic drug delivery systems. A shift to the posterior segment. *Drug Discov Today* 2008, 13, (3-4), 135-143.

[30] Moshfeghi, D. M.; Kaiser, P. K.; Scott, I. U.; Sears, J. E.; Benz, M.; Sinesterra, J. P.; Kaiser, R. S.; Bakri, S. J.; Maturi, R. K.; Belmont, J.; Beer, P. M.; Murray, T. G.; Quiroz-Mercado, H.; Mieler, W. F., Acute endophthalmitis following intravitreal triamcinolone acetonide injection. *Am J Ophthalmol* 2003, 136, (5), 791-796.

[31] Fialho, S. L.; Siqueira, R. C.; Jorge, R.; Silva-Cunha, A., Biodegradable implants for ocular delivery of anti-inflammatory drug. *J Drug Deliv Sci Technol* 2007, 17, (1), 93-97.

[32] Okabe, K.; Kimura, H.; Okabe, J.; Ogura, Y., Ocular tissue distribution of betamethasone after anterior-episcleral, posterior-episcleral, and anterior-intrascleral placement of nonbiodegradable implants. *Retina-the Journal of Retinal and Vitreous Diseases* 2007, 27, (6), 770-777.

[33] Taban, M.; Lowder, C. Y.; Kaiser, P. K., Outcome of Fluocinolone Acetonide Implant (Retisert (Tm)) Reimplantation for Chronic Noninfectious Posterior Uveitis. *Retina-the Journal of Retinal and Vitreous Diseases* 2008, 28, (9), 1280-1288.

[34] Wolf, E. J.; Braunstein, A.; Shih, C.; Braunstein, R. E., Incidence of visually significant pseudophakic macular edema after uneventful phacoemulsification in patients treated with nepafenac. *J Cataract Refract Surg* 2007, 33, (9), 1546-1549.

[35] Labetoulle, M.; Frau, E.; Le Jeunne, C., Systemic adverse effects of topical ocular treatments. *Presse Med* 2005, 34, (8), 589-595.

[36] Schalnus, R., Topical nonsteroidal anti-inflammatory therapy in ophthalmology. *Ophthalmologica* 2003, 217, (2), 89-98.

[37] Awan, M. A.; Agarwal, P. K.; Watson, D. G.; McGhee, C. N. J.; Dutton, G. N., Penetration of topical and subconjunctival corticosteroids into human aqueous humour and its therapeutic significance. *BrJ Ophthalmol* 2009, 93, (6), 708-713.

[38] Anumolu, S. S.; Singh, Y.; Gao, D.; Stein, S.; Sinko, P. J., Design and evaluation of novel fast forming pilocarpine-loaded ocular hydrogels for sustained pharmacological response. *J Control Releaseease* 2009, 137, (2), 152-159.

[39] Bucolo, C.; Spadaro, A., Pharmacological evaluation of anti-inflammatory pyrrole-acetic acid derivative eye drops. *J Ocul Pharmacol Ther* 1997, 13, (4), 353-361.

[40] Adibkia, K.; Shadbad, M. R. S.; Nokhodchi, A.; Javadzedeh, A.; Barzegar-Jalali, M.; Barar, J.; Mohammadi, G.; Omidi, Y., Piroxicam nanoparticles for ocular delivery: Physicochemical characterization and implementation in endotoxin-induced uveitis. *J Drug Target* 2007, 15, (6), 407-416.

[41] Gupta, A. K.; Madan, S.; Majumdar, D. K.; Maitra, A., Ketorolac entrapped in polymeric micelles: preparation, characterisation and ocular anti-inflammatory studies. *Int J Pharm*2000, 209, (1-2), 1-14.

[42] Maxwell, W. A.; Reiser, H. J.; Stewart, R. H.; Cavanagh, H. D.; Walters, T. R.; Sager, D. P.; Meuse, P. A., Nepafenac Dosing Frequency for Ocular Pain and Inflammation Associated with Cataract Surgery. *J Ocul Pharmacol Ther* 2008, 24, (6), 593-599.

[43] Shirasaki, Y., Molecular design for enhancement of ocular penetration. *J Pharm Sci* 2008, 97, (7), 2462-2496.

[44] Unger, W. G., Review: mediation of the ocular response to injury. *J Ocul Pharmacol* 1990, 6, (4), 337-53.

[45] Acosta, M. C.; Luna, C.; Graff, G.; Meseguer, V. M.; Viana, F.; Gallar, J.; Belmonte, C., Comparative effects of the nonsteroidal anti-inflammatory drug nepafenac on corneal sensory nerve fibers responding to chemical irritation. *Invest Ophthalmol Vis Sci* 2007, 48, (1), 182-188.

[46] Stein, R.; Stein, H. A.; Cheskes, A.; Symons, S., Photorefractive keratectomy and postoperative pain. *Am J Ophthalmol* 1994, 117, (3), 403-5.

[47] Heier, J. S.; Topping, T. M.; Baumann, W.; Dirks, M. S.; Chern, S., Ketorolac versus prednisolone versus combination therapy in the treatment of acute pseudophakic cystoid macular edema. *Ophthalmology* 2000, 107, (11), 2034-2038.

[48] Jaanus, S. D.; Lesher, G. A., Anti-inflammatory drugs. In *Clinical ocular pharmacology*, Bartlett J.D., J. S. D., Ed. Butterworth-Heineman: Boston, 1995; pp 303-314.

[49] Campbell, W. B.; Halushka, P. V., Lipid derived autocoids. In *Goodman and Gilman's. The Pharmacological Basis of Therapeutics. 9th ed*, Hardman, J. G. a. L., L.E., Ed. McGraw-Hill: New York, 1990; pp 601-33.

[50] Gaudio, P., A review of evidence guiding the use of corticosteroids in the treatment of intraocular inflammation. *Ocular Immunol Inflamm* 2004, 12, 169-192.

[51] Jaffe, G. J.; Ben-Nun, J.; Guo, H.; Dunn, J. P.; Ashton, P., Fluocinolone acetonide sustained drug delivery device to treat severe uveitis. *Ophthalmology* 2000, 107, (11), 2024-33.

[52] Jaffe, G. J.; Pearson, P. A.; Ashton, P., Dexamethasone sustained drug delivery implant for the treatment of severe uveitis. *Retina* 2000, 20, (4), 402-3.

[53] Samudre, S. S.; Lattanzio, F. A., Jr.; Williams, P. B.; Sheppard, J. D., Jr., Comparison of topical steroids for acute anterior uveitis. *J Ocul Pharmacol Ther* 2004, 20, (6), 533-47.

[54] Recasens, J. F.; Green, K., Effects of endotoxin and anti-inflammatory agents on superoxide dismutase in the rabbit iris. *Ophthalmic Res* 1990, 22, (1), 12-8.

[55] Bron, A.; Denis, P.; T.C., H. X.; P., C.; Hachet, E.; Medhorn, E.; Akingbehin, A., The effects of Rimexolone 1% in postoperative inflammation after cataract extraction. A double-masked placebo-controlled study. *Eur J Ophthalmol* 1998, 8, 16 -21.

[56] Nagelhout, T. J.; Gamache, D. A.; Roberts, L.; Brady, M. T.; Yanni, J. M., Preservation of tear film integrity and inhibition of corneal injury by dexamethasone in a rabbit model of lacrimal gland inflammation-induced dry eye. *J Ocul Pharmacol Ther* 2005, 21, (2), 139-48.

[57] Renfro, L.; Snow, J. S., Ocular effects of topical and systemic steroids. *Dermatol Clin* 1992, 10, (3), 505-12.

[58] O'Brien, T. P., Emerging guidelines for use of NSAID therapy to optimize cataract surgery patient care. *Curr Med Res Opin* 2005, 21, (7), 1131-7.

[59] Reddy, M. S.; Suneetha, N.; Thomas, R. K.; Battu, R. R., Topical diclofenac sodium for treatment of postoperative inflammation in cataract surgery. *Indian J Ophthalmol* 2000, 48, (3), 223-6.

[60] Flach, A. J., Topical nonsteroidal antiinflammatory drugs in ophthalmology. *Int Ophthalmol Clin* 2002, 42, (1), 1-11.

[61] Leonardi, A.; Borghesan, F.; Faggian, D.; Depaoli, M.; Secchi, A. G.; Plebani, M., Tear and serum soluble leukocyte activation markers in conjunctival allergic diseases. *Am J Ophthalmol* 2000, 129, (2), 151-8.

[62] Miyake, K.; Ibaraki, N., Prostaglandins and cystoid macular edema. *Surv Ophthalmol* 2002, 47(Suppl.1), 203-218.

[63] Price, M. O.; Price, F. W., Efficacy of topical ketorolac tromethamine 0.4% for control of pain or discomfort associated with cataract surgery. *Curr Med Res Opin* 2004, 20, (12), 2015-9.

[64] Bandare, B. M.; Sankaridurg, P. R.; Willcox, M. D., Non-steroidal antinflammatory agents decrease bacterial colonization of contact lenses and prevent adhesion to human corneal epithelial cells. *Curr Eye Res* 2004, 29, 245-251.

[65] Walters, T.; Raizman, M.; Ernest, P.; Gayton, J.; Lehmann, R., In vivo pharmacokinetics and in vitro pharmacodynamics of nepafenac, amfenac, ketorolac, and bromfenac. *J Cataract Refract Surg* 2007, 33, (9), 1539-45.

[66] Brauninger, G. E.; Shah, D. O.; Kaufman, H. E., Direct physical demonstration of oily layer on tear film surface. *Am J Ophthalmol* 1972, 73, (1), 132-134.

[67] Malhotra, M.; Majumdar, D. K., In vivo ocular availability of ketorolac following ocular instillations of aqueous, oil, and ointment formulations to normal corneas of rabbits: A technical note. *Aaps Pharmscitech* 2005, 6, (3).

[68] Nanjawade, B. K.; Manvi, F. V.; Manjappa, A. S., In situ.-forming hydrogels for sustained ophthalmic drug delivery. *J Control Release* 2007, 122, (2), 119-134.

[69] Hoar, T. P.; Schulman, J. H., Transparent water-in-oil dispersions the oleopathic hydro-micelle. *Nature* 1943, 152, 102-103.

[70] Lawrence, M. J.; Rees, G. D., Microemulsion-based media as novel drug delivery systems. *Adv Drug Deliv Rev* 2000, 45, (1), 89-121.

[71] Gupta, S.; Moulik, S. P., Biocompatible microemulsions and their prospective uses in drug delivery. *J Pharm Sci* 2008, 97, (1), 22-45.

[72] Alany, R. G.; Rades, T.; Nicoll, J.; Tucker, I. G.; Davies, N. M., W/O microemulsions for ocular delivery: Evaluation of ocular irritation and precorneal retention. *J Control Release* 2006, 111, (1-2), 145-152.

[73] Bonacucina, G.; Cespi, M.; Misici-Falzi, M.; Palmieri, G. F., Colloidal soft matter as drug delivery system. *J Pharm Sci* 2009, 98, (1), 1-42.

[74] Siebenbrodt, I.; Keipert, S., Poloxamer-Systems As Potential Ophthalmics. 2. Microemulsions. *Eur J Pharm Biopharm* 1993, 39, (1), 25-30.

[75] Hasse, A.; Keipert, S., Development and characterization of microemulsions for ocular application. *Eur J Pharm Biopharm* 1997, 43, (2), 179-183.

[76] Fialho, S. L.; Silva-Cunha, A., New vehicle based on a microemulsion for topical ocular administration of dexamethasone. *Clin Experiment Ophthalmol* 2004, 32, (6), 626-632.

[77] Gaudana, R.; Jwala, J.; Boddu, S. H.; Mitra, A. K., Recent perspectives in ocular drug delivery. *Pharm Res* 2009, 26, (5), 1197-1216.

[78] El Aasser, M. S.; Sudol, E. D., Miniemulsions: Overview of research and applications. *Jct Research* 2004, 1, (1), 21-31.

[79] Muchtar, S.; Abdulrazik, M.; FruchtPery, J.; Benita, S., Ex-vivo permeation study of indomethacin from a submicron emulsion through albino rabbit cornea. *J Control Release* 1997, 44, (1), 55-64.

[80] Badawi, A. A.; El-Laithy, H. M.; El Qidra, R. K.; El Mofty, H.; El dally, M., Chitosan based nanocarriers for indomethacin ocular delivery. *Arch Pharm Res* 2008, 31, (8), 1040-9.

[81]   Yamaguchi, M.; Yasueda, S.; Isowaki, A.; Yamamoto, M.; Kimura, M.; Inada, K.; Ohtori, A., Formulation of an ophthalmic lipid emulsion containing an anti-inflammatory steroidal drug, difluprednate. *Int J Pharm* 2005, 301, (1-2), 121-8.

[82]   Tamilvanan, S., Oil-in-water lipid emulsions: implications for parenteral and ocular delivering systems. *Progress in Lipid Research* 2004, 43, (6), 489-533.

[83]   Tamilvanan, S.; Benita, S., The potential of lipid emulsion for ocular delivery of lipophilic drugs. *Eur J Pharm Biopharm* 2004, 58, (2), 357-368.

[84]   Ibrahim, S. S.; Awad, G. A.; Geneidi, A.; Mortada, N. D., Comparative effects of different cosurfactants on sterile prednisolone acetate ocular submicron emulsions stability and release. *Colloids Surf B Biointerfaces* 2009, 69, (2), 225-31.

[85]   Gutierrez, J. M.; Gonzalez, C.; Maestro, A.; Sole, I.; Pey, C. M.; Nolla, J., Nano-emulsions: New applications and optimization of their preparation. *Curr Opin Colloid Interface Sci* 2008, 13, (4), 245-251.

[86]   Solans, C.; Izquierdo, P.; Nolla, J.; Azemar, N.; Garcia-Celma, M. J., Nano-emulsions. *Curr Opin Colloid Interface Sci* 2005, 10, (3-4), 102-110.

[87]   Beilin, M.; Barilan, A.; Amselem, S.; Schwarz, J.; Yogev, A.; Neumann, R., Ocular Retention Time of Submicron Emulsion (Sme) and the Miotic Response to Pilocarpine Delivered in Sme. *Invest Ophthalmol Vis Sci* 1995, 36, (4), S166-S166.

[88]   Mehnert, W.; Mader, K., Solid lipid nanoparticles: production, characterization and applications. *Adv Drug Deliv Rev* 2001, 47, (2-3), 165-196.

[89]   Calvo, P.; Vila-Jato, J. L.; Alonso, M. J., Comparative in vitro evaluation of several colloidal systems, nanoparticles, nanocapsules, and nanoemulsions, as ocular drug carriers. *J Pharm Sci* 1996, 85, (5), 530-6.

[90]   Calvo, P.; Alonso, M. J.; Vila-Jato, J. L.; Robinson, J. R., Improved ocular bioavailability of indomethacin by novel ocular drug carriers. *J Pharm Pharmacol* 1996, 48, (11), 1147-52.

[91]   Gershkovich, P.; Wasan, K. M.; Barta, C. A., A Review of the Application of Lipid-Based Systems in Systemic, Dermal/Transdermal, and Ocular Drug Delivery. *Crit Rev Ther Drug Carrier Syst* 2008, 25, (6), 545-584.

[92]   Rabinovich-Guilatt, L.; Couvreur, P.; Lambert, G.; Dubernet, C., Cationic vectors in ocular drug delivery. *J Drug Target* 2004, 12, (9-10), 623-633.

[93]   Klang, S. H.; Siganos, C. S.; Benita, S.; Frucht-Pery, J., Evaluation of a positively charged submicron emulsion of piroxicam on the rabbit corneum healing process following alkali burn. *J Control Release* 1999, 57, (1), 19-27.

[94]   Klang, S.; Abdulrazik, M.; Benita, S., Influence of emulsion droplet surface charge on indomethacin ocular tissue distribution. *Pharm Dev Technol* 2000, 5, (4), 521-32.

[95]   Yamaguchi, M.; Ueda, K.; Isowaki, A.; Ohtori, A.; Takeuchi, H.; Ohguro, N.; Tojo, K., Mucoadhesive properties of chitosan-coated ophthalmic lipid emulsion containing indomethacin in tear fluid. *Biol Pharm Bull* 2009, 32, (7), 1266-71.

[96]   Meisner, D.; Mezei, M., Liposome Ocular Delivery Systems. *Adv Drug Deliv Rev* 1995, 16, (1), 75-93.

[97]   Bangham, A. D.; Horne, R. W., Negative staining of phospholipids and their structural modification by surface-active agents as observed in the electron microscope. *J Mol Biol* 1964, 8, 660-668.

[98] Ebrahim, S.; Peyman, G. A.; Lee, P. J., Applications of liposomes in ophthalmology. *Surv Ophthalmol* 2005, 50, (2), 167-182.

[99] Mehanna, M. M.; Elmaradny, H. A.; Samaha, M. W., Ciprofloxacin liposomes as vesicular reservoirs for ocular delivery: formulation, optimization, and in vitro characterization. *Drug Dev Ind Pharm* 2009, 35, (5), 583-593.

[100] Bejjani, R. A.; Jeanny, J. C.; Bochot, A.; Behar-Cohen, F., The use of liposomes as intravitreal drug delivery system. *Journal Francais D Ophtalmologie* 2003, 26, (9), 981-985.

[101] Barza, M.; Stuart, M.; Szoka, F., Jr., Effect of size and lipid composition on the pharmacokinetics of intravitreal liposomes. *Invest Ophthalmol Vis Sci* 1987, 28, (5), 893-900.

[102] Liu, K. R.; Peyman, G. A.; Khoobehi, B.; Alkan, H.; Fiscella, R., Intravitreal liposome-encapsulated trifluorothymidine in a rabbit model. *Ophthalmology* 1987, 94, (9), 1155-1159.

[103] Alghadyan, A. A.; Peyman, G. A.; Khoobehi, B.; Milner, S.; Liu, K. R., Liposome-bound cyclosporine: clearance after intravitreal injection. *Int Ophthalmol* 1988, 12, (2), 109-112.

[104] Kawakami, S.; Yamamura, K.; Mukai, T.; Nishida, K.; Nakamura, J.; Sakaeda, T.; Nakashima, M.; Sasaki, H., Sustained ocular delivery of tilisolol to rabbits after topical administration or intravitreal injection of lipophilic prodrug incorporated in liposomes. *J Pharm Pharmacol* 2001, 53, (8), 1157-1161.

[105] Zeng, S.; Hu, C. Z.; Wei, H. R.; Lu, Y. S.; Zhang, Y.; Yang, J. X.; Yun, G. X.; Zou, W. P.; Song, B. P., Intravitreal Pharmacokinetics of Liposome-Encapsulated Amikacin in A Rabbit Model. *Ophthalmology* 1993, 100, (11), 1640-1644.

[106] Wiechens, B.; Grammer, J. B.; Johannsen, U.; Pleyer, U.; Hedderich, J.; Duncker, G. I. W., Experimental intravitreal application of ciprofloxacin in rabbits. *Ophthalmologica* 1999, 213, (2), 120-128.

[107] Wiechens, B.; Krausse, R.; Grammer, J. B.; Neumann, D.; Pleyer, U.; Duncker, G. I. W., Clearance of liposome-incorporated ciprofloxacin after intravitreal injection in rabbit eyes. *Klinische Monatsblatter fur Augenheilkunde* 1998, 213, (5), 284-292.

[108] Wiechens, B.; Neumann, D.; Grammer, J. B.; Pleyer, U.; Hedderich, J.; Duncker, G. I. W., Retinal toxicity of liposome-incorporated and free ofloxacin after intravitreal injection in rabbit eyes. *Int Ophthalmol* 1998, 22, (3), 133-143.

[109] Wiechens, B.; Schutze, D.; Grammer, J. B.; Krause, R.; Pleyer, U.; Duncker, G., Clearance of free and liposome-incorporated Norfloxacin after intravitreal injection. *Invest Ophthalmol Vis Sci* 1999, 40, (4), S87-S87.

[110] Cheng, C. K.; Yang, C. H.; Hsueh, P. R.; Liu, C. M.; Lu, H. Y., Vitrectomy with fluconazole infusion: Retinal toxicity, pharmacokinetics, and efficacy in the treatment of experimental candidal endophthalmitis. *J Ocul Pharmacol Ther* 2004, 20, (5), 430-438.

[111] Taskintuna, I.; Rahhal, F. M.; Arevalo, J. F.; Munguia, D.; Banker, A. S.; DeClercq, E.; Freeman, W. R., Low-dose intravitreal cidofovir (HPMPC) therapy of cytomegalovirus retinitis in patients with acquired immune deficiency syndrome. *Ophthalmology* 1997, 104, (6), 1049-1057.

[112] Cheng, L. Y.; Hostetler, K. Y.; Ozerdem, U.; Gardner, M. F.; Mach-Hofacre, B.; Freman, W. R., Intravitreal toxicology and treatment efficacy of a long acting anti-viral lipid prodrug of ganciclovir (HDP-GCV) in liposome formulation. *Invest Ophthalmol Vis Sci*1999, 40, (4), S872-S872.

[113] Cheng, L. Y.; Hostetler, K. Y.; Toyoguchi, M.; Beadle, J. R.; Rodanant, N.; Gardner, M. F.; Aldern, K. A.; Bergeron-Lynn, G.; Freeman, W. R., Ganciclovir release rates in vitreous from different formulations of 1-O-hexadecylpropanediol-3-phospho-ganciclovir. *J Ocul Pharmacol Ther* 2003, 19, (2), 161-169.

[114] Yasukawa, T.; Kimura, H.; Kunou, N.; Miyamoto, H.; Honda, Y.; Ogura, Y.; Ikada, Y., Biodegradable scleral implant for intravitreal controlled release of ganciclovir. *Graefes Archive for Clinical and Experimental Ophthalmology* 2000, 238, (2), 186-190.

[115] Lallemand, F.; Felt-Baeyens, O.; Besseghir, K.; Behar-Cohen, F.; Gurny, R., Cyclosporine A delivery to the eye: a pharmaceutical challenge. *Eur J Pharm Biopharm* 2003, 56, (3), 307-318.

[116] Kawakami, S.; Harada, A.; Sakanaka, K.; Nishida, K.; Nakamura, J.; Sakaeda, T.; Ichikawa, N.; Nakashima, M.; Sasaki, H., In vivo gene transfection via intravitreal injection of cationic liposome/plasmid DNA complexes in rabbits. *Int J Pharm* 2004, 278, (2), 255-262.

[117] Peeters, L.; Sanders, N. N.; Jones, A.; Demeester, J.; De Smedt, S. C., Post-pegylated lipoplexes are promising vehicles for gene delivery in RPE cells. *J Control Release* 2007, 121, (3), 208-217.

[118] Arakawa, Y.; Hashida, N.; Ohguro, N.; Yamazaki, N.; Onda, M.; Matsumoto, S.; Ohishi, M.; Yamabe, K.; Tano, Y.; Kurokawa, N., Eye-concentrated distribution of dexamethasone carried by sugar-chain modified liposome in experimental autoimmune uveoretinitis mice. *Biomedical Research-Tokyo* 2007, 28, (6), 331-334.

[119] Schaeffer, H. E.; Breitfeller, J. M.; Krohn, D. L., Lectin-Mediated Attachment of Liposomes to Cornea - Influence on Trans-Corneal Drug Flux. *Invest Ophthalmol Vis Sci* 1982, 23, (4), 530-533.

[120] McCalden, T. A.; Levy, M., Retention of Topical Liposomal Formulations on the Cornea. *Experientia* 1990, 46, (7), 713-715.

[121] Monem, A. S.; Ali, F. M.; Ismail, M. W., Prolonged effect of liposomes encapsulating pilocarpine HCl in normal and glaucomatous rabbits. *Int J Pharm* 2000, 198, (1), 29-38.

[122] Mainardes, R. M.; Urban, M. C. C.; Cinto, P. O.; Khalil, N. M.; Chaud, M. V.; Evangelista, R. C.; Gremiao, M. P. D., Colloidal carriers for ophthalmic drug delivery. *Curr Drug Targets* 2005, 6, (3), 363-371.

[123] Singh, K.; Mezei, M., Liposomal Ophthalmic Drug Delivery System. 1. Triamcinolone Acetonide. *Int J Pharm*1983, 16, (3), 339-344.

[124] Taniguchi, K.; Itakura, K.; Yamazawa, N.; Morisaki, K.; Hayashi, S.; Yamada, Y., Efficacy of a liposome preparation of anti-inflammatory steroid as an ocular drug-delivery system. *J Pharmacobiodyn* 1988, 11, (1), 39-46.

[125] Al-Muhammad, J.; Ozer, A. Y.; Hincal, A. A., Studies on the formulation and in vitro release of ophthalmic liposomes containing dexamethasone sodium phosphate. *J Microencapsul* 1996, 13, (2), 123-30.

[126] Al-Muhammed, J.; Ozer, A. Y.; Ercan, M. T.; Hincal, A. A., In-vivo studies on dexamethasone sodium phosphate liposomes. *J Microencapsul* 1996, 13, (3), 293-306.

[127] Sun, K. X.; Wang, A. P.; Huang, L. J.; Liang, R. C.; Liu, K., [Preparation of diclofenac sodium liposomes and its ocular pharmacokinetics]. *Yao Xue Xue Bao* 2006, 41, (11), 1094-8.

[128] Li, N.; Zhuang, C.; Wang, M.; Sun, X.; Nie, S.; Pan, W., Liposome coated with low molecular weight chitosan and its potential use in ocular drug delivery. *Int J Pharm* 2009, 379, (1), 131-8.

[129] Sahoo, S. K.; Diinawaz, F.; Krishnakumar, S., Nanotechnology in ocular drug delivery. *Drug Discovery Today* 2008, 13, (3-4), 144-151.

[130] Nasr, M.; Mansour, S.; Mortada, N. D.; Elshamy, A. A., Vesicular aceclofenac systems: A comparative study between liposomes and niosomes. *J Microencapsul* 2008, 25, (7), 499-512.

[131] Sammour, O. A.; Al Zuhair, H. H.; El Sayed, M. I., Inhibitory effect of liposome-encapsulated piroxicam on inflammation and gastric mucosal damage. *Pharmazeutische Industrie* 1998, 60, (12), 1084-1087.

[132] Trif, M.; Moisei, M.; Roseanu, A., Designing of efficient lipidic nanostructures for the therapy of the inflammatory diseases. *Romanian Journal of Information Science and Technology* 2007, 10, (1), 85-95.

[133] Hagiwara, Y.; Arima, H.; Miyamoto, Y.; Hirayama, F.; Uekama, K., Preparation and pharmaceutical evaluation of liposomes entrapping salicylic acid/gamma-cyclodextrin conjugate. *Chemical & Pharmaceutical Bulletin* 2006, 54, (1), 26-32.

[134] Katare, O. P.; Vyas, S. P.; Dixit, V. K., Enhanced In-Vivo Performance of Liposomal Indomethacin Derived from Effervescent Granule Based Proliposomes. *J Microencapsul* 1995, 12, (5), 487-493.

[135] Bula, D.; Ghaly, E. S., Liposome Delivery Systems Containing Ibuprofen. *Drug Dev Ind Pharm*1995, 21, (14), 1621-1629.

[136] Wang, T.; Deng, Y. J.; Geng, Y. H.; Gao, Z. B.; Zou, H. P.; Wang, Z. Z., Preparation of submicron unilamellar liposomes by freeze-drying double emulsions. *Biochimica et Biophysica Acta-Biomembranes* 2006, 1758, (2), 222-231.

[137] Maestrelli, F.; Gonzalez-Rodriguez, M. L.; Rabasco, A. M.; Mura, P., Effect of preparation technique on the properties of liposomes encapsulating ketoprofen-cyclodextrin complexes aimed for transdermal delivery. *Int J Pharm* 2006, 312, (1-2), 53-60.

[138] Li, J.; Yang, J.; Wang, W. X.; Yu, J. C.; Fu, J. G.; Wang, X. L., A Novel Liposomal Dexamethasone Palmitate Formulation and Anti-inflammatory Effects on Mice. *Chinese Journal of Chemistry* 2009, 27, (7), 1411-1414.

[139] Korting, H. C.; Zienicke, H.; Schaferkorting, M.; Braunfalco, O., Liposome Encapsulation Improves Efficacy of Betamethasone Dipropionate in Atopic Eczema But Not in Psoriasis-Vulgaris. *Eur J Clin Pharmacol* 1990, 39, (4), 349-351.

[140] Piel, G.; Piette, M.; Barillaro, V.; Castagne, D.; Evrard, B.; Delattre, L., Betamethasone-in-cyclodextrin-in-liposome: The effect of cyclodextrins on encapsulation efficiency and release kinetics. *Int J Pharm* 2006, 312, (1-2), 75-82.

[141] Nii, T.; Ishii, F., Encapsulation efficiency of water-soluble and insoluble drugs in liposomes prepared by the microencapsulation vesicle method. *Int J Pharm* 2005, 298, (1), 198-205.

[142] Martins, S.; Sarmento, B.; Ferreira, D. C.; Souto, E. B., Lipid-based colloidal carriers for peptide and protein delivery--liposomes versus lipid nanoparticles. *Int J Nanomedicine* 2007, 2, (4), 595-607.

[143] Wissing, S. A.; Kayser, O.; Muller, R. H., Solid lipid nanoparticles for parenteral drug delivery. *Adv Drug Deliv Rev* 2004, 56, (9), 1257-1272.

[144] Muller, R. H.; Radtke, M.; Wissing, S. A., Solid lipid nanoparticles (SLN) and nanostructured lipid carriers (NLC) in cosmetic and dermatological preparations. *Adv Drug Deliv Rev* 2002, 54, S131-S155.

[145] Pietkiewicz, J.; Sznitowska, M.; Placzek, M., The expulsion of lipophilic drugs from the cores of solid lipid microspheres in diluted suspensions and in concentrates. *Int J Pharm* 2006, 310, (1-2), 64-71.

[146] Westesen, K.; Bunjes, H.; Koch, M. II. J., Physicochemical characterization of lipid nanoparticles and evaluation of their drug loading capacity and sustained release potential. *J Control Release* 1997, 48, (2-3), 223-236.

[147] Bunjes, H.; Westesen, K.; Koch, M. H. J., Crystallization tendency and polymorphic transitions in triglyceride nanoparticles. *Int J Pharm* 1996, 129, (1-2), 159-173.

[148] Muller, R. H.; Radtke, M.; Wissing, S. A., Nanostructured lipid matrices for improved microencapsulation of drugs. *Int J Pharm* 2002, 242, (1-2), 121-128.

[149] Muller, R. H.; Mader, K.; Gohla, S., Solid lipid nanoparticles (SLN) for controlled drug delivery - a review of the state of the art. *Eur J Pharm Biopharm* 2000, 50, (1), 161-177.

[150] Muller, R. H.; Mehnert, W.; Lucks, J. S.; Schwarz, C.; Zurmuhlen, A.; Weyhers, H.; Freitas, C.; Ruhl, D., Solid Lipid Nanoparticles (Sln) - An Alternative Colloidal Carrier System for Controlled Drug-Delivery. *Eur J Pharm Biopharm*1995, 41, (1), 62-69.

[151] Souto, E. B.; Müller, R. H., Lipid nanoparticles (solid lipid nanoparticles and nanostructured lipid carriers) for cosmetic, dermal and transdermal applications. In *Nanoparticulate Drug DelivSystems: Recent Trends and Emerging Technologies*, Thassu, D., Deleers, M., Pathak, Y. (Eds.), CRC Press, Chapter 14, Ed. 2007; pp 213-233.

[152] Souto, E. B.; Müller, R. H., Lipid nanoparticles (SLN and NLC) for drug delivery. In *Nanoparticles for Pharmaceutical Applications*, Domb, A.J., Tabata, Y., Ravi Kumar, M.N.V., Farber, S. (Eds.), American Scientific Publishers, Chapter 5: 2007; pp 103-122.

[153] Cavalli, R.; Bocca, C.; Miglietta, A.; Caputo, O.; Gasco, M. R., Albumin adsorption on stealth and non-stealth solid lipid nanoparticles. *Stp Pharma Sciences* 1999, 9, (2), 183-189.

[154] Bhaskar, K.; Anbu, J.; Ravichandiran, V.; Venkateswarlu, V.; Rao, Y. M., Lipid nanoparticles for transdermal delivery of flurbiprofen: formulation, in vitro, ex vivo and in vivo studies. *Lipids in Health and Disease* 2009, 8.

[155] Han, F.; Li, S.; Yin, R.; Shi, X.; Jia, Q., Investigation of nanostructured lipid carriers for transdermal delivery of flurbiprofen. *Drug Dev Ind Pharm* 2008, 34, (4), 453-458.

[156] Jain, S. K.; Chourasia, M. K.; Masuriha, R.; Soni, V.; Jain, A.; Jain, N. K.; Gupta, Y., Solid lipid nanoparticles bearing flurbiprofen for transdermal delivery. *Drug Deliv* 2005, 12, (4), 207-215.

[157] Castelli, F.; Puglia, C.; Sarpietro, M. G.; Rizza, L.; Bonina, F., Characterization of indomethacin-loaded lipid nanoparticles by differential scanning calorimetry. *Int J Pharm* 2005, 304, (1-2), 231-238.

[158] Chattopadhyay, P.; Shekunov, B. Y.; Yim, D.; Cipolla, D.; Boyd, B.; Farr, S., Production of solid lipid nanoparticle suspensions using supercritical fluid extraction of emulsions (SFEE) for pulmonary delivery using the AERx system. *Adv Drug Deliv Rev* 2007, 59, (6), 444-453.

[159] Ricci, M.; Puglia, C.; Bonina, F.; Di Giovanni, C.; Giovagnoli, S.; Rossi, C., Evaluation of indomethacin percutaneous absorption from nanostructured lipid carriers (NLC): In vitro and in vivo studies. *J Pharm Sci* 2005, 94, (5), 1149-1159.

[160] Puglia, C.; Blasi, P.; Rizza, L.; Schoubben, A.; Bonina, F.; Rossi, C.; Ricci, M., Lipid nanoparticles for prolonged topical delivery: An in vitro and in vivo investigation. *Int J Pharm* 2008, 357, (1-2), 295-304.

[161] Puglia, C.; Filosa, R.; Peduto, A.; de Caprariis, P.; Rizza, L.; Bonina, F.; Blasi, P., Evaluation of alternative strategies to optimize ketorolac transdermal delivery. *Aaps Pharmscitech* 2006, 7, (3).

[162] Joshi, M.; Patravale, V., Formulation and evaluation of nanostructured lipid carrier (NLC)-based gel of Valdecoxib. *Drug Dev Ind Pharm* 2006, 32, (8), 911-918.

[163] Attama, A. A.; Weber, C.; Muller-Goymann, C. C., Assessment of drug permeation from lipid nanoparticles formulated with a novel structured lipid matrix through artificial skin construct bio-engineered from HDF and HaCaT cell lines. *J Drug Deliv Sci Technol* 2008, 18, (3), 181-188.

[164] Xiang, Q. Y.; Wang, M. T.; Chen, F.; Gong, T.; Jian, Y. L.; Zhang, Z. R.; Huang, Y., Lung-targeting delivery of dexamethasone acetate loaded solid lipid nanoparticles. *Arch Pharm Res* 2007, 30, (4), 519-525.

[165] Cavalli, R.; Peira, E.; Caputo, O.; Gasco, M. R., Solid lipid nanoparticles as carriers of hydrocortisone and progesterone complexes with beta-cyclodextrins. *Int J Pharm* 1999, 182, (1), 59-69.

[166] Sivaramakrishnan, R.; Nakamura, C.; Mehnert, W.; Korting, H. C.; Kramer, K. D.; Schafer-Korting, M., Glucocorticoid entrapment into lipid carriers - characterisation by parelectric spectroscopy and influence on dermal uptake. *J Control Release* 2004, 97, (3), 493-502.

[167] Liu, W.; Hu, M. L.; Liu, W. S.; Xue, C. B.; Xu, H. B.; Yang, X. L., Investigation of the carbopol gel of solid lipid nanoparticles for the transdermal iontophoretic delivery of triamcinolone acetonide acetate. *Int J Pharm* 2008, 364, (1), 135-141.

[168] Schafer-Korting, M.; Mehnert, W. G.; Korting, H. C., Lipid nanoparticles for improved topical application of drugs for skin diseases. *Adv Drug Deliv Rev* 2007, 59, (6), 427-443.

[169] Paliwal, R.; Rai, S.; Vaidya, B.; Khatri, K.; Goyal, A. K.; Mishra, N.; Mehta, A.; Vyas, S. P., Effect of lipid core material on characteristics of solid lipid nanoparticles designed for oral lymphatic delivery. *Nanomedicine* 2009, 5, (2), 184-191.

[170] Ruckmani, K.; Sivakumar, M.; Ganeshkumar, P. A., Methotrexate loaded solid lipid nanoparticles (SLN) for effective treatment of carcinoma. *J Nanosci Nanotechnol* 2006, 6, (9-10), 2991-2995.

[171] Cavalli, R.; Gasco, M. R.; Chetoni, P.; Burgalassi, S.; Saettone, M. F., Solid lipid nanoparticles (SLN) as ocular delivery system for tobramycin. *Int J Pharm* 2002, 238, (1-2), 241-5.

[172] Kalam, M. A.; Sultana, Y.; Ali, A.; Aqil, M., Gatifloxacin-loaded solid lipid nanoparticles for topical ocular delivery. *J Pharm Pharmacol* 2009, 61, A75-A75.

[173] Niu, M.; Shi, K.; Sun, Y.; Wang, J.; Cui, F., Preparation of CyA-loaded solid lipid nanoparticles and application on ocular preparations. *J Drug Deliv Sci Technol* 2008, 18, (4), 293-297.

[174] Attama, A. A.; Reichl, S.; Muller-Goymann, C. C., Sustained Release and Permeation of Timolol from Surface-Modified Solid Lipid Nanoparticles through Bioengineered Human Cornea. *Curr Eye Res* 2009, 34, (8), 698-705.

[175] Del Pozo-Rodriguez, A.; Delgado, D.; Solinis, M. A.; Gascon, A. R.; Pedraz, J. L., Solid lipid nanoparticles: formulation factors affecting cell transfection capacity. *Int J Pharm* 2007, 339, (1-2), 261-268.

[176] Friedrich, I.; Reichl, S.; Muller-Goymann, C. C., Drug release and permeation studies of nanosuspensions based on solidified reverse micellar solutions (SRMS). *Int J Pharm* 2005, 305, (1-2), 167-75.

[177] Attama, A. A.; Reichl, S.; Muller-Goymann, C. C., Diclofenac sodium delivery to the eye: in vitro evaluation of novel solid lipid nanoparticle formulation using human cornea construct. *Int J Pharm* 2008, 355, (1-2), 307-13.

[178] Zhang, L. J.; Liu, L.; Qian, Y.; Chen, Y., The effects of cryoprotectants on the freeze-drying of ibuprofen-loaded solid lipid microparticles (SLM). *Eur J Pharm Biopharm* 2008, 69, (2), 750-759.

[179] Park, E. S.; Chang, S. Y.; Hahn, M.; Chi, S. C., Enhancing effect of polyoxyethylene alkyl ethers on the skin permeation of ibuprofen. *Int J Pharm* 2000, 209, (1-2), 109-119.

[180] Casadei, M. A.; Cerreto, F.; Cesa, S.; Giannuzzo, M.; Feeney, M.; Marianecci, C.; Paolicelli, P., Solid lipid nanoparticles incorporated in dextran hydrogels: A new drug delivery system for oral formulations. *Int J Pharm* 2006, 325, (1-2), 140-146.

[181] Long, C. X.; Zhang, L. J.; Qian, Y., Preparation and crystal modification of ibuprofen-loaded solid lipid microparticles. *Chinese Journal of Chemical Engineering* 2006, 14, (4), 518-525.

[182] Pang, X. J.; Zhou, J.; Chen, J. J.; Yu, M. H.; Cui, F. D.; Zhou, W. L., Synthesis of ibuprofen loaded magnetic solid lipid nanoparticles. *Ieee Transactions on Magnetics* 2007, 43, (6), 2415-2417.

[183] Paolicelli, P.; Cerreto, F.; Cesa, S.; Feeney, M.; Corrente, F.; Marianecci, C.; Casadei, M. A., Influence of the formulation components on the properties of the system SLN-dextran hydrogel for the modified release of drugs. *J Microencapsul* 2009, 26, (4), 355-364.

[184] Silva, A. C.; Santos, D.; Ferreira, D. C.; Souto, E. B., Oral delivery of drugs by means of solid lipid nanoparticles. *Minerva Biotecnologica* 2007, 19, (1), 1-5.

[185] Li, X.; Nie, S. F.; Kong, J.; Li, N.; Ju, C. Y.; Pan, W. S., A controlled-release ocular delivery system for ibuprofen based on nanostructured lipid carriers. *Int J Pharm* 2008, 363, (1-2), 177-182.

[186] Barbault-Foucher, S.; Gref, R.; Russo, P.; Guechot, J.; Bochot, A., Design of poly-epsilon-caprolactone nanospheres coated with bioadhesive hyaluronic acid for ocular delivery. *J Control Release* 2002, 83, (3), 365-375.

[187] Calvo, P.; RemunanLopez, C.; VilaJato, J. L.; Alonso, M. J., Development of positively charged colloidal drug carriers: Chitosan coated polyester nanocapsules and submicron-emulsions. *Colloid and Polymer Science* 1997, 275, (1), 46-53.

[188] Shen, J.; Wang, Y.; Ping, Q. N.; Xiao, Y. Y.; Huang, X., Mucoadhesive effect of thiolated PEG stearate and its modified NLC for ocular drug delivery. *J Control Release* 2009, 137, (3-4), 217-223.

[189] Gasco, M. R.; Gallarate, M.; Trotta, M.; Bauchiero, L.; Gremmo, E.; Chiappero, O., Microemulsions as topical delivery vehicles: ocular administration of timolol. *J Pharm Biomed Anal* 1989, 7, (4), 433-9.

[190] Wong, H. L.; Li, Y.-Q.; Bendayan, R.; Rauth, M. A.; Wu, X. Y., Solid Lipid Nanoparticles for Antitumor Drug Delivery. In *Nanotechnology for Cancer Therapy*, Mansoor M. Amiji (Ed.), CRC Press, Chapter 36, 741-776: 2007.

[191] Müller-Goymann, C. C., Physicochemical characterization of colloidal drug delivery systems such as reverse micelles, vesicles, liquid crystals and nanoparticles for topical administration. *Eur J Pharm Biopharm* 2004, 58, (2), 343-356.

[192] Ludwig, A., Ocular Applications of Nanoparticulate Drug-Delivery Systems. In *Nanoparticulate Drug DelivSystems: Recent Trends and Emerging Technologies*, Thassu, D., Deleers, M., Pathak, Y., Ed. CRC Press: 2007; pp 271-280.

[193] Date, A. A.; Joshi, M. D.; Patravale, V. B., Parasitic diseases: Liposomes and polymeric nanoparticles versus lipid nanoparticles. *Adv Drug Deliv Rev* 2007, 59, (6), 505-521.

[194] Siqueira, R. C.; Filho, E. R.; Fialho, S. L.; Lucena, L. R.; Filho, A. M.; Haddad, A.; Jorge, R.; Scott, I. U.; Cunha Ada, S., Pharmacokinetic and toxicity investigations of a new intraocular lens with a dexamethasone drug delivery system: a pilot study. *Ophthalmologica* 2006, 220, (5), 338-42.

[195] Farshi, F. S.; Ozer, A. Y.; Ercan, M. T.; Hincal, A. A., In-vivo studies in the treatment of oral ulcers with liposomal dexamethasone sodium phosphate. *J Microencapsul* 1996, 13, (5), 537-44.

In: Conjunctivitis: Symptoms, Treatment and Prevention   ISBN: 978-1-61668-321-4
Editor: Anna R. Sallinger, pp. 141-160   © 2010 Nova Science Publishers, Inc.

Chapter IV

ALLERGIC CONTACT CONJUNCTIVITIS CAUSED BY OPHTHALMIC PREPARATIONS

Giuseppe Mancuso

Department of Dermatology, Municipal Hospital of Lugo, Ravenna, Italy.

ABSTRACT

Both preservatives and active ingredients of ophthalmic preparations may produce allergic contact conjunctivitis. The number of potential ophthalmic allergens is destined to increase. According to a recent review of the literature, an additional 15 allergenic ingredients were reported between 1997 and 2007.

Preservatives, such as benzalkonium chloride, chlorhexidine and thimerosal, are well-known, frequent sensitizers in eyedrops and in contact lens solutions. Other less frequently reported allergenic ophthalmic preservatives include disodium EDTA, polyquaternium 1, phenylmercuric nitrate, chlorobutanol, parabens, and sorbic acid. Preservative-free monodose containers are now available for the most important ophthalmic preparations.

Active ingredients of the ophthalmic products that may produce contact sensitization include beta- blockers, mydriatics, antibiotics, antiviral drugs, antihistamines, anti-inflammatory drugs, corticosteroids and anesthetics.

Symptoms may be limited to the conjunctiva or may more frequently also involve the periocular skin and the eyelids. Ophthalmologic examination reveals pronounced vasodilation and chemosis of the conjunctiva. Lacrimation and papillary reaction can be present. Corneal involvement is usually limited to punctuate epithelial keratitis. Eyelid dermatitis is not a constant finding.

Allergic contact conjunctivitis may be caused by type IV allergy, although type I allergy, other hypersensitivity mechanisms, or irritation cannot be excluded. Conventional patch testing is sometimes a poor detector of contact allergy from ophthalmic preparations. Some authors have suggested that patch tests should be performed on stripped or scarified skin, or after pricking the skin, and by intradermal testing. Pre-treatment with sodium lauryl sulphate has recently been found to be another effective method of patch testing. The diagnosis of allergic contact conjunctivitis may be confirmed by a conjunctival challenge test with the ophthalmic preparation believed to be responsible for the allergy.

If correctly diagnosed and managed, allergic contact conjunctivitis has a good prognosis as it clears spontaneously when use of the offending allergen is discontinued, without the need in many cases of any other therapy.

INTRODUCTION

Ophthalmic preparations contain a wide range of potential allergens including preservatives, active pharmaceutical ingredients and additives [1-3]. Their number is destined to increase. According to a recent review of the literature, an additional 15 new allergens were reported between 1997 and 2007 [4]. They usually cause delayed contact allergy type IV that is mediated by cellular immunity, but immediate type I reactions (mainly IgE-mediated) are also possible. Initial sensitization requires at least 5 days and can take months or years of exposure to the chemical. In sensitized patients the contact reaction appears within 12-72 hours after the re-exposure to the allergen in delayed hypersensitivity and within seconds or minutes in immediate hypersensitivity. The same ophthalmic component may elicit allergic, irritant or sub-clinical toxic reactions on the conjunctiva, these adverse effects sometimes being present simultaneously [5-7].

ALLERGENIC OPHTHALMIC PRESERVATIVES

Preservatives play a fundamental role in suppressing microbial growth and preventing decomposition of the active drug in multidose ophthalmic preparations [5]. The preservatives, especially thimerosal, are a prominent source of allergic reactions for the ocular surface [2] (Table 1).

Thimerosal (merthiolate) is a mercuy-based oxidative compound that was widely used as a preservative in vaccines, immunoglobulins, intracutaneous test solutions and ophthalmic preparations. It has been reported as one of the most common contact allergens in the general population. Positive patch test reactions to this preservative are frequent, the prevalence varying from 1.3% to 26% depending on the country [8-12]. In many cases a positive patch test to thimerosal should be considered an accidental finding without relevance to current dermatitis [13].

Among the ocular side effects of thimerosal contained in eye drops and in contact lens solutions, redness and irritation were the main clinical manifestations. The delayed allergic reaction to thimerosal-containing eye drops may produce a combination of conjunctivitis and eyelid dermatitis (ACDC or allergic contact dermatoconjunctivitis) [14] or conjunctivitis without eyelid involvement (ACC or allergic contact conjunctivitis) [13]. ACC alone has been described in soft contact lens wearers who were sensitized to thimerosal contained in contact lens solutions [15,16]. In soft contact lens wearers, contact allergy to thimerosal-containing lens solutions induced an ocular inflammatory process and, if not treated, corneal neovascularization [17]. Because of its allergic and toxic effects, in 1998 the FDA banned thimerosal in topical over-the-counter medicaments, including ophthalmic preparations. In Italy thimerosal is still present in some eye drops that can be purchased without a prescription.

Table 1. Chemicals inducing ocular contact allergy in ophthalmic preparations

Group	Substance	References	Group	Substance	References
Preservatives	Thimerosal	[8-17]	**NSAIDs**	Diclofenac	[75,76]
	Phenylmercuric			Ketorolac	[77.78]
	nitr.	[2]			
	Benzalkonium	[18-24]	**Antiviral drugs**	Beta-interferon	[80]
	chl.	[27]		Vidarabine	[81,82]
	Polyquaternium 1	[28]		Idoxuridine	[83-85]
	Chlorobutanol	[29,30]		Trifluoridine	[86,87]
	Parabens	[13,16]		Acyclovir	[87]
	Chlorhexidine	[31]			
	Sorbic acid	[3]	**Antihistamines**	Chlorpheniramine	[88]
	Disodium EDTA			Pheniramine	[89]
				Ketotifen fumarate	[90]
				Cromoglycate	[91.92]
				Amlexanox	[93,94]
				NAAGA	[95]
Beta-blockers	Timolol	[33-35]	**Antibiotics**		
	Levobunolol	[36-40]			
	Befunolol	[41,42]			
	Metipranolol	[43]			
	Carteolol	[44,45]			
	Betaxolol	[46]			
Carbonic anhidrase inhibitor	Dorzolamide	[54-56]			
Prostaglandin analogs	Latanoprost	[57]	**Anestetics**	Benzocaine	[2]
	Bimatoprost	[58]		Procaine	[2]
				Tetracaine	[2,102]
				Propracaine	[101,102]
				Oxybuprocaine	[103]
			Corticosteroids	Dexamethasone	[104]
				Betamethasone	[105]
				Hydrocortisone	[105]
				Prednisolone	[106]
Alfa 2 adrenergic agents	Apraclonidine	[59,60]			
	Brimonidine	[61,62]	**Miscellaneous**	Pilocarpine	[107]
				Bismuth	[108]
				N-acetylcysteine	[109]
Mydriatics and cycloplegics	Phenylephrine	[63-67]		Epsilon-	
	Atropine	[68,69]		aminocaproic acid	[110]
	Cyclopentolate	[70]		Rubidium iodide	[111]
	Dipivefrine	[71,72]		D-penicillamine	[112]
	Tropicamide	[73]		Pirfenexone	[113]
				Trometamol	[114]
				Tegobetaine L7	[115]

Benzalkonium chloride (BAK) is a quaternary ammonium cationic detergent compound with bacteriostatic and bactericide activity. It is present in over 70% of commercially produced eye drops and is the most common preservative used in ophthalmic preparations [13]. BAK is a well-known irritant; a 0.5% aqueous solution gives a mild to moderate irritant reaction in 29% of patch-tested patients [18]. As a preservative for eye drops it is usually well tolerated up to concentrations of 0.02% but is usually used at 0.01%. It is important to stress that BAK is a safe and effective preservative for short-term use in low concentrations; it is its long term use that can no longer be recommended because of toxic sub-clinical corneal and conjunctival changes [5-7]. The recommended patch test concentration for BAK is 0.1% petrolatum or 0.1-0.01% aqueous [13,19]. It has been classified as a weak sensitizer in animal experiments and is not a significant allergen in the average population [20-22]. However, allergy to BAK occurs relatively often in medical professionals and in ophthalmological patients [21-23]. Generalized reactions from systemic administration of chemically-related drugs such as antihypertensives (tetraethylammonium chloride), neuromuscular blockers (deccamethonium bromide) and heparin antagonists (hexadimethrine bromide) have occurred in topically sensitized individuals [24].

Chlorhexidine is a synthetic cationic bis-biguanide antiseptic and disinfectant with antibacterial activity against gram-positive and gram-negative bacteria. It has been reported to induce ACC by its presence as a preservative in contact lens solutions(13,16). Chlorexidine can also induce contact urticarial reactions and anaphylaxis due to type 1 hypersensitivity mechanism [25,26]. Chlorhexidine 0.5% in petrolatum can be used for patch testing.

Other less frequently reported allergenic ophthalmic preservatives include *disodium EDTA*(3), *polyquaternium 1* [27], *phenylmercuric nitrate* [2], *chlorobutanol* [28], *parabens* [29,30], and *sorbic acid* [31]. Sorbic acid has been reported to cause nonimmunologic contact urticaria [31].

In recent years new preservatives have been introduced in ophthalmic preparations, such as stabilized oxychloro complex, the preservative system sofZia, and an oxidative preservative composed of sodium perborate [2,32]. These preservatives have been shown to induce less adverse allergic and toxic effects on the ocular surface compared with more conventional preservatives. Moreover, monodose preservative-free ophthalmic preparations are now available for the most important active ingredients.

ALLERGENIC OPHTHALMIC ACTIVE INGREDIENTS

In addition to preservatives, many active ingredients used in ophthalmic medications may cause sensitization; these include β-blockers, mydriatics, non-steroid anti-inflammatory drugs, antiviral drugs, antihistamines, antibiotics, anesthetics and corticosteroids (Table 1).

Topical *beta-blockers* are widely used in open-angle glaucoma to lower intraocular pressure. Irritant ocular side-effects induced by topical beta-blockers are known and include irritation on instillation, follicular conjunctivitis, dry eye and blurred vision. Though widely prescribed, there are few reports of allergic contact conjunctivitis from beta-blockers. Sensitization may be to a single agent such as timolol [33-35], levobunolol [36-40], befunolol

[41,42], metipranolol [43], carteolol [44,45] and betaxolol [46] or, more rarely, to multiple beta-blockers in a single patient [47-53]. Cross-reactivity among beta-blockers, documented by positive patch tests to other beta-blockers never previously used by the patient, has been described [47-51]. The proposed hypothesis is a cross-reactivity due to the common lateral aliphatic chain, that conditions affinity to the receptor [50]. Giordano-Labadie described a patient who developed, one after another, contact allergy to three beta-blockers including timolol, befunolol and carteolol applied consecutively. According to the author, the similar chemical structure of the beta-blockers cannot be considered as a hapten, the cross-reactivity developing only after metabolism of these drugs to a common aldehyde [51]. In some cases, the reactions to other beta-blockers was found to be multiple concomitant sensitizations rather than cross-reactivity [52,53]. Systemic reactions to the topically applied beta-blockers included exacerbation of asthma, hypotension, bradycardia and congestive heart failure. The risk of side effects in topically sensitized patients when taking oral beta-blockers is unknown [51].

Dorzolamide hydrochloride is a *carbonic anhydrase inhibitor* used for long-term glaucoma therapy. It is a sulfonamide. Though widely prescribed, there have been few cases reported of documented contact allergy [54-56]. In **Shimada's** patient, the patch tests to dorzolamide (5% aqueous solution and 5% in petrolatum) were positive only on tape-stripped skin [55].

Prostaglandin analogs are potent highly effective first-line or adjunctive agents used to treat glaucoma. Latanoprost, a prostaglandin analog that is widely prescribed for the treatment of glaucoma, has been recently reported to cause ACDC [57]. Side effects other than ACDC include conjunctival hyperemia, increased iris pigmentation, and thickening, darkening, lengthening and increased density of lashes and hair in or around the eye being treated [57]. Bimatoprost is a new prostaglandin analog, similar to latanoprost. The drug has been reported to cause documented ACDC with increased pigmentation of the periocular skin [58].

Alfa 2-adrenergic agents are drugs utilized to treat glaucoma in patients who are intolerant to beta-blockers [1] or other antiglaucoma drugs, in cases of uncontrolled pressure despite traditional therapy and when there is a need to postpone glaucoma surgery. They include apraclonidine and brimonidine. Apraclonidine has been reported to cause ACDC in two cases with documented allergy by a 0.5% petrolatum patch test in one [59]. In a retrospective analysis of 64 patients receiving long- term 1% apraclonidine therapy, Butler reported a high incidence of adverse local reactions as 31 patients (48%) were not able to continue the therapy owing to intolerable local side effects. The author believes that these reactions were mainly allergic and not toxic. The presumed allergic reactions were not documented by patch test [60].

Brimonidine also induces ocular contact allergy. Becker reported 4 cases of anterior uveitis and concurrent allergic conjunctivitis associated with long-term use of topical brimonidine tartrate. The allergy to brimonidine was not documented by patch test [61]. In **Sodhi's** patients, brimonidine tartrate induced ACDC with periocular skin pigmentation (two cases confirmed by patch tests) and lichen planus of the right little finger nail (1 case) [62]. Brimonidine may be used in patients allergic to apraclonidine [62]. Its systemic side effects include severe dry mouth, fatigue, central nervous system depression, drowsiness, psychosis and minimal cardiopulmonary adverse effects [62].

Contact allergy from *mydriatics and cycloplegics* is rare despite extensive use by ophthalmologists. Phenylephrine, a sympathomimetic amine with predominantly alpha-receptorial stimulating properties, is responsible for 54-95% of cases of contact allergy induced by mydriatics [63-65]. Erdmann described a case of ACDC from phenylephrine in eye drops; no cross-reactivity with closely related and structurally similar drugs such as epinephrine and ephedrine was observed [66]. In patients allergic to phenylephrine the sensitivity of the conventional patch test is low. In 31 subjects patch tests detected only 68% of those allergic to phenylephrine; 24% of the patients allergic to phenilephrine were detected only by conjunctival challenge test [67]. Ocular contact allergy to atropine, an anticholinergic drug used in ophthalmology as a mydriatic and cycloplegic agent, often occurs after surgery where the drug is used because of its long-acting activity [68,69]; the reactions to chemically-related mydriatic agents such as scopolamine and homatotropine are probably due to cross-reactivity [68]. Cyclopentolate, an antimuscarinic agent [70], and dipivefrine, a sympathomimetic agent [71], are other mydriatic agents reported as causes of delayed contact allergy. A type-1 hypersensitivity mechanism was also hypothesized for allergy to cyclopentolale [3]. Parra suggested cross-reactivity between epinephrine and its prodrug, dipivefrine [72]. Tropicamide, an anti-cholinergic drug utilized for diagnostic procedures, has also been reported to cause contact allergy [73].

The adverse ocular effects of topical *non-steroid anti-inflammatory drugs (NSAIDs)* are well known and include itching, reduction of corneal sensitivity, keratopathy, ulcerations, corneal and scleral thinning and even corneal perforation [74]. Ocular contact allergy to NSAIDs is uncommon. Valsecchi first reported ACDC from eye drops containing diclofenac; contact allergy to diclofenac was confirmed by a 1% concentration in petrolatum patch test. The case demonstrates the lack of cross-reaction between diclofenac and bufexamac, though both are derivatives of phenylcarbon acid [75]. Although both have benzene rings, the different side chains (acetic acid for diclofenac and acetamide for bufexamac) could probably explain the lack of cross-reactivity. Ueda's patient developed a contact ocular allergy to diclofenac with concomitant sensitization to indomethacin without evidence of cross-reactivity [76]. Topical ketorolac tromethamine, a second generation topical NSAID of the pyrrole-pyrrolo group, also induced ACDC with intense follicle-papillar reaction [77]. Topical application of ketorolac may induce bronchial spasm or worsening of asthma in patients who are allergic to NSAIDs or who associate intolerance to aspirin, asthma and nasal polyps [78].

Ocular contact allergy caused by topical *antiviral drugs* is an uncommonly observed occurrence [79]. Pigatto first described a case of ACDC from β-interferon; no cross-reactivity with α-or γ-interferon was found [80]. Vidarabine 3% ophthalmic ointment used for treatment of epithelial keratitis caused by herpes simplex, induced burning, pain, irritation, tearing, superficial punctuate keratitis, photofobia and undocumented contact sensitivity [81,82]. Idoxuridine (IDU) eye drops have been reported to cause ACDC [83,84]; cross-reactivity to brominated and chlorinated, but not fluorinated, pyrimidine analogues has been reported [85]. IDU is probably the most well-known cause of chronic irritative follicular conjunctivitis among antiviral drugs [3]. Trifluoridine 1% ophthalmic solution, utilized in the treatment of ocular herpetic infection, is a sensitizer in ophthalmic preparations [86,87]. In the patient described by Millan-Parilla, no cross-reactivity with idoxuridine was observed [86]. A 5% petrolatum patch test confirmed the allergy [86]. Punctate keratopathy was present in 2 out of 58 patients receiving acyclovir 3% ophthalmic ointment; no other side effects were seen [87].

Contact allergy due to *antihistamines* of the alkylamine group, such as chlorpheniramine and pheniramine, was described mostly in Italy where they are used in various over the counter preparations including eye drops [88,89]. A case of ACDC from eye drops containing ketotifen fumarate, an H1-antihistamine/mast cell stabilizer, is also described. A positive patch test to ketotifen 0.069% aqueous solution was observed[90]. Camarasa reported a case of ACDC from sodium-cromoglycate-containing eye drop. Cromoglycate proved to be allergenic on patch testing (1% concentration in petrolatum) only if associated with benzalkonium chloride, a preservative present in the same eye drop; the two substances were tested separately and gave a negative result (compound allergy) [91]. A possible inhibitory effect of cromoglycate on allergic patch test reaction has also been reported [92]. Amlexanox is a sensitizer in ophthalmic solutions. It is structurally similar to sodium cromoglycate, although there are no reports of cross-reactivity between the two substances [93,94]. N-acetyl-aspartyl glutamic acid (NAAGA), a mast cell stabilizer present in ophthalmic solutions, also induced contact sensitization confirmed with a 1% petrolatum patch test [95].

Aminoglycosides are broad-spectrum *antibiotics* that can be allergenic and toxic to the conjunctiva and corneal epithelium with long-term use. Neomycin, which is included in the standard patch test series, has been reported to cause ocular contact allergy and in most statistics is the most important allergenic medicament [2,3]. The standard patch test concentration is 20% in petrolatum. Neomycin may exhibit late positive patch test reactions, and a delayed reading at 7D is thus recommendable. Cross-sensitivity of neomycin with other aminoglycoside antibiotics (gentamicin, tobramycin and kanamycin) has been described [96]. It is often associated with corticosteroids in ophthalmic preparations and this can sometimes mask contact sensitivity to neomycin because of the corticosteroid anti-inflammatory activity. Gentamicin, present in many ophthalmic preparations, seems to be less allergenic than neomycin, with which it may cross-react [97]. Cross-reaction of gentamicin with kanamycin but not with neomycin was also described [97]. Gentamicin 25% in petrolatum can be used for patch testing. Cross-sensitivity between aminoglycosides is related to the two main structures, neosamine and deoxystreptamine, common to compounds of this antibiotic class except streptomycin [97]. Kanamycin and tobramycin have also been reported as sensitizers [2]. Contact allergy to chloramphenicol is uncommon [98]. Sulphathiazole is still present in ophthalmic preparations, but there are few reports of sensitization [2]. Other antibiotics in ophthalmic preparations, including cefradine, penicillin, oxytetracycline, polymyxin B, vancomycin [99]., tobramycin and sodium colistimethate [100], have been reported as sensitizers [2,4]. Penicillin has been the most important iatrogenic cause of ocular immunologic contact urticaria, although its topical use is now rare [3].

The esters of p-aminobenzoic acid, benzocaine, procaine and tetracaine are allergenic *anesthetics* in ophthalmic preparations [2]. In particular, benzocaine is a common and powerful sensitizer and has been included in the standard series. The standard patch test dilution is 5% in petrolatum. Cross reactions of these anesthetics with each other and with other components of the para-group, e.g., p-phenylenediamine, the most popular of hair dyes, have been described [2] .The topical anesthetic proparacaine, an ester of m-aminobenzoic acid, is a sensitizer in ophthalmic preparations [101]. Dannaker reported a case of ocular contact allergy to proparacaine with concomitant sensitization to tetracaine [102]. The recommended patch test concentration for proparacaine is 2% in petrolatum. Topical proparacaine may also induce ocular immunologic contact urticaria [3] . Another anesthetic in ophthalmic preparations, oxybuprocain, has been reported as a sensitizer [103].

Contact allergy from *corticosteroids* in ophthalmic preparations is rare. Tosti reported two cases of ACC both induced by dexamethasone [104]. Alani described two patients who presented ACDC respectively from betamethasone and hydrocortisone. Hydrocortisone 25% in petrolatum is recommended for patch testing [105]. **Schmoll's** patient presented ACDC caused by prednisolone in an ophthalmic preparation. No cross-reactions were observed to other corticosteroids [106]. Delayed patch test reactions may be observed owing to the anti-inflammatory properties of these compounds, therefore a patch-test reading at 7 days is recommendable.

MISCELLANEOUS

Pilocarpine is a direct-acting cholinergic agonist with a dominant muscarinic action. It is used in the treatment of glaucoma. Helton reported one case of ACDC with photocontact allergy from pilocarpine and with a late positive patch test reaction on day 7. The use test required 3 weeks to become positive [107].

Bismuth is utilized topically for its bacteriostatic activity. A case of contact sensitization to a bismuth compound in an ophthalmic ointment used for atopic eyelid dermatitis has been reported [108].

N-acetylcysteine, a mucolytic agent present in eyedrops used to alleviate the chronic soreness associated with dry eyes, induced ACDC. A 10% aqueous patch test was diagnostic [109].

Epsilon-aminocaproic acid is a potent synthetic fibrolysin. It may produce ACDC as a result of its presence in eye preparations used in Japan to treat cataracts [110].

Rubidium iodide, used in ophthalmic preparations to prevent or retard the formation of cataracts, has been reported as a sensitizer. Patch test was positive to 1% petrolatum [111].

D-penicillamine prevents fibrosis of the cornea after chemical trauma. It has been reported to induce ACDC confirmed in a patient with 1% aqueous patch tests. This can cross-react with penicillin [112].

Pirfenexone, an antioxidant utilized for the treatment of cataracts, has been reported to cause ACDC confirmed with a 0.005% aqueous patch test [113].

Trometamol is a biologically inert amino alcohol, which buffers carbon dioxide and acids in vitro and in vivo. It induced ACDC as a result of its presence in ophthalmologic preparations with patch test positive at 0.5% aqueous solution [114].

Tegobetaine L7 is an amphoteric surfactant usually found in hair shampoos and skin cleansers, but also contained in contact lens solutions. It induced ACDC confirmed by a 1% petrolatum and 1% aqueous patch test [115].

CLINICAL FEATURES AND EVOLUTION

Immediate and delayed allergic contact reaction of the conjunctiva associated with ophthalmic preparations have been described [3,116-118], the clinical features of which are summarized in table 2.

Table 2. Clinical features of allergic contact conjunctivitis

Immediate allergic reaction	Delayed allergic reaction
Appearance of the conjunctival reaction within seconds or minutes after the re-exposure to the allergen	Appearance of the conjunctival reaction within 12-72 hours after the re-exposure to the allergen
Severe itch	Itch
Conjunctival hyperaemia and chemosis	Punctate epithelial erosions of the inferior conjunctiva
Mild papillary hypertrophy	Papillary hypertrophy
Mucoid discharge	Mucoid discharge or mildly mucopurulent discharge
Mild signs/symptoms if chronic	Associated eczematoid lesions of the eyelids and periocular skin
Eosinophils present in conjunctival scrapings	Eosinophils rarely present in conjunctival scrapings
The proof of immediate contact hypersensitivity is obtained mostly by occlusive or open test with reading at 20-30 minutes	The patch test with reading at 48-72 h is the standard confirmatory test

In the immediate allergic reactions the symptoms occurred suddenly (within seconds or minutes) on exposure to the offending allergen. In the acute form the symptomatology includes tearing, itching, and burning [3]. Clinical evaluation reveals conjunctival hyperemia and chemosis, the latter sometimes being the predominant finding masking the concomitant hyperemia. Mucoid discharge is an early symptom. The cornea is not usually involved [3]. In the chronic form the symptoms and signs are less impressive. A mild papillary reaction may be present. Conjunctival scraping is a useful examination, as it can reveal the presence of eosinophils that are characteristic of immediate rather than delayed hypersensitivity [3]. The presence of itching and eosinophils in conjunctival scrapings strongly suggest that the ocular reaction is allergic rather than toxic.

In delayed allergy the symptoms occurred 12-72 hours after contact with the allergen. Ophthalmologic examination reveals papillar conjunctivitis and sometimes chemosis with mucoid or mildly muco-purulent discharge. Initially the conjunctivitis is worse inferonasally and inferiorly, where the topical medicaments tend to gravitate, but it can become more widespread later [3]. In severe cases mild keratinisation of the conjunctiva and punctal edema, stenosis, and occlusion have been observed [3]. Itching is present but is not so prominent as with immediate allergic reactions [3,116]. Although papillary response may occur in both allergic and toxic reactions, this is more frequent in allergy while a follicular response is mainly viral or toxic in nature [117]. However, allergic cell-mediated reactions to eye drop components associated with follicular conjunctivitis have been described [13].

Corneal involvement is present and is limited to punctate epithelial keratitis and erosions; these changes may be widespread but are more frequently localized in the lower two-thirds of the cornea [3]. In severe cases corneal ulcerations and edema may be present [118]. Scrapings from the conjunctiva reveal mononuclear cells, occasional neutrophils, mucus, on rare occasions the presence of eosinophils [3]. The ocular symptoms may be limited to the conjunctiva (ACC) or may also involve the eyelids and periocular skin with eczematiform lesions [edema, hyperemia, and sometimes vesicles] [ACDC]. Eyelid dermatitis from allergenic ophthalmic preparations instilled into the conjunctival sac is not a constant finding [13]. Topical ophthalmic medications that induce eyelid dermatitis usually cause first allergic contact conjunctivitis. Eyelid involvement in the absence of any conjunctival sign indicates that the product [e.g. ophthalmic ointment, eye makeup, airborne allergens, etc.] has only come into contact with the eyelid without having been instilled into the conjunctival sac [3].

The allergic reactions generally improve or clear quickly once the culprit eye drop use is discontinued. In Wilson's patients, the ocular reaction sometimes improved within 2 or 3 days, but 11 or 12 days are needed on average. Some cases, however, show no improvement until more than 1 month has passed. In particular cases, the ocular reactions clear only after several months [3]. In two cases of documented contact allergy to phenylephrine, the ocular changes persisted for 5 and 8 months respectively, despite suspension of the drug, with ophthalmic complications such as keratitis and trichiasis in one case [119].

DIAGNOSTIC PROCEDURES

A diagnosis of ocular contact allergy is reached on the basis of a detailed history and clinical examination followed by skin tests, with assessment of the relevance to the current ACC of any positive reaction. Two-day closed patch testing, applied to the upper back on which patch tests are usually performed, is the "gold standard" confirmatory testing for delayed contact allergy. In clinical practice, when contact allergy to ophthalmic preparation is suspected, a 2-day closed patch test is performed with ophthalmic preparation tested as is, integrated in our experience by an *International Contact Dermatitis Research Group* [ICDRG]standard series and a series of ophthalmic compounds identified from the literature and personal experience [Table 3]. However, for the ophthalmic preparation tested as is, conventional patch testing is sometimes a poor detector of contact allergy, especially when the responsible allergen is a preservative [2] or a beta-blocking agent [120]. False-negative results may be determined by the low concentration or the scarce bioavailability of the potential allergen in the ophthalmic preparation. In addition, ophthalmic preparations may not readily penetrate the healthy thick skin of the back which has different anatomical and physiological properties from the thin, sometimes damaged, conjunctival mucosa. Among possible means employed for enhancing the penetration of substances applied to the skin and increasing sensitivity to test, some authors have suggested that patch tests should be performed on tape-stripped or scarified skin (scratch –patch test), or after pricking the skin, and by intradermal testing with some success [52,120-122]. Enlargement of the patch test area or an increased concentration of allergen have also been suggested [123,124]. Pre-treatment of the patch test area with sodium lauril sulfate, a primary irritant, was also able to elicit a positive patch test reaction to ophthalmic preparations in patients previously negative to conventional patch test [125].

Table 3. Ophthalmic preparation constituents commercially availables tested in addition to the ICDRG standard series

Eye drops constituens	Concentration and vehicle
Ophthalmic preparation	(as is)
Atropine sulfate	1 % pet.
Benzalkonium chloride	0.1 % aq.
Caine mix (dibucaine 1%, tetracaine 1%, benzocaine ** 5%)	7 % pet.
Chlorhexidine digluconate	0.5 % pet.
Chloramphenicol	3 % pet.
Dexamethasone	0.5 % pet.
Ethylenediamine tetra-acetate acid	1 % pet.
Epinephrine	1 % pet.
Gentamycin sulphate	25 % pet.
Hydrocortisone	25 % pet.
Idoxuridine	0.5 % pet.
Phenylephrine hydrochloride*	10 % aq.
Phenylmercuric nitrate	0.01% aq.
Pheniramine	2 % pet.
Pilocarpine *	1 % aq.*
Polymyxin B	3% pet.
Prednisolone	5 % pet.
Sorbic acid	5 % pet.
Thimerosal	0.05 % pet.

All substances apart those marked * are supplied by Firma Diagent, Florence, Italy. Those marked * are commercially available from Trolab Hermal , Reinbeck, Germany. ** benzocaine is present also in the ICDRG standard series.

pet. = petrolatum; aq. = water.

Negative patch test reactions to ophthalmic preparation as is do not exclude the possibility of contact sensitization to one or more of the components of the preparations. To avoid false-negative reactions, each of the components should always be patch tested in patients suspected of having contact allergy, rather than simply relying on a patch test with their eye drops or contact lens solutions as is [126].

Commercially available ophthalmic patch test series may not contain some of the individual components of the ophthalmic preparation being tested, above all some of the active ingredients; in our experience these substances, generally supplied on request by the pharmaceutical manufacturers themselves, are prepared according to general instructions for extempore patch test preparations [127].

Readings of the patch tests are performed after an application period of 2 days, at 2 and 4 days [D] according to the ICDRG criteria. However, late appearing positive patch test reactions to ophthalmic preparations and their ingredients [107] suggests the appropriateness of delayed readings even on D7. A positive reaction [+ - -] is defined as at least homogeneous redness and palpable infiltration in the test area. If vesicles occur, a + + - scoring is used and + + + for a bullous reaction. When patch-testing patients with non-standardized allergens, case control tests [at least 20 control subjects] and serial dilution tests are always required, to detect false positive and clinically non-relevant test results.

Kanerva believes that the majority of patch test reactions disappear within 5-10 days and rarely last longer [128]. Nevertheless, two cases of long-lasting allergic patch test reactions [LLAPTR] to phenylephrine have been described, which persisted for 2-7 months respectively [128]. LLAPTR are by definition those in which the clinical signs of palpable erythema are still present at the allergen application site 2 or more weeks after the test. The pathogenetic mechanism of LLAPTR is still unknown. Interestingly, in the cases described, despite the LLAPTR the ocular symptoms healed rapidly [129].

If the patch tests are negative and the patient has on the other hand a well-founded suspicion of allergy to the substance, a repeated open application test [ROAT] or a conjunctival provocation test is carried out [28,57,126]. In Villareal's patients, the conjunctival challenge test with serial dilutions of the ophthalmic preparation believed to be responsible for the allergy proved to be a valid and safe alternative method to conventional patch tests. In fact, in 24% of the patients with negative conventional patch test results to the mydriatic agent, allergy to phenylephrine was observed only by conjunctival challenge test [67].

Patch-test scoring in itself has no meaning if it is not linked with the clinical features of ocular allergy and exposure history of the patient's ocular allergy. A positive test can in fact refer to a previous, unrelated episode of contact allergy. The relevance can be divided into current and past relevance and each, according Lachapelle, should be assessed and recorded as not traced, doubtful, possible or likely [130]. In order to increase the accuracy of relevance of positive patch tests, additional testing procedures with the suspected allergen include serial dilution patch testing, sequential patch testing, ROAT or use test [130].

The proof of immediate contact hypersensitivity is obtained mostly by occlusive or open test methods on normal skin, with a reading at 20-30 minutes [131,132]. A weal-and-flare reaction is regarded as positive. If these procedure tests are negative, then prick or scratch tests are used, the second being preferable when only non-standardized allergens are available. The conjunctival challenge test has also been used diagnostically. Skin and conjunctival tests are not innocuous and they can cause severe anaphylaxis [3]. Many chemicals can induce urticarial contact reactions followed by a delayed eczematous reaction so a delayed reading at 24-48 hours of the same test used to detect immediate hypersensitivity is recommendable [131].

More detailed information on the procedures, concentrations and vehicles for skin testing is available elsewhere [133-134].

PREVENTION AND PROGNOSIS

A distinction can be made between primary and secondary prevention; the first aims at eliminating all the possibilities of onset of the contact allergy in a population of healthy subjects; the aim of secondary prevention is to prevent already sensitized subjects from experiencing recurrences. Ideal primary prevention is based on the choice, by the pharmaceutical industry, of non-irritant and non-allergenising substances in the formulation of new ophthalmic preparations. In order to prevent primary sensitization from ophthalmic preparations they must be prescribed with care since inappropriate administration can lead to a risk of sensitization. It is advisable to prescribe products with components that have little or no haptenic potential.

Secondary prevention is based on identification and avoidance of the offending chemical[s]. Allergy tests [patch test, prick test, challenge test, repeated open application test, etc.] integrate the clinical examination in the search for the offending allergen and in identification of alternative chemicals tolerated by the patient. The same active ingredients and, even more frequently, the same preservatives can be present in various different ophthalmic preparations which makes prevention difficult and relapses a fairly common occurrence in long-term treatment. The problem is further complicated by the cross-reactivity between substances containing common antigenic determinants.

It is essential, moreover, to provide the patient with detailed and understandable information concerning the chemical[s] to which he is allergic, including all known names of the chemical [e.g. thimerosal also known as merthiolate] and alternative chemicals to those which have caused the allergy. This information is important since some ophthalmic preparations are available over the counter and can thus be used with no medical control.

If correctly diagnosed and managed, ACC has a good prognosis as it clears spontaneously when use of the offending chemical is discontinued, without the need in many cases of any other therapy [3].

REFERENCES

[1]   Rietschel RL, Fowler JF. Medications and medical devices, and implications for the medical community. In: *Fisher's Contact Dermatitis.*, 6th edition. Hamilton: BC Decker; 2008: 125-174.

[2]   Brandão FM, Goossens AN, Tosti A. Topical drugs In: *Textbook of Contact Dermatitis.* Rycroft RJG, Menné T, Frosch PJ, Lepoittevin JP, eds. 3th edition. Berlin: Springer-Verlag 2001: 687-723.

[3]   Wilson FM. Adverse external ocular effects of topical ophthalmic medications. *Surv Ophthalmol* 1979;24: 57-88.

[4]   Chaudhari PR, Maibach HI. Allergic contact dermatitis from ophthalmics: 2007. *Contact Dermatitis* 2007; 57:11-13.

[5]   Noecker RJ, Herrigers LA, Anwaruddin R. Corneal and conjunctival changes caused by commonly used glaucoma medications. *Cornea* 2004;23; 490-496.

[6]   Baudouin C, Allergic reaction to topical eyedrops. *Curr Opin Allergy Clin Immunol* 2005; 5: 459-463.

[7]   Mietz H, Niesen U, Krieglstein GK. The effect of preservatives and antiglaucomatous medication on the histopathology of the conjunctiva. *Arch Clin Exp Ophthalmol* 1994; 232: 561-565.

[8]   Hjorth N. Sensitivity to organic mercury compounds. *Contact Dermatitis Newsletter* 1967;1:15

[9]   Hansson H, Möller H. Patch test reactions to merthiolate in healthy young subjects. *Br J Derm* 1970; 83: 349-356.

[10] Möller H. Merthiolate allergy: a nationwide iatrogenic sensitization. *Acta Derm Venereol* 1977; 57: 509-517.

[11] Melino M, Antonelli C, Barone M. Contact dermatitis from merthiolate. *Contact Dermatitis* 1986; 14: 125.

[12] Emmons WW, Marks JG. Immediate and delayed reactions to cosmetic ingredients. *Contact Dermatitis* 1985; 13: 258-265.

[13] Tosti A, Tosti G. Thimerosal: a hidden allergen in ophthalmology. *Contact Dermatitis* 1988; 18: 268-273.

[14] Fregert S, Hjorth H. In: Rook AJ, Wilkinson DS, Ebling JFG, eds. Textbook of dermatology. Oxford. Blackwell, 1972:333.

[15] Pedersen NB. Allergic conjunctivitis from Merthiolate in soft contact lenses. *Contact Dermatitis* 1978; 4:165.

[16] Van Ketel WG. Melzer-Van Riemsdijk FA. Conjunctivitis due to soft lens solutions. *Contact Dermatitis* 1980;6:321-324.

[17] Rietschel RL. Wilson LA. Ocular inflammation in patients using soft contact lenses. *Arch Dermatol* 1982; 118:147-149.

[18] Willis CM, Stephens JM, Wilkinson JD. Experimentally-induced irritant contact dermatitis. Determination of optimum irritant concentrations. *Contact Dermatitis* 1988; 18: 20-24.

[19] Andersen KE, Rycroft RJG. Recommended patch test concentrations for preservatives, biocides and antimicrobials. *Contact Dermatitis* 1991; 25: 1-18.

[20] Kanerva L. Skin disease from dental materials. In: *Textbook of Contact Dermatitis*. Rycroft RJG, Menné T, Frosch PJ, Lepoittevin JP (eds):, Third edition. Berlin; Springer-Verlag, 2001: 841-881.

[21] Schnuch A. Benzalkoniumchloride. *Dermatosen* 1997; 45: 179-180.

[22] Fuchs T, Meinert A, Aberer W, Bahmer FA et al. Benzalkonium chloride - a relevant contact allergen or irritant? Results of a multicentre study conducted by the German Contact Allergy Group. *Hautarzt* 1993; 44:699-702.

[23] Fisher AA. Allergic contact dermatitis and conjunctivitis from benzalkonium chloride. *Cutis* 1987; 39: 381-383.

[24] Huriez C, Agache P, Martin S et al. Frequence de sensibilizations aux ammoniums quaternaries. *Bull Soc Fr Dermatol Syphilol* 1965;72; 106-114

[25] Okano M, Nomura M, Hata S, Okada N, Sato K, Kitano Y, Tashiro M, Yoshimoto Y, Hama R, Aoki T. Anaphylactic symptoms due to chlorhexidine gluconate.*Arch Dermatol* 1989; 125: 50-52.

[26] Krautheim AB, Jermann THM, Bircher AJ. Chlorhexidine anaphylaxis: case report and review of the literature. *Contact Dermatitis* 2004 50: 113-116.

[27] Ooi KGJ, Adler PA, Goldberg I. Trabeculectomy trapdoor separation with allergic periorbital dermatitis: an unusual late-onset complication of guarded filtration surgery. *Clin Experiment Ophthalmol* 2007; 35: 578-579.

[28] Garcia-Medina JJ, Garcia-Medina M, Zanon-Moreno VC, Scalerandi G, Pinazo-Duran MD. Conjunctival provocation test for the diagnosis of ocular hypersensitivity to chlorobutanol. *Cornea* 2007; 26:94-97.

[29] Vilaplana J, Romaguera C. Contact dermatitis from parabens as preservatives in eyedrops. *Contact Dermatitis* 2000; 43:248.

[30] Sher MA. Contact dermatitis of the eyelids. S Afr Med J 1979; 55: 511-513.

[31] Podmore P, Storrs FJ. Contact lens intolerance; allergic conjunctivitis ?. *Contact Dermatitis* 1989; 20:98-103.

[32] Pflugfelder SC. Ophthalmic preservatives: the past, present, and future. CME. Candeo Clinical/Science Communications 2008; 1-8.

[33] Romaguera C. Grimalt F, Vilaplana J. Contact dermatitis by timolol. *Contact Dermatitis* 1986; 14:248.

[34] Fernandez –Vozmediano JM, Blasi NA, Romero-Cabrera MA, Carrascosa –Cerquero A. Allergic contact dermatitis to timolol. *Contact Dermatitis* 1986; 14:252.

[35] Cameli N, Vincenzi C, Tosti A. Allergic contact conjunctivitis due to timolol in eyedrops. *Contact Dermatitis* 1991; 25:129-130.

[36] Schultheiss E. Hypersensitivity to levobunolol. *Derm Beruf Umwelt* 1989; 37:185-186.

[37] Van der Meeren HL, Meurs PJ. Sensitization to levobunolol eyedrops. *Contact Dermatitis* 1993; 28: 41-42.

[38] Di Lernia V, Albertini G, Bisighini G. Allergic contact dermatitis from levobunolol eyedrops. *Contact Dermatitis* 1995; 33:57.

[39] Garcia F, Blanco J, Juste S, Garces MM, Alonso L, Marcos ML, Carretero P, Perez R. Contact dermatitis due to levobunolol in eyedrops. *Contact Dermatitis* 1997;36:230.

[40] Erdmann S, Hertl M, Merk HF.Contact dermatitis from levobunolol eyedrops. *Contact Dermatitis* 1999; 41: 44-46.

[41] Kanzaki T, Kato N, Kabasawa Y, Mizuno N, Yuguchi M, Majima A. Contact dermatitis due to the beta-blocker befunolol in eyedrops. *Contact Dermatitis* 1988; 19:388.

[42] Mancuso G. Allergic contact dermatitis due to befunolol in eyedrops. *Contact Dermatitis* 1992; 27: 198.

[43] De Groot AC, Conemans J. Contact allergy to metipranolol. *Contact Dermatitis* 1988; 18:107-108.

[44] Holdiness MR. Contact dermatitis to topical drugs for glaucoma. Am J Contact Dermat 2001; 12: 217-219.

[45] Sanchez-Perez J, Cordoba S, Bartolomé B, Garcia-Diez A. Allergic contact dermatitis due to the β-blocker carteolol in eyedrops. *Contact Dermatitis* 1999;41:298.

[46] O'Donnel BF, Foulds IS. Contact allergy to beta-blocking agents in ophthalmic preparations. *Contact Dermatitis* 1993; 28: 121-122.

[47] Quiralte J, Florido F, de San Pedro BS. Allergic contact dermatitis from carteolol and timolol in eyedrops. *Contact dermatitis* 2000; 42:245.

[48] Jappe U, Uter W, Menezes de Padua CA, Herbst RA, Schnuch A. Allergic contact dermatitis due to β-blockers in eye drops: a retrospective analysis of multicentre surveillance data 1993-2004. *Acta Derm Venereol* 2006; 86: 509-514.

[49] Nino M, Suppa F, Ayala F, Balato N. Allergic contact dermatitis due to the β-blocker befunolol in eyedrops, with cross-sensitivity to carteolol. *Contact Dermatitis* 2001; 44:369.

[50] Corazza M, Virgili A. Mantovani L, Taddei Masieri L. Allegic contact dermatitis from cross-reacting beta-blocking agents. *Contact Dermatitis* 1993; 28:188-189.

[51] Giordano-Labadie F, Lepoittevin JP, Calix I, Bazex J. Allergie de contact aux β bloquers des collyres: allergie croisée ? *Ann Dermatol Venereol* 1997; 124: 322-324.

[52] Koch P. Allergic contact dermatitis due to timolol and levobunolol in eyedrops, with no cross-sensitivity to other ophthalmic β-blockers. *Contact Dermatitis* 1995; 33:140-141

[53] Zucchelli V, Silvani S, Vezzani C, Lorenzi S, Tosti A. Contact dermatitis from levobunolol and befunolol. *Contact dermatitis* 1995; 33: 66-67

[54] Aalto-Korte K, Contact allergy to dorzolamide eyedrops. *Contact Dermatitis* 1998; 39:206

[55] Shimada M, Higaki Y, Kawashima M. Allergic contact dermatitis due to dorzolamide eyedrops. *Contact Dermatitis* 2001; 45:52.

[56] Mancuso G, Berdondini RM. Allergic contact blepharoconjunctivitis from dorzolamide. *Contact Dermatitis* 2001; 45:243.

[57] Jerstad KM, Warshaw E. Allergic contact dermatitis to latanoprost. *Am J Contact Dermatitis* 2002; 13: 39-41.

[58] Sodhi PK, Verma L, Ratan SK. Contact dermatitis from topical bimatoprost. *Contact Dermatitis* 2004; 50:50.

[59] Armisen M, Vidal C, Quintans R, Suarez A, Castroviejo M. Allergic contact dermatitis from apraclonidine. *Contact Dermatitis* 1998; 39:193.

[60] Butler P, Mannschreck M. Lin S. Hwang I, Alvarado J. Clinical experience with the long-term use of 1% apraclonidine. Incidence of allergic reactions. *Arch Ophthalmol* 1995; 113:293-296.

[61] Becker HI, Walton RC, Diamant JI, Zegans ME. Anterior uveitis and concurrent allergic conjunctivitis associated with long-term use of topical 0.2% brimonidine tartrate. *Arch Ophthalmol* 2004; 122: 1063-1066.

[62] Sodhi PK, Verma L, Ratan J. Dermatological side effects of brimonidine: a report of three cases. *The Journal of Dermatology* 2003; 30: 697-700.

[63] Camarasa JG. Contact dermatitis to phenylephrine. *Contact Dermatitis* 1984; 10:182.

[64] Ducombs G, Casamayor J, Verin HP, Maleville J. Allergic contact dermatitis to phenylephrine. *Contact Dermatitis* 1986. 15: 107-108.

[65] Almeida L, Ortega N, Dumpierrez AG, Castillo R, Blanco C, Navarro L, Carrillo T. Conjunctival allergic contact hypersensitivity. *Allergy* 2001; 56: 785.

[66] Erdmann SM, Sachs B, Merk HF. Allergic contact dermatitis from phenilephrine in eyedrops. *Am J Contact Dermatitis* 2002; 13: 37-38.

[67] Villarreal O. Reliability of diagnostic tests for contact allergy to mydriatic eyedrops. *Contact Dermatitis* 1998; 38: 150-154.

[68] Decraene T, Goossens A. Contact allergy to atropine and other mydriatic agents in eye drops. *Contact Dermatitis* 2001; 45: 309-310.

[69] De Misa RF, Suarez J, Feliciano L, Lopez B. Allergic periocular contact dermatitis due to atropine. *Clin Exp Dermatol* 2003; 28: 97-98.

[70] Camarasa JG, Pla C. Allergic contact dermatitis from cyclopentolate. *Contact Dermatitis* 1996; 35; 368-369.

[71] Vilaplana J, Zaballos P, Romaguera C. Contact dermatitis by dipivefrine. *Contact Dermatitis* 2005; 52:169-170.

[72] Parra A, Casas L, Tombo MJ, Yanez M, Vila L. Contact dermatitis from dipivefrine with possibile cross-reaction to epinephrine. *Contact Dermatitis* 1998;39:325-326.

[73] Boukhman MP, Maibach HI. Allergic contact dermatitis from tropicamide ophthalmic solution. *Contact Dermatitis* 1999;41: 47-48.

[74] Aragona P, Tripodi G, Spinella R, Laganà E, Ferreri G,. The effects of the topical administration of non-steroidal anti-inflammatory drugs on corneal epithelium and corneal sensitivity in normal subjects. *Eye* 2000; 14: 206-210.

[75] Valsecchi R, Pansera B, Leghissa P, Reseghetti A. Allergic contact dermatitis of the eyelids and conjunctivitis from diclofenac. *Contact Dermatitis* 1996,34: 150-151.

[76] Ueda K, Higashi N, Kume A, Ikushima-Fujimoto M, Ogiwara S. Allergic contact dermatitis due to diclofenac and indomethacin. *Contact Dermatitis* 1998; 39: 323.

[77] Rodriguez NA, Abarzuza R, Cristobal JA, Sierra J, Minguez E, Del Buey MA. Eyelid contact allergic eczema caused by topical ketorolac tromethamine 0.5%. *Arch Soc Esp Oftalmol* 2006; 81: 213-216.

[78] Sitenga GL, Ing EB, Van Dellen RG, Younge RB, Leavitt JA. Asthma caused by topical application of ketorolac. *Ophthalmology* 1996; 103:890-892.

[79] Holdiness MR. Contact dermatitis from topical antiviral drugs. *Contact Dermatitis* 2001; 44:265-269.

[80] Pigatto PD, Bigardi A, Legori A, Altomare GF, Riboldi A. Allergic contact dermatitis from beta-interferon in eyedrops. *Contact Dermatitis* 1991; 25: 199-200.

[81] Pavan–Langston D, Current trends in the therapy of ocular herpes simplex: experimental and clinical studies. *Adv Ophthal* 1979 ; 38:82-88.

[82] Wood MJ, Geddes AM. Antiviral therapy. *Lancet* 1987; 2:1189-1193.

[83] Stern GA, Killingsworth DW. Complications of topical antimicrobial agents. *Int Ophthalmol* 1989;29: 137-142.

[84] McGill J, Williams H, McKinnon J, Holt-Wilson AD, Jones BR. Reassesment of idoxuridine therapy of herpetic keratitis. *Trans Ophthal Soc UK* 1974; 94: 542-551.

[85] Amon RB, Lis AW, Hanifin JM. Allergic contact dermatitis caused by idoxuridine. Patterns of cross reactivity with other pyrimidine analogues. *Arch Dermatol* 1975; 111: 1581-1584.

[86] Millan-Parrilla F, De La Cuadra J. Allergic contact dermatitis from trifluoridine in eye drops. *Contact Dermatitis* 1990; 22: 289.

[87] Naito T, Shiota H, Mimura Y. Side effects in the treatment of herpetic keratitis. *Curr Eye Res* 1987; 6: 237-239.

[88] Tosti A, Bardazzi F, Piancastelli E. Contact dermatitis due to chlorpheniramine maleate in eyedrops. *Contact Dermatitis* 1990; 21:55.

[89] Parente G, Pazzaglia M, Vincenti C, Tosti A. Contact dermatitis from pheniramine maleate in eyedrops. *Contact Dermatitis* 1999; 40: 338.

[90] Niizeki H, Inamoto N, Nakamura K, Nakanoma I,Nakano T. Contact dermatitis from ketotifen fumarate eyedrops. *Contact Dermatitis* 1994; 31: 266.

[91] Camarasa JG, Serra-Baldrich E, Monreal P, Soller J. Contact dermatitis from sodium-cromoglycate-containing eyedrops. *Contact Dermatitis* 1997, 36: 160-161.

[92] Meffert H, Wischnewski Gunther W. Disodium cromoglycate inhibits allergic patch test reactions. *Contact Dermatitis* 1985; 12:18-20.

[93] Yamashita H, Kawashima M. Contact dermatitis from amlexanox eyedrops. *Contact Dermatitis* 1991; 25:255-256.

[94] Kabasawa Y, Kanzaki T. Allergic contact dermatitis from amlexanox (Elics) ophthalmic solution. *Contact Dermatitis* 1991; 24: 148.

[95] Blanco R, Quirce S, Pedraza L, Diez-Gomez ML. Allergic conjunctivitis from eyedrops. *Allergy* 1997;52: 686-687.

[96] Kimura M, Kawada A. Contact sensitivity induced by neomycin with cross-sensitivity to other aminoglycoside antibiotics. *Contact Dermatitis* 1998; 39: 148-150.

[97] Sanchez-Pérez J, Lopez MP, De Vega Haro MJM, Garcia-Diez A. Allergic contact dermatitis from gentamycin in eyedrops, with cross-reactivity to kanamycin but not neomycin. *Contact Dermatitis* 2001; 44: 54.

[98] Le Coz CJ, Santinelli F. Facial contact dermatitis from chloramphenicol with cross-sensitivity to thiamphenicol. *Contact Dermatitis* 1998; 38: 108-109.

[99] Hwu JJ, Chen KH, Hsu WM, Lai JY, Li YS. Ocular hypersensitivity to topical Vancomycin in a case of chronic endophthalmitis. *Cornea* 2005; 24:754-756.

[100] Sasaki S, Mitsuhashi Y, Kondo S. Contact dermatitis due to sodium colistimethate. *J Dermatol* 1998; 25: 415-417.

[101] March C, Greenwood MA. Allergic contact dermatitis to proparacaine. *Arch Opthalmol* 1968; 79: 159-160

[102] Dannaker CJ, Maibach HI, Austin E. Allergic contact dermatitis to proparacaine with subsequent cross-sensitization to tetracaine from ophthalmic preparations. *Am J Contact Dermatitis* 2001;12: 177-179.

[103] Blaschke V. Fuchs T. Relevant allergens by periorbital allergic contact dermatitis. Oxybuprocain, an underestimated allergen. *Opthalmologe* 2003;100: 628-632.

[104] Tosti A, Tosti G. Allergic contact conjunctivitis due to ophthalmic solutions. In: *Current Topics in Contact Dermatitis*. Frosch PJ, Dooms-Goossens A, Lachapelle JM, Rycroft RJG, Scheper RJ, eds. Berlin: Springer Verlag 1989; p. 269-272.

[105] Alani SD, Alani MD. Allergic contact dermatitis and conjunctivitis to corticosteroids. *Contact Dermatitis* 1976; 2:301-304.

[106] Schmoll M, Hausen BM. Allergic contact dermatitis to prednisolone-21-trimethyl acetate. *Z Hautkr* 1988; 63: 311-313.

[107] Helton J, Storrs FJ. Pilocarpine allergic contact and photocontact dermatitis. *Contact Dermatitis* 1991; 25: 133-134.

[108] Wictorin A, Hansson C. Allergic contact dermatitis from a bismuth compound in an eye ointment. *Contact Dermatitis* 2001; 45:318.

[109] Davison SC, Wakelin SH. Allergic contact dermatitis from N-acetylcysteine eyedrops. *Contact Dermatitis* 2002; 47:238.

[110] Miyamoto H, Okajima M. Allergic contact dermatitis from epsilon-aminocaproic acid. *Contact Dermatitis* 2000; 42:50.

[111] Cameli N, Bardazzi F, Morelli P, Tosti A. Contact dermatitis from rubidium iodide in eyedrops. *Contact Dermatitis* 1990; 23:377-378.

[112] Coenraads PJ,Woest TE, Blanksma LJ, Houtman WA. Contact allergy to d-penicillamine. *Contact Dermatitis* 1990;23: 371-372.

[113] Inui S, Ozawa K, Song M, Itami S, Katayama I. Contact dermatitis due to pirfenoxone. *Contact Dermatitis* 2004;50: 375-376.

[114] Bohn S, Hurni M, Bircher AJ. Contact allergy to trometamol. *Contact Dermatitis* 2001; 44:319.

[115] Cameli N, Tosti G, Venturo N, Tosti A. Eyelid dermatitis due to cocamidropropylbetaine in a hard contact lens solution. *Contact Dermatitis* 1991; 25: 261-262.

[116] Broadway D, Grierson I, Hitchings R. Adverse effects of topical antiglaucomatous medications on the conjunctiva. *Br J Ophthalmol* 1993;77: 590-596.

[117] Ziskind A. Allergic conjunctivitis. *Current Allergy and Clin Immunol* 2006; 19: 56-59.

[118] Friedlaender MH. Ocular allergy. *Seminars in Ophthalmology* 1996; 11: 69-78.

[119] Peyron NR, Du Thanh A, Demoly P, Guillot B. Long-lasting allergic contact blepharoconjunctivitis to phenilephrine eyedrops. *Allergy* 2009;64 :657-658.

[120] Frosch PJ, Weickel R, Schmitt T, Krastel H. Nebenwirkungen von ophthalmologischen Externa. *Z Hautkr* 1988;63:126-136

[121] Akita H, Akamatsu H, Matsunaga K. Allergic contact dermatitis due to phenylephrine hydrochloride, with an unusual patch test reaction. *Contact Dermatitis* 2003; 49:232-235.

[122] Wilkinson M. False-negative patch test with levobunolol. *Contact Dermatitis* 2001; 44: 264.

[123] Gailhofer G, Ludvan M. "Beta-blockers": sensitizers in periorbital allergic contact dermatitis. *Contact Dermatitis* 1990; 23:262.

[124] De Groot AC, Van Ginkel CJ, Bruynzeel DP, Smeenk G, Conemans JM. Contact allergy to eyedrops containing beta-blockers Ned-Tijdschr Geneeskd 1998; 142:1034-1036.

[125] Corazza M, Virgili A. Allergic contact dermatitis from ophthalmic products: can pre-treatment with sodium lauryl sulfate increase patch test sensitivity ? *Contact Dermatitis* 2005; 52: 239-241.

[126] Statham BN. Failure of patch testing with levobunolol eyedrops to detect contact allergy. *Contact Dermatitis* 2000; 43: 365-366.

[127] Nava C. Le preparazioni per prove epicutanee.In: Le allergopatie professionali. Nava C, ed. Masson Italia, Milano 1987. Pag. 259-282.

[128] Kanerva l, Estlander T, Jolanki R. Immunohistochemistry of lymphocytes and Langerans 'cells in long-lasting allergic patch test. *Acta dermato-Venereologica* 1988; 68:116-122.

[129] Mancuso G, Reggiani M, Staffa M. Long-lasting allergic patch test reaction to phenylephrine. *Contact Dermatitis* 1997; 36: 110 -111.

[130] Lachapelle JM. A proposed relevance scoring system for positive allergic patch test reactions. Practical implications and limitations. *Contact Dermatitis* 1997; 36: 39-43.

[131] Rietschel RL, Fowler JF. Contact urticaria. In: *Fisher's Contact Dermatitis.* 6th edition. Hamilton: DC Decker; 2008: 615-640.

[132] Hannuskela M. Skin tests for immediate hypersensitivity. In: *Textbook of Contact Dermatitis.* Rycroft RJG, Menné T, Frosch PJ, Lepoittevin JP, eds. Third edition. Springer-Verlag 2001: 519-526.

[133] Rietschel RL, Fowler JF. Practical aspects of patch testing. In: *Fisher's Contact Dermatitis,* 6th edition. Hamilton: DC Decker; 2008: 11-29.

[134] Wahlberg JE. Patch Testing. In: *Textbook of Contact Dermatitis.* Rycroft RJG, Menné T, Frosch PJ, Lepoittevin JP, eds. Third edition. Springer-Verlag 2001: 435-468.

Chapter V

STEVENS-JOHNSON SYNDROME WITH OCULAR COMPLICATIONS

Mayumi Ueta[1,2,*]

[1]Kyoto Prefectural University of Medicine, Kyoto, Japan;
[2]Doshisha University, Kyoto, Japan.

ABSTRACT

Stevens-Johnson syndrome (SJS) and toxic epidermal necrolysis (TEN) are acute inflammatory vesiculobullous reactions of the skin and mucous membranes. Drugs are the suspected etiologic factor in SJS/TEN. SJS/TEN patients often experience the prodromata, including nonspecific fever, coryza, and sore throat, that closely mimic upper respiratory tract infections treated with antibiotics.

IκBζ, is important for Toll-like receptor (TLR)/IL-1 receptor signaling and essential for innate immune responses; knockout (KO) mice exhibit severe, spontaneous ocular surface inflammation with the loss of goblet cells, and perioral inflammation.

As findings in IκBζ-KO mice suggested that dysfunction/abnormality of innate immunity can result in ocular surface inflammation, we posited that it may play a role in human ocular surface inflammatory disorders. Under the hypothesis of a disordered innate immune response we performed gene expression analysis of CD14[+] cells from peripheral blood of SJS/TEN patients with ocular complications. We found that IL-4R gene expression differed between SJS/TEN patients and the controls; upon LPS stimulation, it was down-regulated in patients and slightly up-regulated in the controls. We also found that the expression of 2 genes, IκBζ and IL-1α, was significantly down-regulated in SJS/TEN. Single nucleotide polymorphism (SNP) association analysis of candidate genes associated with innate immunity, allergy, or apoptosis revealed that TLR3 SNP (rs.3775296 and rs.3775290), IL4R SNP Gln551Arg (rs.1801275), IL13 SNP Arg110Gln (rs.20541), and FasL SNP (rs.3830150 and rs.2639614) were significantly

---

* Correspondence concerning this article should be addressed to: Dr. Mayumi Ueta, Department of Ophthalmology, Kyoto Prefectural University of Medicine, Hirokoji, Kawaramachi, Kamigyoku, Kyoto 602-0841, Japan. Phone: 81-75-251-5578; Fax: 81-75-251-5663; e-mail: mueta@koto.kpu-m.ac.jp.

associated with SJS/TEN with ocular complications. SJS/TEN may be different from allergic diseases since in both Arg110Gln of IL-13- and Gln551Arg of IL-4R polymorphisms the ratio of each allele was the inverse of that reported for atopy and asthma. IL-4R and FasL may play a role in innate immunity which reportedly able to regulate allergy and apoptosis.

We hypothesized that viral infection and/or drugs may trigger a disorder in the host innate immune response and that this event is followed by aggravated inflammation of the mucosa, ocular surface, and skin.

Ophthalmologists and dermatologists documented that the HLA-B12 (HLA-Bw44) antigen was significantly increased in Caucasian SJS patients; in our Japanese study population there was no such association. Although HLA-A*0206 was strongly associated with SJS/TEN with ocular complications in the Japanese, it is absent in Caucasian populations, suggesting strong ethnic differences in the HLA-SJS/TEN association.

Genetic and environmental factors may play a role in an integrated etiology of SJS/TEN and there may be an association between SJS/TEN with ocular complications and disordered innate immunity.

STEVENS-JOHNSON SYNDROME (SJS)

SJS, an acute inflammatory vesiculobullous reaction of the skin and mucous membranes, was first described in 1922 by the American pediatricians Stevens and Johnson [1]. They reported 2 boys aged 7 and 8 who presented with "an extraordinary, generalized eruption with continued fever, inflamed buccal mucosa and severe purulent conjunctivitis" that progressed to severe visual disturbance. By careful inquiry that showed that no drugs had been administered to either patient, they ruled out that the skin eruption was due to drug ingestion. Other pediatricians subsequently claimed that SJS was associated with infectious agents such as Mycoplasma pneumoniae [2] or a viral etiology involving herpes simplex-, Epstein-Barr-, cytomegalo-, and varicella zoster virus [3].

On the other hand, dermatologists reported that SJS and its severe variant, toxic epidermal necrolysis (TEN), are life-threatening severe adverse drug reactions characterized by high fever, rapidly developing blistering exanthema of macules, and target-like lesions accompanied by mucosal involvement and skin detachment [4]. The number of causative drugs was estimated to exceed 100 [5].

Although erythema multiforme (EM), SJS, and TEN were formerly accepted as part of a single "EM spectrum", a retrospective analysis of the type and distribution of skin lesions and the extent of epidermal detachment identified EM major and SJS/TEN as 2 separate clinical entities that differed with respect to histopathologic changes and etiology [6]. The annual incidence of SJS and TEN has been estimated as 0.4-1 and 1-6 cases per million persons, respectively [6,7]; the mortality rate is 3 and 27%, respectively [8]. Although rare, these reactions carry high morbidity and mortality rates and often result in severe and definitive sequelae such as vision loss. The pathobiological mechanisms underlying the onset of SJS/TEN have not been fully established. The extreme rarity of cutaneous and ocular surface reactions due to drug therapies led us to suspect individual susceptibility.

In Europe and the USA, a consensus classification was proposed. Accordingly, in bullous EM, less than 10% of the body surface area (BSA) is detached and localized typical- or raised atypical targets are present. Patients with SJS manifest detachment of less than 10% of BSA and widespread erythematous or purpuric macules or flat atypical targets. In overlapping SJS/TEN detachment involves 10 - 30% of BSA and there are widespread purpuric macules or flat atypical targets. TEN with spots shows more than 30% detachment with widespread purpuric macules or flat atypical targets. Lastly, patients with TEN without spots exhibit more than 10% detachment, large epidermal sheets, and no purpuric macules [5,6].

In Japan, SJS is diagnosed when patients manifest less than 10% BSA detachment, widespread blistering exanthema of macules, and atypical target-like lesions accompanied by mucosal involvement. A diagnosis of TEN is made when BSA detachment exceeds that seen in SJS [9].

Dermatologists tend to see patients with SJS/TEN in the acute stage while many patients encountered by ophthalmologists present in the chronic stage. Of our 71 SJS/TEN patients, 77% were in the chronic-, 10% in the subacute-, and 13% in the acute stage when they first reported to our hospital. It is difficult for ophthalmologists to render a differential diagnosis of SJS or TEN when patients present in the chronic stage because the vesiculobullous skin lesion expressed in the acute- have healed by the chronic stage. Thus, ophthalmologists tend to report both SJS and TEN as "SJS" in a broad sense. Our diagnosis of SJS/TEN (SJS in the broad sense) was based on a confirmed history of acute-onset high fever, serious mucocutaneous illness with skin eruptions, and involvement of at least 2 mucosal sites including the ocular surface [10-16].

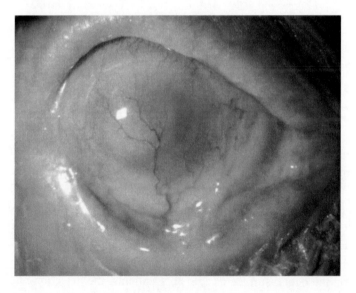

Figure 1. Ocular surface sequelae in SJS. In this 54-year old woman, the ocular surface sequelae of SJS, i.e. conjunctival invasion into the cornea and symblepharon, persisted 25 years after disease onset.

In the acute stage, SJS/TEN patients manifest severe conjunctivitis, alolpecia, and corneal/conjunctival epithelial defects with vesiculobullous skin lesions. Without adequate treatment, persistent epithelial defects occur and often progress to corneal melting and perforation. In the chronic stage, ocular surface complications such as conjunctival invasion into the cornea due to corneal epithelial stem cell deficiency, symblepharon, ankyloblepharon, dry eye, trichiasis, and in some instances, keratinization of the ocular surface, persist despite the healing of the skin lesions (Figure 1) [10]. The conjunctival invasion into the cornea results in severe visual disturbance. SJS/TEN is one of the most devastating ocular surface diseases leading to corneal damage and loss of vision. Moreover, we observed that more than 95% of patients with SJS/TEN with ocular complications had lost their fingernails in the acute- or subacute stage and that some continue to have transformed nails even after healing of the skin lesions (Figure 2) [11,14]. The reported incidence of ocular complications in SJS/TEN is 50-68% [7,8].

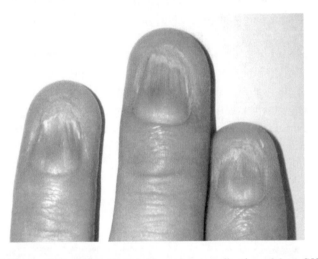

Figure 2. Transformed fingernails in SJS patients with ocular complications. Many SJS/TEN patients with ocular complications lost their fingernails during the acute stage and some continue to have transformed nails even after healing of the skin lesions.

SJS AND DISORDERED INNATE IMMUNITY

Drugs are probably the most widely accepted etiologic factor in SJS/TEN [4,5,17]. SJS/TEN patients often had the prodromata, including nonspecific fever, coryza, and sore throat, that closely mimic upper respiratory tract infections commonly treated with antibiotics [7,14]. These prodromata were evident from the clinical records of our SJS/TEN patients [14]. In fact, 55 of 71 patients we examined (77.5%) developed SJS after drug treatment for the common cold with antibiotics, cold remedies, and/or non-steroid anti-inflammatory drugs. Only 4 of our 71 patients (5.6%) developed SJS after drug treatment to prevent convulsion.

Moreover, on the ocular surface of SJS/TEN patients, the detection rate for methicillin-resistant Staphylococcus aureus (MRSA) or methicillin-resistant Staphylococcus epidermidis (MRSE) was higher than in other devastating ocular surface disorders [18].

Given the association between the onset of SJS/TEN and infections, and the opportunistic infection of ocular surfaces by bacteria such as MRSA or MRSE, we considered the possibility that there is an association between SJS/TEN and a disordered innate immune response [11,14]. We postulated that viral infection and/or drugs may trigger a disorder in the host's innate immune response and that this event is followed by aggravated inflammation of the mucous membranes, ocular surface, and skin and that the ocular surface inflammation of SJS is attributable to anomalies in mucosal innate immunity.

We previously reported that IκBζ-/- mice with a 129/Ola×C57BL/6 background expressly exhibit severe, spontaneous ocular surface inflammation accompanied by the eventual loss of almost all goblet cells [19]. Moreover, Balb/c background IκBζ KO mice showed not only spontaneous ocular surface- but also perioral inflammation (Figure 3) [20]. Thus, we propose IκBζ-/- mice as a suitable model for SJS because they manifest the loss of goblet cells seen in human SJS (Figure 3) [19]. IκBζ is induced by diverse pathogen-associated molecular patterns (PAMPs) and regulates NF-κB activity [21]. Thus, IκBζ is important for Toll like receptor signaling, which is essential for the innate immune response. The spontaneous ocular surface inflammation in IκBζ KO mice suggests the possibility that dysfunction/abnormality of innate immunity can lead to ocular surface inflammation.

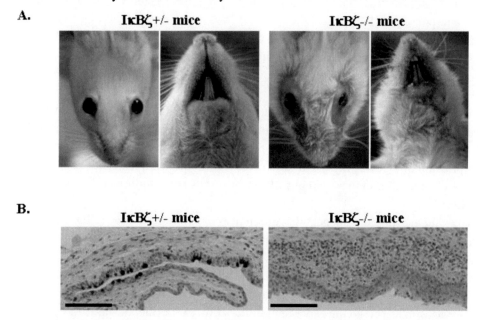

Figure 3. A. The inflammatory phenotype in the eyes and perioral skin of IκBζ-/- mice.The photographs show the face and perioral skin of 29-week-old IκBζ+/- and IκBζ-/- mice (23 weeks post-onset). B. Histological analysis of the eyelids of IκBζ-/- mice.The eyelids of 13-week-old IκBζ+/- and IκBζ-/- mice 8 weeks after symptom onset. Goblet cells were stained purple by PAS stain. Each bar represents a length of 100 μm.

Based on these considerations we postulated that dysfunction/abnormality of innate immunity may be present in human ocular surface inflammatory disorders. The ocular surface epithelium neither responds to commensal bacteria nor does it induce inflammation against them. However, a hyper-inflammatory reaction against bacteria may induce ocular surface inflammation. Even the healthy ocular surface harbors commensal bacteria such as *S. epidermidis* and *P. acnes* and under normal conditions there is no inflammation despite the presence of resident commensal bacteria. Whereas elderly people who are hospitalized do not exhibit ocular surface inflammation even when MRSA or MRSE reside on their ocular surface, SJS patients often have severe ocular surface inflammation when these bacteria are detected on their ocular surface. Moreover, the ocular surface inflammation of patients with SJS is greatly reduced after treatment with antibiotics against MRSA or MRSE. Although the role of acquired immunity in the pathogenicity of SJS/TEN has been reported, to date the critical role of innate immunity in the pathophysiology of SJS/TEN, i.e. the bridging between the acute response to invading non-self molecules and chronic local immune inflammation, has not been recognized.

SJS AND INNATE IMMUNITY

Under the hypothesis of a disordered innate immune response, we performed gene expression- and SNP association analysis to examine the existence of a disordered innate immune response in SJS/TEN.

For gene expression analysis we used monocytes derived from peripheral blood because these cells are essential for innate immunity. First we subjected CD14$^+$ cells from peripheral blood of 4 SJS/TEN patients and 3 normal volunteers to gene expression analysis; the cells were cultured for 1 hr with or without LPS. We found that IL-4R gene expression was different in SJS/TEN patients and the controls; upon LPS stimulation, it was down-regulated in the patients and slightly up-regulated in the controls despite large individual differences with respect to LPS reactivity. Our study of 7 SJS/TEN patients and 6 controls showed that the expression of 2 genes, IκBζ and IL-1α was significantly lower in SJS/TEN patients than the controls after 1-hr culture without LPS. Our results were confirmed by quantitative RT-PCR assay.

Together, our findings suggest that differences in IL-4R gene expression and the reduced expression of the IκBζ and IL-1α genes may play an important role in the pathophysiology of SJS/TEN.

According to Correia et al. [22] IL-1α was significantly lower in the blister fluid of TEN- than burn patients. Our study detected a significant difference between SJS/TEN patients and the controls with respect to the expression of IL-1α by CD14$^+$ monocytes.

IκBζ induced by diverse PAMPs regulates NF-κB activity [21] possibly to prevent excessive inflammation in the presence of bacterial components [19,20,23]. Our preliminary report documented ocular surface inflammation in IκBζ KO mice [19,20]. We previously reported that virus dsRNA-mimic polyI:C, a TLR3 ligand, elicited the elevated expression of human IκBζ-specific mRNA in primary corneal epithelial cells [24]. Considering the induction of IκBζ by TLRs [21,24], the ocular surface inflammation seen in SJS/TEN patients may be related to innate PAMP-amplified immune responses to microbes.

Although SJS/TEN can be induced by drugs, not all patients treated with these drugs develop SJS/TEN and relatively few individuals present with SJS/TEN. To test the hypothesis that there is a genetic predisposition in individuals who develop SJS/TEN we subjected SJS/TEN patients with ocular complications to SNP association analysis. Here we show the results of our SNP analysis of 71 patients with SJS/TEN with ocular complications and 160 healthy controls. All study subjects provided prior informed written consent and all participants and volunteers were ethnically Japanese and resided in Japan.

First we examined the two genes, IκBζ and IL1α, for which there were differences between SJS/TEN patients and the controls in our gene expression analysis. With respect to IκBζ, we analyzed 7 polymorphisms reported in the Japanese Single Nucleotide Polymorphisms database (JSNP) (rs.2305991, rs.622122, rs.14134, rs.3217713, rs.595788, rs.677011, rs.3821727); we found no significant association in these 7 polymorphisms. For IL1α, we analyzed 5 SNPs reported in the JSNP database (rs.1609682, rs.1894399, rs.2071373, rs.2071375, rs.2071376), again there was no significant association in these 5 SNPs.

Next we examined the TLR2 closely related to *S. aureus* or *S. epidermidis* including MRSA and MRSE, because opportunistic infections of the ocular surface by MRSA and MRSE have been recognized in SJS/TEN patients with ocular complications [18]. For TLR2 we analyzed 3 SNPs reported in the JSNP (rs.3840100, rs.3840099, rs.3840097). There was no significant association in these 3 SNPs.

Moreover, we studied TLR3, because there is an association between the onset of SJS/TEN and infections; many SJS/TEN patients had prodromata including nonspecific fever, coryza, and sore throat that closely mimic upper respiratory tract infections commonly treated with antibiotics [14]. Elsewhere we documented that the human ocular surface epithelium harbors messages for most TLRs, that TLR3 is the most highly expressed TLR, and that the cell-surface TLR3 of human corneal epithelial cells responds to virus dsRNA-mimic polyI:C to generate pro-inflammatory cytokines and IFN-β [24]. Therefore, we performed SNP association analysis of the TLR3 gene. Our study of 7 SNPs reported in the JSNP database (rs.3775290, rs.3775291, rs.3775292, rs.3775293, rs.3775294, rs.3775295, rs.3775296), SNP rs.3775296T/G manifested a significant association under a recessive model (rs.3775296 T/G + G/G vs T/T, raw p-value = 0.00006, corrected p-value = 0.0004, OR = 0.18) and a weak inverse association with allele frequency (G vs T, raw p value = 0.01, corrected p value = 0.07, OR = 0.59). When we corrected the p-value for the 7 alleles tested, the results ceased to be significant. SNP rs.3775290A/G also showed a weak inverse association under a recessive model (rs.3775290 A/G + G/G vs A/A, raw p-value = 0.02, corrected p-value = 0.12, OR = 0.43). Analysis of the genotype pattern of SNPs rs.3775296T/G and rs.3775290A/G revealed a strong association between rs.3775290A/A - rs.3775296T/T and SJS/TEN in Japanese patients (χ^2 test, p = 0.00007, OR = 6.3, 95% CI = 2.3 -17.2). Our results suggest that polymorphisms in the TLR3 gene may be associated with SJS/TEN in the Japanese [14]. According to the International HapMap project, rs.3775296 SNP exists not only in Japanese- (G/G 0.386, G/T 0.500, T/T 0.114) but also in Han Chinese- (G/G 0.659, G/T 0.295, T/T 0.046) and Caucasian (G/G 0.719, G/T 0.263, T/T 0.018) populations, indicating that it is important to examine TLR3 SNPs in non-Japanese populations.

We hypothesized that viral infection and/or drugs may trigger a disorder in the host innate immune response and that this event is followed by aggravated inflammation of the mucosa, ocular surface, and skin [14]. Therefore, genetic and environmental factors may play a role in an integrated etiology of SJS/TEN [11-16] and there is a possible association between SJS/TEN and a disordered innate immunity.

SJS AND ALLERGY

We also examined the SNPs of IL-4R genes because in our GeneChip analysis IL-4R gene expression was different in SJS/TEN patients and the controls.

The IL-4R gene is an important allergy-related gene. As its well-documented polymorphisms include Ile50Val (rs.1805010), Ser478Pro (rs.1805015), and Gln551Arg (rs.1801275), we compared these polymorphisms between Japanese patients with SJS/TEN and healthy Japanese volunteers. Among the 3 SNPs of IL-4R, Gln551Arg showed a significant association with allele frequency (A vs G, raw p value = 0.0016, corrected p value = 0.0048, OR = 3.5) and the dominant model (A/A vs A/G + G/G, raw p value = 0.0021, corrected p value = 0.0065, OR = 3.6) [11,13]. With respect to Gln551Arg polymorphisms, although Arg551 alleles were significantly increased in atopy [25] and asthma [26], in SJS/TEN patients Gln551- but not Arg551 alleles were significantly increased. SJS/TEN was associated with Gln551Arg, shown to have no effect on IgE synthesis [27], but not with Ile50Val and Ser478Pro associated with IgE synthesis [27,28]. Next we investigated the relationship between serum IgE and SJS/TEN; we assayed both total- and antigen-specific IgE. There was no significant difference between SJS/TEN patients and the controls with respect to the incidence of high total serum IgE [11]. In addition, assessment of positivity for antigen-specific IgE showed no marked difference between the 2 groups [11]. Our results indicate that serum IgE was not associated with SJS/TEN and they coincide with the finding that it was associated with Gln551Arg, which has no effect on IgE synthesis.

A strong genetic predisposition underlies the manifestation of allergic diseases [25-28]. IL-4R is representative of the candidate genes for atopy and asthma. Our results show that in Japanese patients with SJS/TEN there might be an association with IL-4R gene polymorphisms. However, based on our findings we posit that SJS/TEN is different from allergic diseases such as atopy and asthma because the ratio of each allele of the polymorphisms was the opposite of the ratio reported in atopy and asthma.

It has been suggested that the pathogenesis of TEN involves cytotoxic CD8[+] lymphocytes [29]. As CD8[+] T-cells involve Th1 cytokine-driven inflammatory mechanisms, such mechanisms may play a role in the skin inflammation seen in the acute stage of SJS/TEN. In contrast, Th2 cytokine-driven inflammatory mechanisms may play a role in the inflammation seen in allergic diseases such as atopy and asthma [25-28].

Ophthalmologically, the ocular surface inflammation seen in SJS/TEN is quite different from allergic inflammation. In SJS/TEN, goblet cells in the conjunctiva are remarkably decreased or disappear [30], whereas in allergic diseases their number is increased [31]. IL-4 induces the differentiation of IL-4R-expressing epithelium into mucous goblet cells [32]. We confirmed IL-4R-specific mRNA expression in conjunctival epithelial cells. It is possible that IL-4R on the ocular surface plays an important role in the ocular surface inflammation seen in not only allergic diseases but also SJS/TEN. In the acute- or subacute stage, the discharge from the ocular surface of SJS/TEN patients consists primarily of neutrophils [11]; in patients with allergic- and atopic conjunctivitis it is mainly comprised of eosinophils. Thus, based on both dermatologic and ophthalmologic findings, SJS/TEN is quite different from allergic diseases.

Our finding that in human corneal epithelial cells IL-4R-specific mRNA was down-regulated upon stimulation with PolyI:C that mimics viral components, suggests that IL-4R is linked with innate immunity.

IL-4Rα is a component of not only the IL-4- but also the IL-13 receptor and is essential for both IL-4 and IL-13 signaling. The type-I IL-4 receptor is composed of 2 subunits, an α subunit (IL-4Rα) that binds IL-4 and transduces its growth-promoting and transcription-activating functions, and a γc subunit common to several cytokine receptors that amplifies signaling of IL-4Rα. The IL-13 receptor (IL-13R) is composed of the IL-4Rα chain (IL-4Rα) and the IL-13Rα1 chain (IL-13Rα1) [33]. As IL-4 is able to bind to this receptor, it is also called type-II IL-4R [33]. There exists another IL-13 binding unit, the IL-13Rα2 chain (IL-13Rα2); it acts as a decoy receptor [33].

Since there is an association between SJS/TEN and IL4Rα polymorphism, we speculated that there might be an association between IL-4- and/or IL-13 signaling and SJS/TEN. Therefore, we examined IL-4- and IL-13 gene polymorphisms and their combination with IL-4R polymorphism.

With respect to IL-4 gene polymorphisms, a variant of the promoter region of the IL-4 gene, -590C/T, has been shown to be related to asthma [34-36]. Regarding IL-13 gene polymorphisms, a variant of the promoter region of the IL-13 gene, -1111C/T [28,37] and a variant of Arg110Gln were reportedly associated with asthma [38].

We examined polymorphisms of the promoter -590C/T (rs.2243250) in the IL-4 gene, and of -1111C/T (rs.1800925) and Arg110Gln (rs.20541) in the IL-13 gene in Japanese SJS/TEN patients with ocular complications and healthy volunteers. We also assayed their plasma IL-13 level since Arg110Gln in the IL-13 gene affects the serum level of IL-13 [39].

In the promoter -590C/T SNP of the IL-4 gene related to higher IgE levels [34] there was no significant association [13], nor was there a significant association in the promoter -1111C/T SNP of the IL-13 gene related to asthma [28,37]. Gln110Arg SNPs of IL-13 exhibited a significant association with allele frequency (G vs A, raw p-value = 0.017, corrected p-value = 0.034, OR =1.8) even when we corrected the p-value for the number of alleles detected in IL13 SNPs (n=2) [13]. It also exhibited a weak association with the recessive model (G/G +G/A vs A/A, raw p-value = 0.046, corrected p-value = 0.092, OR = 4.1); correction of the p-value for the number of alleles detected (n=2) rendered the result not significant [13]. These findings contrast with those of Heinzmann et al. [38] who reported that Gln110 was significantly increased in human asthma. We detected a significant increase in Arg110 in our SJS/TEN patients [13].

We also studied the plasma IL-13 level in our SJS/TEN patients because these levels were reportedly higher in individuals with Gln110 [39]. Comparison of plasma IL-13 in Arg110Arg and Arg110Gln genotypes showed that its level was significantly higher in SJS/TEN patients with the Arg110Gln- than the Arg110Arg genotype [13]. Plasma IL-13 levels tended to be lower in SJS/TEN patients than the controls, however, the difference was not statistically significant [13]. Our results are in accord with findings that SJS/TEN with ocular surface complications is associated with Arg110Gln, which affects the plasma IL-13 level. In SJS/TEN there is a significant increase in the Arg110 allele; this increase may result in lower serum IL-13 levels than controls.

We also analyzed the genotype pattern of IL-4R SNP Arg551Gln and IL-13 SNP Arg110Gln. We found that the Gln551Gln(A/A) – Arg110Arg(G/G) genotype pattern also associated with SJS/TEN in Japanese patients (χ^2 test, p = 0.0009, OR = 2.6, 95% CI = 1.5 - 4.6) [13], suggesting that IL-4R and IL-13 polymorphisms exert combined effects.

SJS/TEN is different from allergic diseases such as atopy and asthma because the ratio of each allele of the IL-13 SNP Arg110Gln was the opposite of the ratio in atopy and asthma. Namely, in SJS/TEN, Arg110- rather than Gln110 alleles, which are significantly increased in asthma [38], showed a significant increase. Arima et al. [39] reported that the Gln110 variant of Gln110Arg decreased the affinity with IL-13Rα2, a decoy receptor, and enhanced its stability as a protein, resulting in the up-regulation of the IL-13 concentration *in vivo*. The results we obtained by polymorphism analysis were supported by our findings that the plasma IL-13 level tended to be lower in patients with SJS/TEN.

Dermatologists who examined the IL-13 levels in the serum or skin lesions of acute-phase SJS/TEN patients reported that the expression of IL-13 was up-regulated [40]. They also found that the serum IL-13 levels normalized in all 3 STN/TEN patients tested after the resolution of the cutaneous disease. We assayed serum IL-13 in SJS/TEN patients in the chronic- or sub-acute phase whose cutaneous disease was resolved. We propose that the baseline serum IL-13 level in the chronic- or sub-acute-, but not in the acute phase, tends to be lower in SJS/TEN patients with ocular complications than in the controls because the Arg110Arg genotype, in which the IL-13 level was reportedly lower than in Arg110Gln, was significantly increased in SJS/TEN patients with ocular complications.

SJS AND FasL

In the acute stage of SJS/TEN the skin lesions were histologically characterized by marked keratinocyte apoptosis in the epidermis with dermo-epidermal separation, resulting in bullae [41]. Moreover, in the acute stage, SJS/TEN patients manifested increased Fas Ligand (FasL) serum levels [42,43]. The activation of Fas through FasL was an important first step leading to the diffuse death of epidermal cells in SJS/TEN [42,43]. Therefore, we performed SNP association analysis of the FasL gene. We examined 4 SNPs of FasL reported in the JSNP database (rs.929087, rs.3830150, rs.2639614, rs.2859247).

SNP rs.3830150 A/G exhibited a significant strong inverse association with allele frequency (A vs G, raw and corrected p-value 0.004 and 0.016, respectively; OR = 0.49) and with the dominant model (A/A vs A/G + G/G, raw and corrected p-value = 0.001 and 0.005, respectively; OR = 0.39). SNP rs.2639614 G/A had a significant inverse association with allele frequency (G vs A, raw p-value = 0.020; OR = 0.51) and with the dominant model (G/G vs G/A + A/A, raw p value = 0.017; OR = 0.46), although the results ceased to be significant when we corrected the p-value for the number of alleles tested (n=4). Analysis of the genotype pattern of SNPs rs.3830150 and rs.2639614 (rs.3830150 A/A - rs.2639614 G/G) showed a strong inverse association with SJS/TEN in Japanese patients (χ^2 test, p = 0.0006, OR = 0.37, 95% CI = 0.2 - 0.7).

Our results suggest that polymorphisms in the FasL gene may be associated with SJS/TEN in the Japanese population. According to the International HapMap project, rs.3830150 and rs.2639614 SNP, which showed a significant association with SJS/TEN, exist not only in Japanese- but also in Han Chinese- and Caucasian populations, indicating that it is important to examine FasL SNPs in non-Japanese populations.

In the mouse eye FasL is expressed by the corneal epithelium and endothelium [44]. To maintain the cornea as a transparent barrier, the Fas-FasL pathway has a special significance in corneal immune privilege and in limiting inflammation [45]. However, the role of Fas/FasL-induced apoptosis in the pathogenesis of ocular complications in SJS patients has not been described and the part played by Fas/FasL signaling in chronic ocular surface inflammation remains unknown.

As apoptosis can reportedly be regulated by innate immunity [46], we considered the possibility that there is an association between SJS/TEN and a disordered innate immune response.

SJS AND HLA

Regarding SJS and HLA, 2 studies reported by American ophthalmologists [47] and French dermatologists [48] showed that the HLA-B12 (HLA-Bw44) antigen was significantly increased in Caucasian SJS patients. However, in our Japanese study population we did not find an association with HLA-B12, probably because in Caucasians the HLA-B12 antigen is primarily coded by HLA-B*4402 whereas in Japanese it is almost exclusively coded by HLA-B*4403 [16]. On the other hand, HLA-A*0206 was strongly associated with SJS/TEN with ocular complications in the Japanese (Table 2) [15, 16] although HLA-A*0206 is absent in Caucasians. Moreover, HLA-DQB1*0601 is reportedly associated with Caucasian SJS patients with ocular complications [49]. We, on the other hand, did not detect an association between SJS/TEN and HLA-DQB1*0601 in Japanese SJS patients with ocular complications [16], suggesting that there are strong ethnic differences in the HLA-SJS/TEN association.

With respect to the connection between drugs and severe cutaneous adverse reactions (SCAR) including SJS and TEN, there appears to be an association between the HLA-B*1502 allele and carbamazepine-induced SJS/TEN [50, 51] and between the HLA-B* 5801 allele and allopurinol-induced SCAR [52,53].

In Han Chinese-, but not in Caucasian patients, there was a strong carbamazepine-specific association between HLA-B*1502 and carbamazepine-induced SJS/TEN [50, 51, 53]. We attribute our failure to detect HLA-B*1502 in Japanese SJS/TEN patients and controls [16] to the very low allele frequency of HLA-B*1502 in the Japanese. We posit that the carbamazepine-specific association between HLA and carbamazepine-induced SJS is specific for certain ethnic groups.

As the allopurinol-specific association between HLA-B* 5801 and allopurinol-induced SCAR was detected in all Han Chinese- [52], in Caucasian- [53], and in Japanese patients [54], the strong allopurinol-specific association between HLA-B*5801 and allopurinol-induced SCAR (including SJS, TEN and Drug-induced Hypersensitivity Syndrome(DIHS)) may be universal. However, it is noteworthy that our 71 Japanese SJS/TEN patients with ocular complications included no patients in whom SJS/TEN was related to allopurinol (unpublished data). It is possible that allopurinol-induced SCAR does not tend to result in serious sequelae on the ocular surface.

Table 1. SNPs of Japanese SJS/TEN patients with ocular surface complications

	Control (%) (N=160)	SJS/TEN (%) (N=71)	Allele 1 v.s. Allele 2 P-value(χ^2) OR (95%CI)	Genotype 11 vs 12+22 P-value(χ^2) OR (95%CI)	Genotype 11+12 vs 22 P-value(χ^2) OR (95%CI)
Genes related to innate immunity					
TLR3 gene SNPs					
rs.3775290					
11 GG	63 (39.4)	26 (36.6)	0.13	0.69	**0.02**
12 GA	78 (48.8)	28 (39.4)	-	-	**0.43**
22 AA	19 (11.9)	17 (23.9)	(-)	(-)	**(0.20-0.88)**
rs.3775296					
GG	77 (48.1)	30 (42.3)	**0.01**	0.41	**0.00006**
GT	75 (46.9)	25 (35.2)	**0.59**	-	**0.18**
22 TT	8 (5.0)	16 (22.5)	**(0.39-0.90)**	(-)	**(0.07-0.45)**
Allergy-related genes					
IL4R					
Gln(A)551Arg(G) (rs.1801275)					
AA	115(71.9)	64(90.1)	**0.0016**	**0.0021**	0.18
AG	41(25.6)	7(9.9)	**3.5**	**3.6**	-
22 GG	4(2.5)	0(0)	**(1.5-7.9)**	**(1.5-8.4)**	(-)
IL13					
Arg(G)110Gln(A) (rs.20541)					
11 GG	77(48.1)	44(62.0)	**0.017**	0.051	**0.046**
12 GA	66(41.2)	25(35.2)	**1.8**	-	**4.1**
22 AA	17(10.6)	2(2.8)	**(1.1-2.8)**	(-)	**(0.9-18.3)**
Apoptosis-related gene					
FasL					
rs.3830150					
AA	118 (73.8)	37 (52.1)	**0.004**	**0.001**	0.92
AG	40 (25.0)	33 (46.5)	**0.49**	**0.39**	-
GG	2 (1.3)	1 (1.4)	**(0.3-0.8)**	**(0.2-0.7)**	(-)
rs.2639614					
GG	131(81.9)	48(67.6)	**0.020**	**0.017**	0.55
GA	28 (17.5)	22 (31.0)	**0.51**	**0.46**	-
AA	1 (0.6)	1 (1.4)	**(0.3-0.9)**	**(0.2-0.9)**	(-)

Drugs are probably the most widely accepted etiologic factor in SJS/TEN [4,5,17]. It is worth noting that SJS/TEN patients often experienced the prodromata, including nonspecific fever, coryza, and sore throat, that closely mimic upper respiratory tract infections commonly treated with antibiotics [7,14]. We ascertained that our patients manifested these prodromata by carefully reviewing their medical records [14].

Table 2.

HLA-A alleles	Carrier frequency				Gene frequency			
	SJS (n=71)	Normal (n=160)	p-value (χ^2)	Odds Ratio	SJS (n=142)	Normal (n=320)	p-value (χ^2)	Odds Ratio
*0101	0.0% (0/71)	1.9% (3/160)	0.25	-	0.0% (0/142)	0.9% (3/320)	0.25	-
*0201	26.8% (19/71)	19.4% (31/160)	0.21	-	15.5% (22/142)	10.1% (34/320)	0.14	-
*0206	42.3% (30/71)	16.9% (27/160)	0.00004 *	3.6	22.5% (32/142)	8.4% (27/320)	0.00003 *	3.1
*0207	7.0% (5/71)	8.1% (13/160)	0.78	-	3.5% (5/142)	4.1% (13/320)	0.78	-
*0210	0.0% (0/71)	0.6% (1/160)	0.50	-	0.0% (0/142)	0.3% (1/320)	0.51	-
*0301	1.4% (1/71)	0.0% (0/160)	0.13	-	0.7% (1/142)	0.0% (0/320)	0.13	-
*0302	0.0% (0/71)	0.6% (1/160)	0.50	-	0.0% (0/142)	0.3% (1/320)	0.51	-
*1101	5.6% (4/71)	20.0% (32/160)	0.005	0.24	2.8% (4/142)	10.0% (32/320)	0.008	0.26
*2402	52.1% (37/71)	58.8% (94/160)	0.35	-	29.6% (42/142)	35.6% (114/320)	0.20	-
*2601	9.9% (7/71)	10.0% (16/160)	0.97	-	4.9% (7/142)	5.0% (16/320)	0.97	-
*2602	5.6% (4/71)	3.1% (5/160)	0.36	-	2.8% (4/142)	1.9% (6/320)	0.52	-
*2603	1.4% (1/71)	9.4% (15/160)	0.03	0.14	0.7% (1/142)	4.7% (15/320)	0.03	0.14
*2605	0.0% (0/71)	0.6% (1/160)	0.50	-	0.0% (0/142)	0.3% (1/320)	0.51	-
*2901	0.0% (0/71)	2.5% (4/160)	0.18	-	0.0% (0/142)	1.3% (4/320)	0.18	-
*3001	1.4% (1/71)	0.0% (0/160)	0.13	-	0.7% (1/142)	0.0% (0/320)	0.13	-
*3101	9.9% (7/71)	21.3% (34/160)	0.04	0.41	4.9% (7/142)	11.3% (36/320)	0.03	0.41
*3201	0.0% (0/71)	0.6% (1/160)	0.50		0.0% (0/142)	0.3% (1/320)	0.51	-
*3303	22.5% (16/71)	10.0% (16/160)	0.01	2.6	11.3% (16/142)	5.0% (16/320)	0.01	2.4

*; The p-value corrected for the number of alleles detected (n=18) is significant.

Yetiv et. al. [7], who performed a retrospective analysis of the etiologic factors in 54 SJS patients diagnosed at Johns Hopkins between 1996 and 1976, concluded that drugs and infections were especially suspect as etiologic agents in SJS. They stated that although they were able to review information on the administered drugs, they could not conclude that these drugs were in fact the etiologic factors because the prodromata of SJS (nonspecific fever, coryza, sore throat, and malaise) involve symptoms that closely mimic upper respiratory tract infections commonly treated with antibiotics. They warned that although SJS is frequently attributed to antibiotics, it is impossible to state unequivocally that SJS developed as a result of the drug treatment because the possibility that the prodromata would have progressed to full-blown SJS in the absence of the drugs cannot be ruled out.

In our series, 55 of 71 patients (77.5%) presented with SJS after receiving antibiotics, cold remedies, and/or non-steroid anti-inflammatory drugs to treat the common cold. On the other hand, only 4 of 71 patients (5.6%) developed SJS after undergoing drug treatment for the prevention of convulsion.

According to a group of dermatologists, allopurinol, a uric acid-lowering drug (17.4%), anticonvulsants such as carbamazepine (8.2%), nevirapine (5.5%), phenobarbital (5.3%), phenytoin (5.0%), and lamotrigine (3.7%) were frequently associated with SJS or TEN, as was cotrimoxazole (6.3%), an antibiotic [52]. We suspect that dermatologists and ophthalmologists encounter different subsets of SJS or TEN patients.

In summary, genetic and environmental factors may play a role in an integrated etiology of SJS/TEN and SJS/TEN with ocular complications may be associated with disordered innate immunity.

REFERENCES

[1] Stevens AM, Johnson FC. A new eruptive fever associated with stomatitis and opthalmia: report of two cases in children. *Am J Dis Child* 1922; 24:526-33.
[2] Leaute-Labreze C, Lamireau T, Chawki D, Maleville J, Taieb A. Diagnosis, classification, and management of erythema multiforme and Stevens-Johnson syndrome. *Arch Dis Child* 2000; 83:347-52.
[3] Forman R, Koren G, Shear NH. Erythema multiforme, Stevens-Johnson syndrome and toxic epidermal necrolysis in children: a review of 10 years' experience. *Drug Saf* 2002; 25:965-72.
[4] Roujeau JC, Kelly JP, Naldi L, Rzany B, Stern RS, Anderson T, et al. Medication use and the risk of Stevens-Johnson syndrome or toxic epidermal necrolysis. *N Engl J Med* 1995; 333:1600-7.
[5] Wolf R, Orion E, Marcos B, Matz H. Life-threatening acute adverse cutaneous drug reactions. *Clin Dermatol* 2005; 23:171-81.
[6] Auquier-Dunant A, Mockenhaupt M, Naldi L, Correia O, Schroder W, Roujeau JC. Correlations between clinical patterns and causes of erythema multiforme majus, Stevens-Johnson syndrome, and toxic epidermal necrolysis: results of an international prospective study. *Arch Dermatol* 2002; 138:1019-24.
[7] Yetiv JZ, Bianchine JR, Owen JA, Jr. Etiologic factors of the Stevens-Johnson syndrome. *South Med J* 1980; 73:599-602.

[8] Power WJ, Ghoraishi M, Merayo-Lloves J, Neves RA, Foster CS. Analysis of the acute ophthalmic manifestations of the erythema multiforme/Stevens-Johnson syndrome/toxic epidermal necrolysis disease spectrum. *Ophthalmology* 1995; 102:1669-76.

[9] Yamane Y, Aihara M, Ikezawa Z. Analysis of Stevens-Johnson syndrome and toxic epidermal necrolysis in Japan from 2000 to 2006. *Allergol Int* 2007; 56:419-25.

[10] Sotozono C, Ang LP, Koizumi N, Higashihara H, Ueta M, Inatomi T, et al. New grading system for the evaluation of chronic ocular manifestations in patients with Stevens-Johnson syndrome. *Ophthalmology* 2007; 114:1294-302.

[11] Ueta M, Sotozono C, Inatomi T, Kojima K, Hamuro J, Kinoshita S. Association of IL4R polymorphisms with Stevens-Johnson syndrome. *J Allergy Clin Immunol* 2007; 120:1457-9.

[12] Ueta M, Sotozono C, Inatomi T, Kojima K, Hamuro J, Kinoshita S. Association of Fas Ligand gene polymorphism with Stevens-Johnson syndrome. *Br J Ophthalmol* 2008; 92:989-91.

[13] Ueta M, Sotozono C, Inatomi T, Kojima K, Hamuro J, Kinoshita S. Association of combined IL-13/IL-4R signaling pathway gene polymorphism with Stevens-Johnson syndrome accompanied by ocular surface complications. *Invest Ophthalmol Vis Sci* 2008; 49:1809-13.

[14] Ueta M, Sotozono C, Inatomi T, Kojima K, Tashiro K, Hamuro J, et al. Toll-like receptor 3 gene polymorphisms in Japanese patients with Stevens-Johnson syndrome. *Br J Ophthalmol* 2007; 91:962-5.

[15] Ueta M, Sotozono C, Tokunaga K, Yabe T, Kinoshita S. Strong Association Between HLA-A*0206 and Stevens-Johnson Syndrome in the Japanese. *Am J Ophthalmol* 2007; 143:367-8.

[16] Ueta M, Tokunaga K, Sotozono C, Inatomi T, Yabe T, Matsushita M, et al. HLA class I and II gene polymorphisms in Stevens-Johnson syndrome with ocular complications in Japanese. *Mol Vis* 2008; 14:550-5.

[17] Halevy S, Ghislain PD, Mockenhaupt M, Fagot JP, Bouwes Bavinck JN, Sidoroff A, et al. Allopurinol is the most common cause of Stevens-Johnson syndrome and toxic epidermal necrolysis in Europe and Israel. *J Am Acad Dermatol* 2008; 58:25-32.

[18] Sotozono C, Inagaki K, Fujita A, Koizumi N, Sano Y, Inatomi T, et al. Methicillin-resistant Staphylococcus aureus and methicillin-resistant Staphylococcus epidermidis infections in the cornea. *Cornea* 2002; 21:S94-101.

[19] Ueta M, Hamuro J, Yamamoto M, Kaseda K, Akira S, Kinoshita S. Spontaneous ocular surface inflammation and goblet cell disappearance in I kappa B zeta gene-disrupted mice. *Invest Ophthalmol Vis Sci* 2005; 46:579-88.

[20] Ueta M, Hamuro J, Ueda E, Katoh N, Yamamoto M, Takeda K, et al. Stat6-independent tissue inflammation occurs selectively on the ocular surface and perioral skin of IkappaBzeta-/- mice. *Invest Ophthalmol Vis Sci* 2008; 49:3387-94.

[21] Yamamoto M, Yamazaki S, Uematsu S, Sato S, Hemmi H, Hoshino K, et al. Regulation of Toll/IL-1-receptor-mediated gene expression by the inducible nuclear protein IkappaBzeta. *Nature* 2004; 430:218-22.

[22]Correia O, Delgado L, Roujeau JC, Le Cleach L, Fleming-Torrinha JA. Soluble interleukin 2 receptor and interleukin 1alpha in toxic epidermal necrolysis: a comparative analysis of serum and blister fluid samples. *Arch Dermatol* 2002; 138:29-32.

[23]Yamazaki S, Muta T, Takeshige K. A novel IkappaB protein, IkappaB-zeta, induced by proinflammatory stimuli, negatively regulates nuclear factor-kappaB in the nuclei. *J Biol Chem* 2001; 276:27657-62.

[24]Ueta M, Hamuro J, Kiyono H, Kinoshita S. Triggering of TLR3 by polyI:C in human corneal epithelial cells to induce inflammatory cytokines. *Biochem Biophys Res Commun* 2005; 331:285-94.

[25]Oiso N, Fukai K, Ishii M. Interleukin 4 receptor alpha chain polymorphism Gln551Arg is associated with adult atopic dermatitis in Japan. *Br J Dermatol* 2000; 142:1003-6.

[26]Rosa-Rosa L, Zimmermann N, Bernstein JA, Rothenberg ME, Khurana Hershey GK. The R576 IL-4 receptor alpha allele correlates with asthma severity. *J Allergy Clin Immunol* 1999; 104:1008-14.

[27]Mitsuyasu H, Yanagihara Y, Mao XQ, Gao PS, Arinobu Y, Ihara K, et al. Cutting edge: dominant effect of Ile50Val variant of the human IL-4 receptor alpha-chain in IgE synthesis. *J Immunol* 1999; 162:1227-31.

[28]Howard TD, Koppelman GH, Xu J, Zheng SL, Postma DS, Meyers DA, et al. Gene-gene interaction in asthma: IL4RA and IL13 in a Dutch population with asthma. *Am J Hum Genet* 2002; 70:230-6.

[29]Correia O, Delgado L, Ramos JP, Resende C, Torrinha JA. Cutaneous T-cell recruitment in toxic epidermal necrolysis. Further evidence of CD8+ lymphocyte involvement. *Arch Dermatol* 1993; 129:466-8.

[30]Ohji M, Ohmi G, Kiritoshi A, Kinoshita S. Goblet cell density in thermal and chemical injuries. *Arch Ophthalmol* 1987; 105:1686-8.

[31]Foster CS, Rice BA, Dutt JE. Immunopathology of atopic keratoconjunctivitis. *Ophthalmology* 1991; 98:1190-6.

[32]Dabbagh K, Takeyama K, Lee HM, Ueki IF, Lausier JA, Nadel JA. IL-4 induces mucin gene expression and goblet cell metaplasia in vitro and in vivo. *J Immunol* 1999; 162:6233-7.

[33]Izuhara K, Arima K. Signal transduction of IL-13 and its role in the pathogenesis of bronchial asthma. *Drug News Perspect* 2004; 17:91-8.

[34]Basehore MJ, Howard TD, Lange LA, Moore WC, Hawkins GA, Marshik PL, et al. A comprehensive evaluation of IL4 variants in ethnically diverse populations: association of total serum IgE levels and asthma in white subjects. *J Allergy Clin Immunol* 2004; 114:80-7.

[35]Noguchi E, Shibasaki M, Arinami T, Takeda K, Yokouchi Y, Kawashima T, et al. Association of asthma and the interleukin-4 promoter gene in Japanese. *Clin Exp Allergy* 1998; 28:449-53.

[36]Walley AJ, Cookson WO. Investigation of an interleukin-4 promoter polymorphism for associations with asthma and atopy. *J Med Genet* 1996; 33:689-92.

[37]Kabesch M, Schedel M, Carr D, Woitsch B, Fritzsch C, Weiland SK, et al. IL-4/IL-13 pathway genetics strongly influence serum IgE levels and childhood asthma. *J Allergy Clin Immunol* 2006; 117:269-74.

[38]Heinzmann A, Mao XQ, Akaiwa M, Kreomer RT, Gao PS, Ohshima K, et al. Genetic variants of IL-13 signalling and human asthma and atopy. *Hum Mol Genet* 2000; 9:549-59.

[39]Arima K, Umeshita-Suyama R, Sakata Y, Akaiwa M, Mao XQ, Enomoto T, et al. Upregulation of IL-13 concentration in vivo by the IL13 variant associated with bronchial asthma. *J Allergy Clin Immunol* 2002; 109:980-7.

[40]Quaglino P, Caproni M, Osella-Abate S, Torchia D, Comessatti A, Del Bianco E, et al. Serum interleukin-13 levels are increased in patients with Stevens-Johnson syndrome/ toxic epidermal necrolysis but not in those with erythema multiforme. *Br J Dermatol* 2008; 158:184-6.

[41]Paul C, Wolkenstein P, Adle H, Wechsler J, Garchon HJ, Revuz J, et al. Apoptosis as a mechanism of keratinocyte death in toxic epidermal necrolysis. *Br J Dermatol* 1996; 134:710-4.

[42]Abe R, Shimizu T, Shibaki A, Nakamura H, Watanabe H, Shimizu H. Toxic epidermal necrolysis and Stevens-Johnson syndrome are induced by soluble Fas ligand. *Am J Pathol* 2003; 162:1515-20.

[43]Viard I, Wehrli P, Bullani R, Schneider P, Holler N, Salomon D, et al. Inhibition of toxic epidermal necrolysis by blockade of CD95 with human intravenous immunoglobulin. *Science* 1998; 282:490-3.

[44]Griffith TS, Brunner T, Fletcher SM, Green DR, Ferguson TA. Fas ligand-induced apoptosis as a mechanism of immune privilege. *Science* 1995; 270:1189-92.

[45]Niederkorn JY. See no evil, hear no evil, do no evil: the lessons of immune privilege. *Nat Immunol* 2006; 7:354-9.

[46]Jiang D, Liang J, Fan J, Yu S, Chen S, Luo Y, et al. Regulation of lung injury and repair by Toll-like receptors and hyaluronan. *Nat Med* 2005; 11:1173-9.

[47]Mondino BJ, Brown SI, Biglan AW. HLA antigens in Stevens-Johnson syndrome with ocular involvement. *Arch Ophthalmol* 1982; 100:1453-4.

[48]Roujeau JC, Bracq C, Huyn NT, Chaussalet E, Raffin C, Duedari N. HLA phenotypes and bullous cutaneous reactions to drugs. *Tissue Antigens* 1986; 28:251-4.

[49]Power WJ, Saidman SL, Zhang DS, Vamvakas EC, Merayo-Lloves JM, Kaufman AH, et al. HLA typing in patients with ocular manifestations of Stevens-Johnson syndrome. *Ophthalmology* 1996; 103:1406-9.

[50]Chung WH, Hung SI, Hong HS, Hsih MS, Yang LC, Ho HC, et al. Medical genetics: a marker for Stevens-Johnson syndrome. *Nature* 2004; 428:486.

[51]Lonjou C, Thomas L, Borot N, Ledger N, de Toma C, LeLouet H, et al. A marker for Stevens-Johnson syndrome.: ethnicity matters. *Pharmacogenomics* J 2006; 6:265-8.

[52]Hung SI, Chung WH, Liou LB, Chu CC, Lin M, Huang HP, et al. HLA-B*5801 allele as a genetic marker for severe cutaneous adverse reactions caused by allopurinol. *Proc Natl Acad Sci U S A* 2005; 102:4134-9.

[53]Lonjou C, Borot N, Sekula P, Ledger N, Thomas L, Halevy S, et al. A European study of HLA-B in Stevens-Johnson syndrome and toxic epidermal necrolysis related to five high-risk drugs. *Pharmacogenet Genomics* 2008; 18:99-107.

[54]Dainichi T, Uchi H, Moroi Y, Furue M. Stevens-Johnson syndrome, drug-induced hypersensitivity syndrome and toxic epidermal necrolysis caused by allopurinol in

patients with a common HLA allele: what causes the diversity? *Dermatology* 2007;
215:86-8.

In: Conjunctivitis: Symptoms, Treatment and Prevention   ISBN: 978-1-61668-321-4
Editor: Anna R. Sallinger, pp. 179-193   © 2010 Nova Science Publishers, Inc.

Chapter VI

OCULAR ADNEXAL MUCOSA-ASSOCIATED LYMPHOID TISSUE LYMPHOMA; ETIOLOGY, PATHOLOGY, CAUSATIVE FACTORS, AND TREATMENT

Yoshihiro Yakushijin and Toshio Kodama
Cancer Center of Ehime University Hospital,
Ehime Graduate School of Medicine
Division of Ophthalmology,
Matsuyama Red Cross Hospital, Japan.

INTRODUCTION

Although the involvement of systemic malignant lymphoma in the ocular region is rare, primary ocular lymphoma and reactive lymphoid hyperplasia (pseudo-lymphoma) have been increasing recently. These lymphoproliferative diseases in the ocular region exist in ocular adnexa such as conjunctiva, the adjoining orbit, and the lachrymal gland [1,2]. In conjunctiva, lymphocytes and plasma cells are found in the layer of substantia propria, which is designated mucosa-associated lymphoid tissue (MALT). When a long-standing inflammatory condition, such as toxic reaction, allergy, or infection, appears in the MALT, true follicles with visible germinal centers will be provoked [3]. Especially, the palpebral conjunctiva has lymphoid tissues containing components for immune responses, suggesting the term 'conjunctiva-associated lymphoid tissue' (CALT) [4]. In contrast, the orbit that mainly consists of fat, extrinsic muscles, and the lachrymal gland, has no distinct lymph node. Since the lachrymal gland, located in the lachrymal fossa in the anterior lateral portion of the roof of the orbit, possesses migrating lymphocytes and plasma cells in the interstitium of lobes after inflammatory stimulation, reactive pseudo-tumors (Figure 1), pseudo-lymphomas, and malignant lymphomas (Figure 2) are often observed there. In the current article, we discuss the incidence, etiology, diagnosis, and treatment of ocular adnexal MALT lymphoma, and focus on the possibility of microorganisms as pathogenetic factors in ocular adnexal MALT lymphoma, especially chlamydial infections.

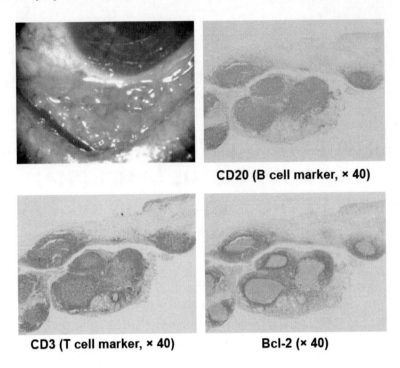

Figure 1. A case of pseudo-tumor; Lymphoid hyperplasia.

OCULAR ADNEXAL MALT LYMPHOMA IN EXTRANODAL MARGINAL ZONE B-CELL LYMPHOMA

The extra-nodal marginal zone (ENMZ) B-cell lymphoma of MALT is a distinct B-cell lymphoma that develops in extra-nodal sites and usually has an indolent clinical course as a localized disease. This lymphoma which accounts for 7-8% of adult non-Hodgkin lymphomas (NHL) was first recognized as a separate clinical pathologic entity by Isaacson and Wright in 1983 [5], and is presently featured in the World Health Organization (WHO) classification as a distinct lymphoma among the mature B-cell neoplasms [6]. These lymphoid tumor cells that possess a mature monocytoid appearance grow in extra-nodal lymphoid tissue and exist in epithelial tissue, and it is often difficult to distinguish malignant lymphoid tissue from benign inflammation. In approximately 12% of these ENMZ B-cell lymphomas, the presentation occurs in the orbital fat, conjunctiva, eyelid, lachrymal gland and sac [7]. This type of ENMZ B-cell lymphoma in ocular adnexa recently has been designated as ocular adnexal lymphoma of the MALT type or ocular adnexal MALT lymphoma (OAML). It is quite often misunderstood that ENMZ B-cell lymphoma and nodal marginal zone (NMZ) B-cell lymphoma are the same condition, which is simply appearing in different anatomical sites such as lymph nodes or extra lymph nodes. This is not correct. The

WHO classification defines NMZ B-cell lymphoma as "a primary nodal B-cell neoplasm that morphologically resembles lymph nodes involved by marginal zone lymphomas of extranodal or splenic types, but without evidence of extranodal or splenic disease", a distinct entity. This indicates that the OAML is never diagnosed as NMZ B-cell lymphoma, even if it is involved in lymph nodes after disease progression. Taken together, the disease prognosis is quite different for NMZ and ENMZ B-cell lymphomas, suggesting that they are clinically different types of disease entry [8].

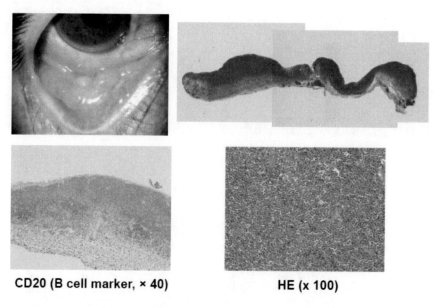

CD20 (B cell marker, × 40)   **HE (x 100)**

Figure 2. A case of ocular adnexal MALT lymphoma (OAML).

ETIOLOGY OF OCULAR ADNEXAL MALT LYMPHOMA

MALT lymphoma is the third most common NHL, and develops in extra-nodal sites such as the gastrointestinal (GI) tract, pharynx, salivary glands, lungs, and thyroid [9]. In this NHL, gastric MALT lymphoma is the most common and well-characterized. In contrast, OAML is a relatively rare disease and somewhat unfamiliar for hematologists and oncologists, because the majority of cases are first treated by ophthalmologists and radiologists. However, recent well-researched papers have reported that about 40-60% of cases of lymphoid tumors involving ocular adnexa are MALT lymphomas in Western countries [10-14], while in Asian countries such as Japan and Korea the percentage is about 80-90% [15]. OAML is not an excessively rare disease. The incidence of OAML is rapidly increasing with annual rates over 6% and no evidence of peaking [16]. This lymphoma arises in females after middle age with a higher prevalence [14,17]. The primary site of OAML is usually presented in ocular fat as tumors (Figure 3) in about 45-75% of cases [14]. The second site as a primary of OAML is the sub-conjunctiva or lachrymal gland (Figure 4-A, B). The involvement of the eyelid and lachrymal sac is rare as a primary disease site [14,18]. Bilateral involvement has occurred in 10-15% of cases [14,17], however, this tumor usually localizes in the primary site and distant tumor metastasis is rare at the first diagnosis. Clinical presentation usually consists of a slowly growing single mass with no pain as a stage I disease under the Ann Arbor classification.

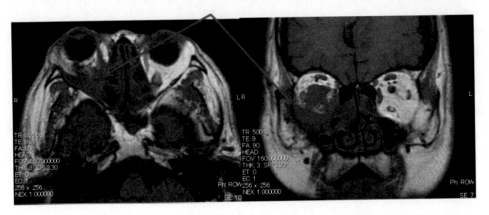

Figure 3. Magnetic Resonance (MR) imaging indicated the primary site of OAML presented in orbital fat as a tumor.

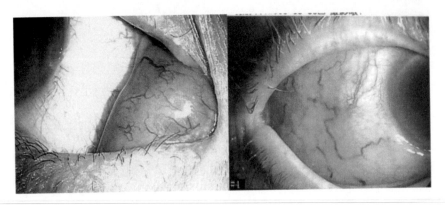

Figure 4-A. A case of OAML in subconjunctiva.

PATHOLOGICAL FEATURES OF OCULAR ADNEXAL MALT LYMPHOMA

An OAML shows a classical histopathology profile of most common MALT lymphomas, indicating that the tumor cells infiltrate around reactive follicles external to a preserved follicle mantle zone. The characteristic OAML cells are heterogeneous small to medium-sized cells with slightly irregular nuclei and moderately dispersed chromatin and have relatively abundant pale cytoplasm resembling centrocytes. The accumulation of more pale-staining cytoplasma may lead to a monocytoid appearance. Tumor cells may be heterogeneous in appearance, since centrocyte-like cells, monocytoid cells, or small-sized lymphocytes may coexist in the same tissue, albeit with different proportions varying from case to case. In glandular tissues the epithelium is often invaded and destroyed by discrete aggregates of tumor cells, resulting in the so-called lympho-epithelial lesions (Figure 5). It is worthwhile to distinguish between neoplastic and non-neoplastic tissues in the ocular adnexa. However, none of the pathological features are unique to OAML but can be found in other types of lymphomas also.

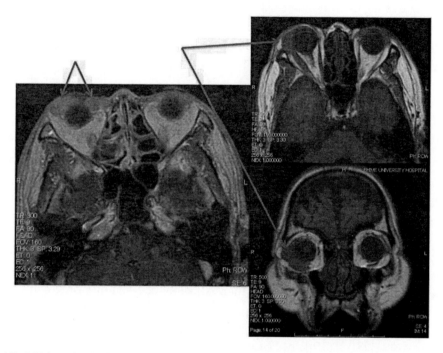

Figure 4-B. MR imaging indicated the primary site of OAML presented in subconjunctiva and lachrymal gland.

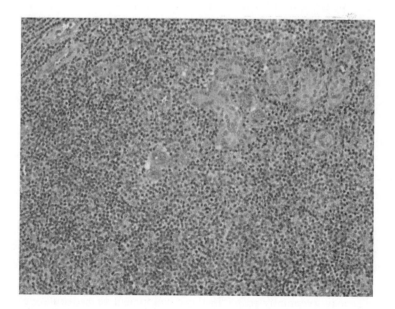

Figure 5. A case of OAML; The lymphoma cells infiltrate around lachrymal gland showing lymphoepithelial lesions.

The typical tumor cells of OAML express IgM, and less often IgA or IgG, and show light chain restriction. Immunophenotypic analysis indicates that tumor cells typically comprise a marginal zone B-cell phenotype, such as CD19+, CD20+, CD21+, CD23-, CD38+, CD3-, CD5-, CD10-, bcl-2+, bcl-6-, cyclin D1-, MUM1-, PAX5+, bcl-10+ in two-thirds of cases [17,20]. There is no specific immunophenotypic marker for OAML at present. The lack of CD5 is useful for the differential diagnosis when distinguishing between other types of small-sized lymphoma, such as mantle cell and small lymphocytic lymphoma. However, a few cases (3-10%) of OAML express CD5 [10], so that both CD23 and cyclin D1 staining should be necessary for its diagnosis.

MOLECULAR FEATURES AND CYTOGENETICS OF OCULAR ADNEXAL MALT LYMPHOMA

Chromosomal abnormalities associated with common MALT lymphoma including t(11;18)(q21;q21) (API2-MALT1), t(14;18)(q32;q21) (IGH-MALT1), t(1;14)(p22;q32) (bcl10-IGH), t(3;14)(p147.1;q32) (FOXP1-IGH), trisomy 3, and trisomy 18 have been identified and reported by several groups [21-27]. T(11;18)(q21;q21) creates a chimeric API2 (an apoptosis inhibitor protein) - MALT1 (a paracaspase-like protein) gene fusion and corresponding oncoprotein. This translocation is mainly detected in gastric and pulmonary MALT lymphoma. In contrast, t(14;18)(q32;q21), which is a deregulation of the MALT1 gene by translocation to the IGH (immunoglobulin heavy-chain gene) locus, is more common in OAML cases [28]. T(3;14)(p147.1;q32) resulting in the FOXP1 (a forkhead family transcription factor) - IGH gene fusion has been reported to be less common in OAML [28]. Somatic hypermutation has been reported in two-thirds of OAML cases [29], indicating that the majority of OAMLs represents a clonal expansion of post-germinal-center memory B cells origin. However, these cytogenetic data also indicated that no specific marker of OAML genetics has been identified.

PATHOGENESIS OF OCULAR ADNEXAL MALT LYMPHOMA

Recent clinicopathological studies suggest a strong relation between MALT lymphoma and inflammatory diseases of the epithelium, such as autoimmune diseases and infections. The best-known example of lymphoid malignancy linked with inflammation is the connection between MALT lymphoma in the stomach and infection with *Helicobacter pylori* (*H. pylori*) [30]. Gastric MALT lymphomas may be dependent on antigen stimulation by *H. pylori* since malignant lymphoid cells respond specifically to *H. pylori* antigens, and the lymphoma has been shown to regress with eradication of the infection. In the cases of the salivary and thyroid glands, the antigenic stimulation may be a component of autoimmune disease, Sjögren syndrome [31] and Hashimoto thyroiditis [32], respectively. Subsequent oncogenic events may eventually result in the development of a distinctive type of B-cell lymphoma that resembles the MALT lymphoma. In fact, patients with Sjögren syndrome and

Hashimoto thyroiditis have a 40-70-fold increased risk of B-cell lymphoma in their anatomical sites of autoimmune diseases [33, 34]. Recently, molecular techniques using PCR analysis of immunoglobulin heavy-chain genes have revealed that VH3 and VH4 family genes were predominantly utilized in OAML, the same as with gastric and thyroid MALT lymphoma. However salivary MALT lymphoma is characteristically restricted to the VH1 family which is thought to be associated with the rheumatoid factor [35,-37]. Moreover, about 10-15% of OAML had bilateral involvement of the ocular adnexa [14,17], although distant tumor metastasis is rare at the first diagnosis of OAML [17]. These clinical and laboratory observations suggest that the patients with bilateral OAMLs seem to have the same physiologic condition or immunologic stimulation in the ocular adnexa on both sides, and these stimulations from antigens such as chronic inflammation, infection, or autoimmune processes preceding OAML may have the same pattern as gastric and thyroid MALT lymphoma.

CHLAMYDIAL INFECTION AND OCULAR ADNEXAL MALT LYMPHOMA

In 2004, an Italian group evaluated a set of MALT lymphomas in the ocular adnexa for infection with *Chlamydophila psittaci* (*C. psittaci*) using the PCR-based technique [38]. In this report, 66% of their specimens showed evidence of the existence of *C. psittaci* DNA, and their immunocytochemical staining using monoclonal antibodies against chlamydial lipopolysaccharide indicated chlamydial infection in OAMLs. Moreover, they have shown the therapeutic efficacy of eradication of chlamydial infections with doxycycline in patients with OAMLs [39]. Since then, one Korean group [40], one Cuban group [41], one Austrian group [42], and one international group [43] have also reported the tight association between OAML and *C. psittaci* infection by using the same PCR technique as the Italian group. However, in contrast, four American groups [44-47], one Dutch group [48], one French group [49], one Austrian group [50], one German group [51], and four Japanese groups [17,52-54] have reported a negative correlation between OAML and *C. psittaci* infection. This controversy about *C. psittaci* infection as a causative factor for OAML is still an ongoing hot topic among researchers of this disease.

POSITIVE OR NEGATIVE CORRELATION BETWEEN OCULAR ADNEXAL MALT LYMPHOMA AND CHLAMYDIAL INFECTION

Positive or negative correlations between OAML and chlamydial infections indicate several possible explanations. The first point to be considered regards the diagnosis of OAML. The major lymphoid tumor disease in the ocular adnexa should be MALT lymphoma (Figure 2). In contrast, polyclonal lymphoid hyperplasias (Figure 1) arising from various inflammations and infections are diseases that also occur in the ocular adnexa at a certain rate (20-30%) [55]. Also, clear immunophenotypic and cytogenetic markers for the diagnosis of

OAML have not been identified so far. Classical genetic analyses, such as Southern blot or PCR amplification for IGH rearrangement, or flowcytemetric analysis, should be necessary for accurate diagnosis of OAML. However, it might be difficult to obtain sufficient amounts of tissue samples for those analyses because of the tumor size and the disease site of primary onset. FISH (fluorescence *in situ* hybridization) or PCR analysis using t(14;18) (q32;q21) involving IGH and MALT1 genes, whose genetic abnormality is expressed in about 3-24% cases of patients with OAML [56,57], may be necessary. However, this analysis is also non-disease-specific and it may be difficult to do it for a routine clinical examination. To accumulate accurate data on this type of NHL, it is necessary to check on whether benign tumors caused by inflammation, especially caused by chlamydial infections, are excluded.

The second problem is derived from the methodological biases for analysis. For instance, compared to other types of chlamydias, the genome of *C. psittaci* is differentiated in several distinct clusters [58,59], so that a careful interpretation should be necessary to select and design PCR primers for the target chlamydial sequences for the removal of non-specific gene amplification. As another aspect of biases, the sensitivity of PCR-based analysis should be discussed. Chlamydial DNAs are easily detected in peripheral blood and vascular tissue samples by PCR [60-62], suggesting that the contamination of chlamydial DNAs could be possible. Taking into consideration the above biases, new types of examinations should be considered in the discussion about the relation between OMAL and *C. psittaci* infection [63-66].

The last factor to be pointed out is the epidemiology of diseases in a general population. It is often stated that there is a clear regional difference between Europe and North America among populations positive for antibodies against HCV in patients with NHL [67-71]. The same regional difference is discussed in the relation between *Borrelia burgdorferi* and NHL [72]. It may be possible that such epidemiological differences with chlamydial infections provide more misleading "noise" regarding the relation between OAML and chlamydial infections. Recently, several clinical papers have been discussing other causative factors and infectious agents involved in OAML pathology. However, it is also true that none of those reports suggests other possible causative factors except *C. psittaci* [17,73-79].

TREATMENT OF OCULAR ADNEXAL MALT LYMPHOMA

Any universal guidelines for the treatment of OAML do not exist yet, because this type of indolent lymphoma has a long clinical course and sometimes exhibits a slow progression and remains stable as a disease. Clinicians or oncologists have treated their OAML patients while subject to several variable factors related to the patient situation (age or performance status), disease status (anatomical sites in ocular adnexa or pathological grade such as the ratio of large cell component or Ki-67 staining), therapy-related toxicities, and their own experiments. Recently some informative clinical reviews discussed the management of this type of indolent lymphoma from the above viewpoints [80-82]. Based on our experiments, the indolent nature of the disease in most cases of OAML makes a conservative approach advisable provided that strict hemato-oncologic follow-up is conducted. We would like to express our approach and opinion about the treatment of OAML below.

The first point is that surgical resection should be considered in all cases of OAML, when the tumor would be encapsulated and the complications would be acceptable. However, the reports that the *extent* of surgical resection does not influence patient survival [83,84] should be remembered, and it is also important that surgical resection requires dexterous surgical oculists. Second, if the patient is elderly or has poor performance status that is not related to the existence of OAML, a 'wait-and-see' approach or corticosteroid therapy is optional [83,85]. Also, bacteria-eradicating therapy (doxycycline or tetracycline) may be considered for some patients [39, 86] when those patients have serum antibodies against chlamydias. On the other hand, though no therapeutic effect of 'blind' antibiotic treatment against OAML has been reported [87], this easy and non-toxic therapy with antibiotics may be one treatment option for the OAML patients who do not have physical conditions requiring any radical therapies. Third, in cases where patients are not elderly or when they have enough performance status for the treatment, radiotherapy (30.6 to 32.4 Gy in a daily fraction of 1.8 Gy) [88] should be considered for the initial therapy. Rituximab, an active immunotherapy for CD20 antigen, can also be considered as a mono-therapy or a combined therapy with radiation. However, it has been reported that in gastric MALT lymphoma the response duration of rituximab as a mono-therapy is usually short and the relapse rate is higher [89]. Late adverse effects of radiotherapy such as cataracts, xerophthalmia, glaucoma, and other retinal disorders [90] should be kept in mind when the treatment would be carried out in younger patients.

Several groups have reported the effectiveness of chemotherapy for OAML, such as a combined chemotherapy, CVP [91], chlorambucil [92,93], fludarabine [94], cladribine [95] [96,97], interferon-alpha [98], and so on. All trials were pilot and single armed studies, and some were retrospective. These chemotherapies are usually selected as second lines or experimental treatments for the disseminated disease stage of OAML. The usage of anthracycline-combined chemotherapy does not have any advantages in a first-line treatment of the localized disease because of its toxicity for this type of indolent lymphoma. All the above therapeutic strategies are depended on efficacy and toxicities, which need to be carefully weighed.

CONCLUSION

OAML is a distinct disease entry in ENML and presents an indolent nature and specific characteristics. Patients with OAML require hematopathologic diagnosis and concomitant clinical management with case-specific treatment. Prospective collaborative studies enrolling sufficient numbers of patients with OAML are needed to compare etiology, pathogenesis, and treatment. Applying a team approach involving pathologists, ophthalmologists, and hematologists should be encouraged, and this strategy would make clear the true features of OAML.

REFERENCES

[1] Bardenstein DS. Orbital and adnexal lymphoma. In: Singh AD, Damato BE, Pe'er J, et al. *Clinical Ophthalmic Oncology* Saunders Elsevier, Philadelphia, 2007; 565-570.

[2] Bardenstein DS. Ocular adnexal lymphoma: Classification, clinical disease, and molecular biology. *Ophthalmol Clin Nor Am* 2005; 18: 187-197.

[3] Records RE. Conjunctiva and lacrimal system. In: Records RE, et al. *Physiology of the Human Eye and Visual System* Harper&Row, Hagerstown, 1979; 25-46.

[4] Knop N and Knop E. Conjunctiva-associated lymphoid tissue in the human eye. *Invest Ophthalmol Vis Sci* 2000; 41: 1270-1279.

[5] Isaacson PG and Wright DH. Malignant lymphoma of mucosa-associated lymphoid tissue. A distinctive type of B-cell lymphoma. *Cancer* 1983; 52: 1410-1416.

[6] Isaacson PG, Chott A, Nakamura S, et al. Extranodal marginal zone B-cell lymphoma of mucosa-associated lymphoid tissue (MALT lymphoma). In: Swerdlow SH, Campo E, Harris NL, et al. *Tumours of Haematopoietic and Lymphoid Tissue 4th Edition, Lyon IARC* 2008: 214-217.

[7] Thieblemont C, Berger F, Dumontet C, et al. Mucosa-associated lymphoid tissue lymphoma is a disseminated disease in one third of 158 patients analyzed. *Blood* 2000; 95: 802-806.

[8] Conconi A, Bertoni F, Pedrinis E, et al. Nodal marginal zone B-cell lymphomas may arise from different subsets of marginal zone B lymphocytes. *Blood* 2001; 98: 781–786.

[9] The non-Hodgkin's lymphoma classification project. A clinical evaluation of the International Lymphoma Study Group classification of non-Hodgkin's lymphoma. *Blood* 1997; 89: 3909-3918.

[10] Coupland SE, Krause L, Delecluse HJ, et al. Lymphoproliferative lesions of the ocular adnexa. Analysis of 112 cases. *Ophthalmology* 1998; 105: 1430-1441.

[11] Jenkins C, Rose GE, Bunce C, et al. Histological features of ocular adnexal lymphoma (REAL classification) and their association with patient morbidity and survival. *Br J Ophthalmol* 2000; 84: 907-913.

[12] McKelvie PA, McNab A, Francis IC, et al. Ocular adnexal lymphoproliferative disease: a series of 73 cases. *Clin Exp Ophthalmol* 2001; 29: 387-393.

[13] Fung VY, Tarbell NJ, Lucarelli SI, et al. Ocular adnexal lymphoma: clinical behavior of distinct World Health Organization classification subtypes. *Int J Radiat Oncol Biol Phys* 2003; 57: 1382-1391.

[14] Ferry JA, Fung CY, Zukerberg L, et al. Lymphoma of the ocular adnexa: a study of 353 cases. *Am J Surg Pathol* 2007; 2: 170-184.

[15] Mannami T, Yoshino T, Oshima K, et al. Clinical, histopathological, and immunogenetic analysis of ocular adnexal lymphoproliferative disorders: characterization of MALT lymphoma and reactive lymphoid hyperplasia. *Mod Pathol* 2001; 14: 641-649.

[16] Moslehi R, Devesa SS, Schaier C, et al. Rapidly increasing incidence of ocular non-Hodgkin lymphoma. *J Natl Cancer Inst* 2006; 98: 936-939.

[17] Yakushijin Y, Kodama T, Takaoka I, et al. Absence of chlamydial infection in Japanese patients with ocular adnexal lymphoma of mucosa-associated lymphoid tissue. *Int J Hematol* 2007; 85: 223-230.

[18]Lagoo AS, Haggerty C, Kim Y, et al. Morphologic features of 115 lymphomas of the orbit and ocular adnexa categorized according to the World Health Organization classification: are marginal zone lymphomas in the orbit mucosa-associated lymphoid tissue-type lymphomas? *Arch Pathol Lab Med.* 2008; 132: 1405-16.

[19]Adachi A, Tamaru JI, Kaneko K, et al. No evidence of a correlation between BCL10 expression and API2-MALT1 gene rearrangement in ocular adnexal MALT lymphoma. *Pathol Int* 2004; 54: 16-25.

[20]Ferreri AJ, Dolcetti R, Du MQ, at al. Ocular adnexal MALT lymphoma: an intriguing model for antigen-driven lymphoma-genesis and microbial-targeted therapy. *Ann Oncol* 2008; 19: 835-846.

[21]Isaacson PG and Du MQ. MALT lymphoma: from morphology to molecules. *Nat Rev Cancer* 2004; 4: 644–653.

[22]Du MQ. MALT lymphoma: recent advances in aetiology and molecular genetics. *J Clin Exp Hematop* 2007; 47: 31–42.

[23]Remstein ED, James CD, and Kurtin PJ. Incidence and subtype specificity of API2-MALT1 fusion translocations in extranodal, nodal, and splenic marginal zone lymphomas. *Am J Pathol* 2000; 156: 1183–1188.

[24]Motegi M, Yonezumi M, Suzuki H et al. API2-MALT1 chimeric transcripts involved in mucosa-associated lymphoid tissue type lymphoma predict heterogeneous products. *Am J Pathol* 2000; 156: 807-812.

[25]Remstein ED, Kurtin PJ, Einerson RR, et al. Primary pulmonary MALT lymphomas show frequent and hetero-geneous cytogenetic abnormalities, including aneuploidy and translocations involving API2 and MALT1 and IGH and MALT1. *Leukemia* 2004; 18: 156–160.

[26]Lucas PC, Yonezumi M, Inohara N, et al. Bcl10 and MALT1, independent targets of chromosomal translocation in malt lymphoma, cooperate in a novel NF-kappa B signaling pathway. *J Biol Chem* 2001; 276: 19012–19019.

[27]Streubel B, Vinatzer U, Lamprecht A, et al. T(3;14)(p14.1;q32) involving IGH and FOXP1 is a novel recurrent chromosomal aberration in MALT lymphoma. *Leukemia* 2005; 19: 652–658.

[28]Remstein ED, Dogan A, Einerson RR, et al. The incidence and anatomic site specificity of chromosomal translocations in primary extranodal marginal zone B-cell lymphoma of mucosa-associated lymphoid tissue (MALT lymphoma) in North America. *Am J Surg Pathol* 2006; 30: 1546-1553.

[29]Coupland SE, Foss HD, Anagnostopoulso I, et al. Immunoglobulin VH gene expression among extranodal marginal zone B-cell lymphoma of the ocular adnexa. *Invest Ophthalmol Vis Sci* 1999; 40: 555-562.

[30]Wotherspoon AC, Ortiz-Hidalgo C, Falzon MR, et al. *Helicobacter pylori*-associated gastritis and primary B-cell gastric lymphoma. *Lancet* 1991; 338: 1175-1176.

[31]Hyjck E, Smith WJ, and Isaacon PG. Primary B cell lymphoma of salivary glands and its relationship to myoepithelial sialadenitis. *Hum Pathol* 1988; 19: 766-776.

[32]Hyjck E and Isaacon PG. Primary B cell lymphoma of the thyroid and its relationship to Hashimoto's thyroiditis. *Hum Pathol* 1988; 19: 1315-1326.

[33] Holm LE, Blomgren H, and Lowhagen T. Cancer risks in patients with chronic lymphocytic thyroiditis. *N Eng J Med* 1985; 312: 601-604.

[34] Aozasa K. Hashimoto thyroiditis as a risk factor of thyroid lymphoma. *Acta Pathol Jpn* 1990; 40: 459-468.

[35] Coupland SE and Foss HD, Anagnostopoulos I, et al. Immunoglobulin V(H) gene expression among extranodal marginal zone B-cell lymphomas of the ocular adnexa. *Invest Ophthal Vis Sci* 1999; 40: 555-562.

[36] Mannami T, Yoshino T, Oshima K, et al. Clinical, histopathological, and immunogenetic analysis of ocular adnexal lymphoproliferative disorders: characterization of MALT lymphoma and reactive lymphoid hyperplasia. *Mod Pathol* 2001; 14: 641-649.

[37] Sato Y, Nakamura N, Nakamura S, et al. Deviated VH4 immunoglobulin gene usage is found among thyroid mucosa-associated lymphoid tissue lymphomas, similar to the usage at other sites, but is not found in thyroid diffuse large B-cell lymphomas. *Mod Pathol* 2006; 19: 1578-1584.

[38] Ferreri AJ, Guidoboni M, Ponzoni M, et al. Evidence for an association between *Chlamydia psittaci* and ocular adnexal lymphomas. *J Natl Cancer Inst* 2004; 96: 586-594.

[39] Ferreri AJ, Ponzoni M, Guidoboni M, et al. Regression of ocular adnexal lymphoma after *Chlamydia psittaci*-eradicating antibiotic therapy. *J Clin Oncol* 2005; 23: 5067-5073.

[40] Yoo C, Ryu M, Huh J, et al. *Chlamydia psittaci* infection and clinicopathologic analysis of ocular adnexal lymphomas in Korea *Am J Hematol* 2007; 82: 821-823.

[41] Gracia E, Frosch P, Mazzucchelli L, et al. Low prevalence of *Chlamydia psittaci* in ocular adnexal lymphomas from Cuban patients. *Leuk and Lymphoma* 2007; 48: 104-108.

[42] Aigelsreiter A, Leitner E, Deutsch JAA et al. *Chlamydia psittaci* in MALT lymphomas of ocular adnexals: The Austrian experience. *Leuk Res* 2008; 32: 1292-1294.

[43] Chanudet E, Zhou Y, Bacon C, et al. *Chlamydia psittaci* is variably associated with ocular adnexal MALT lymphoma in different geographical regions. *J Pathol* 2006; 209: 344–51.

[44] Rosado MF, Byrne GEJ, Ding F, et al. Ocular adnexal lymphoma: a clinicopathologic study of a large cohort of patients with no evidence for an association with *Chlamydia psittaci*. *Blood* 2006; 107: 467-472.

[45] Vargas RL, Fallone E, Felgar RE, et al. Is there an association between ocular adnexal lymphoma and infection with *Chlamydia psittaci*?: The University of Rochester experience. *Leuk Res* 2006; 30: 547-551.

[46] Zhang GS, Winter JN, Variakojis D, et al. Lack of an association between *Chlamydia psittaci* and ocular adnexal lymphoma. *Leuk Lymphoma* 2007; 48: 577-583.

[47] Matthews JM, Moreno LI, Dennis J, et al. Ocular adnexal lymphoma: no evidence for bacterial DNA associated with lymphoma pathogenesis. *Br J Haematol* 2008; 142: 246-249.

[48] Mulder MMS, Heddema ER, Pannekoek Y, et al. No evidence for an association of ocular adnexal lymphoma with *Chlamydia psittaci* in a cohort of patients from the Netherlands. *Leuk Res* 2006; 30: 1305-1307.

[49]DeCremoux P, Subtil A, Ferreri AJ, et al. Evidence for an association between *Chlamydia psittaci* and ocular adnexal lymphomas. *J Natl Cancer Inst* 2006; 98: 365-366.

[50]Ruiz A, Reischl U, Swerdlow SH, et al. Extranodal marginal zone B-cell lymphomas of the ocular adnexa: Multiparameter analysis of 34 cases including interphase molecular cytogenetics and PCR for *Chlamydia psittaci*. *Am J Surg Pathol* 2007; 31: 792-802.

[51]Goebel N, Serr A, Reinhard T, et al. *Chlamydia psittaci, Helicobacter pylori* and ocular adnexal lymphoma is there an association? The German experiment. *Leuk Res* 2007; 31: 1450-1452.

[52]Daibata M, Nemoto Y, Togitani K, et al. Absence of *Chlamydia psittaci* in ocular adnexal lymphoma from Japanese patients. *Br J Haematol* 2006; 132: 651-652.

[53]Liu YC, Ohyashiki JH, Ito Y, et al. *Chlamydia psittaci* in ocular adnexal lymphoma: Japanese experience. *Leuk Res* 2006; 30: 1587-1589.

[54]Yoshida T, Yoshikawa H, Ishibashi T. Relationship between ocular adnexal lymphoma and *Chlamydia psittaci* infection. *Jap J Clin Ophthal* 2007; 61: 1549-1553.

[55]Knowles DM, Jakobiec FA, McNally L, et al. Lymphoid hyperplasia and malignant lymphoma occurring in the ocular adnexa (orbita, conjunctiva, and eyelids): a prospective multiparametric analysis of 108 cases during 1977 to 1987. *Hum Pathol* 1990; 21: 959-973.

[56]Streubel B, Lamprecht A, Dierlamm J, et al. T(14;18)(q32;q21) involving IGH and MALT1 is a frequent chromosomal aberration in MALT lymphoma. *Blood* 2003; 101: 2335-2339.

[57]Tanimoto K, Sekiguchi N, Yokota Y, et al. Fluorescence in situ hybridization (FISH) analysis of primary ocular adnexal MALT lymphoma. *BMC Cancer* 2006; 6: 249.

[58]Meijer A, Morre SA, van den Brule AJC, et al. Genomic relatedness of *Chlamydia* isolates determined by amplified fragment length polymorphism analysis. *J Bacteriol* 1999; 181: 4469-4475.

[59]Fukushi PH, Ochiai Y, Yamaguchi T, et al. Phylogenetic analysis of the genus *Chlamydia* based on the 16S rRNA gene sequences. *Int J Syst Bacteriol* 1997; 47: 425-431.

[60]Ferreri AJ, Dolcetti R, Dognini GP, et al. *Chlamydophila psittaci* is viable and infectious in the conjunctiva and peripheral blood of patients with ocular adnexal lymphoma: Results of a single-center prospective case-control study. *Int J Cancer* 2008; 123: 1089-1093.

[61]Taylor-Robinson D. Chlamydia pneumoniae in vascular tissue. *Atherosclerosis* 1998; 140: S21-24.

[62]Schenker OA and Hoop RK. Chlamydiae and atherosclerosis: can psittacine cases support the link? *Avian Dis* 2007; 51: 8-13.

[63]Bahler DW, Szankasi P, Kulkarni S, et al. Use of similar immunoglobulin VH gene segments by MALT lymphomas of the ocular adnexa. *Mod Pathol* 2009; 22: 833-838.

[64]Matthews JM, Moreno LI, Dennis J, et al. Ocular adnexal lymphoma: no evidence for bacterial DNA associated with lymphoma pathogenesis. *Br J Haematol* 2008; 142: 246-249.

[65] Husain A, Roberts D, Pro B, et al. Meta-analyses of the association between *Chlamydia psittaci* and ocular adnexal lymphoma and the response of ocular adnexal lymphoma to antibiotics. *Cancer* 2007; 110: 809-815.

[66] Schiby G, Polak-Charcon S, Mardoukh C, et al. Orbital marginal zone lymphomas: an immunohistochemical, polymerase chain reaction, and fluorescence in situ hybridization study. *Hum Pathol* 2007; 38: 435-442.

[67] Ferri C, Caracciolo F, Zignego AL, et al. Hepatitis C virus infection in patients with non-Hodgkin's lymphoma. *Br J Haematol* 1994; 88: 392-394.

[68] Mazzaro C, Zagonel V, Monfardini S, et al. Hepatitis C virus and non-Hodgkin's lymphomas. *Br J Haematol* 1996; 94: 544-550.

[69] Sève P, Renaudier P, Sasco AJ, et al. Hepatitis C virus infection and B-cell non-Hodgkin's lymphoma: A cross-sectional study in Lyon, France. *Eur J Gastroenterol Hepatol* 2004; 16: 1361-1365.

[70] Morgensztern D, Rosado M, Silva O, et al. Prevalence of hepatitis C infection in patients with non-Hodgkin's lymphoma in South Florida and review of the literature. *Leuk Lymh* 2004; 45: 2459-2464.

[71] Waters L, Stebbing J, Mandalia S, et al. Hepatitis C infection is not associated with systemic HIV-associated non-Hodgkin's lymphoma: A cohort study. *Int J Cancer* 2005; 116: 161-163.

[72] Roggero E, Zucca E, Mainetti C, et al. Eradication of *Borrelia burgdorferi* infection in primary marginal zone B-cell lymphoma of the skin. *Hum Pathol* 2000; 31: 263-268.

[73] Ferreri AJ, Ernberg I, and Copie-Bergman C. Infectious agents and lymphoma development: molecular and clinical aspects. *J Intern Med* 2009; 265: 421-438.

[74] Sjö LD. Ophthalmic lymphoma: epidemiology and pathogenesis. *Acta Ophthalmol* 2009; 87: 1-20.

[75] Ponzoni M, Ferreri AJ, Guidoboni M, et al. Chlamydia infection and lymphomas: Association beyond ocular adnexal lymphomas highlighted by multiple detection methods. *Clin Cancer Res* 2008; 14: 5794-5800.

[76] Decaudin D, Dolcetti R, de Cremoux P, et al. Variable association between Chlamydophila psittaci infection and ocular adnexal lymphomas: Methodological biases or true geographical variations? *Anti-cancer Drugs* 2008; 19: 761-765.

[77] Verma V, Shen D, Sieving PC, et al. The role of infectious agents in the etiology of ocular adnexal neoplasia. *Surv Ophthalmol* 2008; 53: 312-331.

[78] Cohen VM, Sweetenham J, and Singh AD. Ocular adnexal lymphoma. What is the evidence for an infectious aetiology? *Br J Ophthalmol* 2008; 92: 446-448.

[79] Chan CC, Shen D, Mochizuki M, et al. Detection of *Helicobacter pylori* and *Chlamydia pneumoniae* genes in primary orbital lymphoma. *Trans Am Ophthalmol Soc* 2006; 104: 62-70.

[80] Ferreri AJ, Dolcetti R, Du MQ, et al. Ocular adnexal MALT lymphoma: An intriguing model for antigen-driven lymphomagenesis and microbial-targeted therapy. *Ann Oncol* 2008; 19: 835-846.

[81] Decaudin D, De Cremoux P, Vincent-Salomon A, et al. Ocular adnexal lymphoma: a review of clinicopathologic features and treatment options. *Blood* 2006; 108: 1451-1460.

[82]Stefanovic A and Lossos IS. Extranodal marginal zone lymphoma of the ocular adnexa. *Blood* 2009; 114: 501-510.

[83]Tanimoto K, Kaneko A, Suzuki S, et al. Primary ocular adnexal MALT lymphoma: a long-term follow-up study of 114 patients. *Jpn J Clin Oncol* 2007; 37: 337-344.

[84]Tanimoto K, Kaneko A, Suzuki S et al. Long-term follow-up results of no initial therapy for ocular adnexal MALT lymphoma. *Ann Oncol* 2006; 17: 135-140.

[85]Matsuo T, Yoshino T. Long-term follow-up results of observation or radiation for conjunctival malignant lymphoma. *Ophthalmology* 2004; 111: 1233-1237.

[86]Ferreri AJM, Dognini GP, Ponzoni M, et al. *Chlamydia psittaci*-eradicating antibiotic therapy in patients with advanced-stage ocular adnexal MALT lymphoma. *Ann Oncol* 2008; 19: 194-195.

[87]Grünberger B, Hauff W, Lukas J, et al. 'Blind' antibiotic treatment targeting Chlamydia is not effective in patients with MALT lymphoma of the ocular adnexa. *Ann Oncol* 2006; 17: 484-487.

[88]Le QT, Eulau SM, George TI, et al. Primary radiotherapy for localized orbital MALT lymphoma. *Int J Radiat Oncol Biol Phys* 2002; 52: 657-663.

[89]Sasai K, Yamabe H, Dodo Y, et al. Non-Hodgkin's lymphoma of ocular adnexa. *Acta Oncol* 2001; 40: 485-490.

[90]Ejima Y, Sasaki R, Okamoto Y, et al. Ocular adnexal mucosa-associated lymphoid tissue lymphoma treated with radiotherapy. *Radiother Oncol* 2006; 78: 6-9.

[91]Song EK, Kim SY, Kim TM, et al. Efficacy of chemotherapy as a first-line treatment in ocular adnexal extranodal marginal zone B-cell lymphoma. *Ann Oncol* 2008; 19: 242-246.

[92]Ben Simon GJ, Cheung N, McKelvie P, et al. Oral chlorambucil for extranodal, marginal zone, B-cell lymphoma of mucosa-associated lymphoid tissue of the orbit. *Ophthalmology* 2006; 113: 1209-1213.

[93]Rigacci L, Nassi L, Puccioni M, et al. Rituximab and chlorambucil as first-line treatment for low-grade ocular adnexal lymphomas. *Ann Hematol* 2007; 86: 565-568.

[94]Zinzani PL, Stefoni V, Musuraca G et al. Fludarabine-containing chemotherapy as frontline treatment of nongastrointestinal mucosa-associated lymphoid tissue lymphoma. *Cancer* 2004; 100: 2190-2194.

[95]Jäger G, Neumeister P, Quehenberger F, et al. Prolonged clinical remission in patients with extranodal marginal zone B-cell lymphoma of the mucosa-associated lymphoid tissue type treated with cladribine: 6 year follow-up of a phase II trial. *Ann Oncol* 2006; 17: 1722-1723.

[96]Armitage JO, Tobinai K, Hoelzer D, et al. Treatment of indolent non-Hodgkin's lymphoma with cladribine as single-agent therapy and in combination with mitoxantrone. *Int J Hematol* 2004; 79: 311-321.

[97]Jäger G, Neumeister P, Brezinschek R, et al. Treatment of extranodal marginal zone B-cell lymphoma of mucosa-associated lymphoid tissue type with cladribine: a phase II study. *J Clin Oncol* 2002; 20: 3872-3877.

[98]Blasi MA, Gherlinzoni F, Calvisi G, et al. Local chemotherapy with interferon-alpha for conjunctival mucosa-associated lymphoid tissue lymphoma: a preliminary report. *Ophthalmology* 2001; 108: 559-562.

In: Conjunctivitis: Symptoms, Treatment and Prevention   ISBN: 978-1-61668-321-4
Editor: Anna R. Sallinger, pp. 195-203   © 2010 Nova Science Publishers, Inc.

Chapter VII

CONJUNCTIVITIS:
SYMPTOMS, TREATMENT AND PREVENTION

Munish Ahuja[1] and Dipak K. Majumdar[2],*

[1] Department of Pharmaceutical Sciences, Guru Jambheshwar University of Science and
Technology, Haryana -125 001, India;
[2] Delhi Instiute of Pharmaceutical Sciences and Research, University of Delhi, New
Delhi-110 017, India.

ABSTRACT

Conjunctivitis is the inflammation of conjunctiva, which is manifested as
vasodilatation/hyperemia, edema and exudation. Conjunctivitis may arise due to bacterial
or viral infections or due to allergy or injury by chemical or physical agents. A number of
chemical mediators like prostaglandins and leukotrienes derived from arachidonic acid
cascade, histamine released from mast cells, and cytokines from lymphocytes, monocytes
and macrophages have been implicated in the mediation of inflammatory response.
Topical management of conjunctivitis involves the treatment of underlying cause and
associated inflammation. The differential clinical diagnosis of bacterial and viral
conjunctivitis is very difficult. Acute bacterial conjunctivitis is self-limiting, but the use
of topical antibiotics improves the rate of clinical recovery. Conventionally topical
corticosteroids were employed in management of inflammation but because of their
tendency to raise the intraocular pressure, facilitate infection and cataract formation, they
have been replaced by the safer non-steroidal anti-inflammatory drugs (NSAIDs).
Current treatment modalities for allergic conjunctivitis include topical mast cell
stabilizers / antihistaminic, and NSAIDs.

---

* Correspondence concerning this article should be addressed to: Dipak K. Majumdar, E-mail:
dkmajumdaar@yahoo.com, dkmajumdar@gmail.com.

INTRODUCTION

Conjunctiva is a thin protective vascularized mucous membrane, which covers the sclera (bulbar conjunctiva) and lines the inside of the eyelid (palpebral conjunctiva). Conjunctiva also contributes to the defense mechanisms of the eye by partial secretion of some components of tear film. Injury to conjunctival surface results in conjunctivitis, an inflammation of conjunctiva. Conjunctival injury, may be inflicted by chemical or physical agents, invasion of pathogens, (bacterial, fungal, viral or protozoal) and excessive (allergic) or inappropriate operation of immune mechanisms (autoimmunity) [1,2].

Conjunctival inflammation facilitates the immune response and the subsequent removal of antigenic material and damaged conjunctival tissue. As soon as the injury is recognized, the mechanisms to localize and clear foreign substances and damaged tissues are initiated. Further, the response is amplified by activation of inflammatory cells and production of chemical mediators like vasoactive amines (histamine, serotonin), acidic lipids (prostaglandins, thromboxanes, leukotrienes); cytokines etc [1].

Interaction of allergens with conjunctival mast cell-bound IgE, results in release of chemical mediators like histamine, serotonin etc. Histamine, which is the primary mediator of inflammation in allergic conjunctivitis, causes vasodilatation and increases vascular permeability to produce clinical signs of allergy. Mast cell stabilizers prevent the release of histamine, while histamine H_1 receptor antagonists prevent the histamine-mediated response [3].

Acidic lipids are produced in the arachidonic cascade. Arachidonic acid is released from the phospholipid component of the cell membrane by the action of phospholipase A_2. The arachidonic acid (5, 8, 11, 14 eicosatetraenoic acid) so produced enters either the cyclooxygenase or lipoxygenase pathway. Activation of cyclooxygenase pathway results in formation of prostaglandins (PGs) and thromboxanes, while the lipoxygenase pathway yields hydroxyeicosatetraenoic acid and leukotrienes. PGs cause vasodilation and increased vascular permeability resulting in polymorphonuclear leukocytes migration to tear fluid [4]. PGE_1 & E_2 have been found to be extremely pruritogenic [5]. PGE_2 in synergy with histamine and bradykinin dilates pre-capillary arterioles, contributing to the redness and increased blood flow in areas of acute inflammation. PGE_2 also potentiates the histamine and bradykinin-induced increase in permeability of post-capillary venules, and bradykinin-induced sensitization of afferent C fibres to cause pain [6]. Corticosteroids, the potent anti-inflammatory agents elicit their action by blocking the enzyme phospholipase A_2 to inhibit arachidonic acid production, thereby preventing the synthesis of all the PGs, thromboxanes and eicosanoids. On the other hand, non-steroidal anti-inflammatory drugs (NSAIDs) exert their anti-inflammatory action by inhibiting the enzymes cyclooxygenase (COX 1 & COX 2) [4].

Cytokines are the small soluble proteins secreted by variety of cells like lymphocytes, granulocytes, macrophages, and mast cells. Some of the prominent cytokines are interleukins, interferons, tumor necrosis factor, transforming growth factor and chemokines. Cytokines play vital role in mediating and regulating immune response. Histamine by binding with H_1 receptors on conjunctival epithelial cells causes the release of pro-inflammatory cytokines IL-

6 and IL-8. H_1 receptor antagonists prevent the release of histamine-mediated cytokine release [3].

CLINICAL SIGNS OF CONJUNCTIVITIS

Conjunctivitis is usually manifested as hyperemia, oedema, discharge, follicles, membranes and pseudomembranes [7].

Hyperemia is the redness of the bulbar conjunctiva, which arises due to vasodilation of blood vessels.

Oedema or chemosis is a translucent swelling of tissues, which occurs due to, increased vascular permeability.

Discharge is an abnormal production of external ocular secretions comprising of tears, mucus and debris of epithelial and inflammatory cells. Discharge may be watery, mucoid, purulent or mucopurulent depending upon the relative proportion of different components. The type of discharge helps in differential diagnosis of conjunctivitis e.g., watery discharge is usually associated with viral conjunctivitis, mucoid with allergic conjunctivitis, while mucopurulent or purulent discharge is indicative of bacterial etiology.

Membranes and *pseudomembranes* represent a coagulum of necrotic cells, inflammatory exudates, and other serum components on the conjunctival surfaces. In case of membrane, coagulum is firmly attached and it results in stripping of epithelium and bleeding, while in pseudomembranes, coagulum is only superficially attached to epithelium and its removal is healed without sequelae.

Follicles are smooth grayish-white, dome shaped elevations found in the palpebral conjunctiva. Follicles comprise of lymphoid and sub epithelial cells. Follicular reactions occur commonly in acute viral or chronic chlamydial infections and drug toxicity, while presence of follicles in lower fornices is a normal feature in children.

Papillae are polygonal elevations of conjunctival tissue comprising of fibrovascular core infiltrated by inflammatory cells. Papillae are generally found on the palpebral conjunctiva conferring it a velvety appearance. Large papillae occur frequently in vernal keratoconjunctivitis, chronic foreign body irritation and in contact lens-induced giant papillary conjunctivitis. On the other hand, small papillae are non-specifically found in conjunctival inflammation due to any cause.

TYPES OF CONJUNCTIVITIS

Based on the etiology, conjunctivitis may be classified broadly as- infective conjunctivitis and non-infective conjunctivitis [8-10].

Infective Conjunctivitis

Among the various infectious agents, bacteria, viruses and chlamydia are the most frequent causes, while fungi and parasites are the less common. Differential diagnosis of infectious conjunctivitis is very critical for appropriate treatment.

Bacterial Conjunctivitis [8, 10, 11]

It has been observed that microorganisms responsible for bacterial conjunctivitis tend to vary by age. In adults, *Staphylococcus aureus*, *Hemophilus influenzae*, coagulase negative *Staphylococci*, and *Streptococcus pneumoniae* are the most frequent cause, while *Moraxella lacunata* and *Branhamella catarrhalis* are less frequent. In children, *H. influenzae*, *S. pneumoniae* and *S. aureus* are the most frequent cause. In case of neonates, *Chlamydia trachomonatis* is the most common cause of conjunctivitis, apart from *S. aureus*, *H. influenzae* and *S. pneumoniae*. Bacterial conjunctivitis may be clinically manifested as hyperacute, acute or chronic bacterial conjunctivitis.

Hyperacute bacterial conjunctivitis is characterized by rapid onset of hyperemia, lid oedema, abundant purulent discharge, chemosis, discomfort and pain. The most common cause of hyperacute bacterial conjunctivitis is *Neisseria gonorrhoeae*, and the patients are usually neonates or sexually active adults with associated *N. gonorrhoeae* infection, which is often asymptomatic.

Acute bacterial conjunctivitis is characterized by hyperemia in the fornices, lid oedema, and copious green-yellow muco-purulent or purulent discharge without significant eye pain, discomfort or photophobia. Papillae or follicles are inconspicuous.

Chronic bacterial conjunctivitis presents with mild sectoral hyperemia, chronic scanty and sticky mucopurulent discharge and discomfort. Papillae or follicles may also be present.

Viral Conjunctivitis [8, 10]

In adults, viral conjunctivitis is usually more common than the bacterial conjunctivitis. Viral conjunctivitis is of acute onset, self-limiting and seldom found to be responsible for chronic inflammation. Adenoviruses and Coxsackie viruses induce acute bilateral conjunctivitis of epidemic nature. *Herpes zoster* and *Herpes simplex* cause severe unilateral conjunctivitis. In addition, acute viral conjunctivitis may be observed associated with chicken pox, mumps, measles and infectious mononucleosis. Viral conjunctivitis typically presents with acute onset of hyperemia, excessive watery discharge, itching, photophobia, foreign body sensation, and follicles in the lower palpebral conjunctiva. Mucoid discharge causing matting or crusting of eyelids in the morning is the most prominent feature of viral conjunctivitis. Conjunctival ulcers are observed during chicken pox infections while hemorrhagic manifestations are frequent in epidemic Coxsackie virus infections.

Fungal Conjunctivitis

Fungal infections of conjunctiva are very rare and usually observed in immunocompromised patients. *Candida*, *Coccidioides immitis*, *Sporotrichum schenckii*, *Blastomyces dermatitides*, *Rhinosporidium seeberi*, *Fusarium* and *Aspergillus* species have been found to be associated with fungal infections of conjunctiva [12-14]. Fungal conjunctivitis is usually associated with mycotic infections of eyelids, and is characterized by chronic hyperemia, scanty mucopurulent discharge and mild follicular hypertrophy.

Parasitic Conjunctivitis

It is the extremely rare condition. However, protozoa, nematodes, cestodes and trematodes have been found to be associated with parasitic infestations of conjunctiva [15-18]. Parasitic conjunctivitis is characterized by acute onset of foreign body sensations, itching, eyelid oedema, hyperemia, follicles or papillae. Larvae may often be observed moving under the conjunctival surface (ophthalmomyiasis externa) or penetrated intraocularly (ophthalmomyiasis interna). Conjunctival ulcers or cyst may be seen in severe cases.

Non-Infective Conjunctivitis

Allergic Conjunctivitis

Allergic conjunctivitis is usually found concomitantly with allergic rhinitis, atopic dermatitis and asthma. Allergic conjunctivitis typically presents with symptoms of intense bilateral itching, watery, red, sore and swollen eyes, but without pain [3]. Allergic conjunctivitis may be classified into seasonal allergic conjunctivitis, perennial allergic conjunctivitis, atopic keratoconjunctivitis, vernal kerato conjunctivitis and giant papillary conjunctivitis [3,9,19-21].

Seasonal allergic conjunctivitis (SAC) and *perennial allergic conjunctivitis* (PAC) are the most common forms of ocular allergic disorders caused by direct exposure of conjunctiva to allergens. SAC is mainly provoked by seasonal (outdoor) allergens such as grass pollens or ragweed, while perennial (indoor) allergens like dust mites or animal dander trigger PAC. PAC is generally found to be associated with other allergic conditions such as persistent allergic rhinitis.

Atopic keratoconjunctivitis (AKC) is a severe and chronic inflammatory condition, which commonly involves lower tarsal conjunctiva and frequently cornea. AKC may even lead to blindness. AKC is not directly associated with allergens but usually related to history of atopic dermatitis or allergic asthma. AKC clinically presents with symptoms of itchy, red, eyelid eczema, burning and tearing which tends to be more severe than in SAC or PAC.

Vernal keratoconjunctivitis (VKC) is a severe, recurrent chronic inflammatory disorder which has also not been directly associated with allergens but its association has sometimes been found with seasonal allergic rhinitis, atopic dermatitis and asthma. VKC primarily involves upper tarsal conjunctiva and is characterized by intense bilateral itching, photophobia, hyperemia, and foreign body sensations. Discharge in VKC is a characteristic ropy discharge comprising of thick, sticky, mucous filaments. Papillae of size 7-8 mm known as cobblestone papillae on the upper tarsal conjunctiva are another characteristic feature of VKC. Apart from IgE-mediated processes, other inflammatory mediators have also been implicated in pathogenesis of VKC and AKC.

Giant papillary conjunctivitis (GPC) is most commonly seen in contact lens wearers. Ocular prostheses and sutures may also induce GPC. It arises as a response to chronic mechanical irritation or due to allergic response to lens and prostheses deposits or due to irritating effects of contact lens solutions. GPC typically presents with itching, tearing, ocular discomfort and giant papillae on the upper palpebral conjunctiva.

Iatrogenic Conjunctivitis

This is the type of conjunctivitis, which is induced by drugs, administered either topically or systemically. Inflammation induced by topical agents may arise due to hypersensitivity to medication or additives of the formulation, particularly preservatives. Further, the response may be manifested as acute or delayed hypersensitivity reaction. Systemically administered medications may also induce conjunctivitis, either by interfering with tear film formation or by other non-specific immune mechanisms or as Stevens-Johnson syndrome [22]. Stevens-Johnson syndrome is an acute inflammatory disease, which arises due to immunological hypersensitivity to drugs or microorganisms. Stevens-Johnson syndrome affects predominantly the skin and mucosal membrane including ocular surface. The ocular manifestations of Stevens-Johnson syndrome include severe pseudomembranous conjunctivitis and corneal ulceration [23-24].

TREATMENT AND PREVENTION

Acute bacterial conjunctivitis is self-limiting and usually resolves spontaneously. Earlier studies have shown that 65-70% of cases of acute bacterial conjunctivitis resolve without any treatment within a week. However, the use of topical antibiotics hastens the rate of clinical recovery, and reduces the chances of rare complications and transmission of infection [25-26]. Topical antibiotics commonly used are tetracycline, chloramphenicol, gentamicin, tobramycin, bacitracin, polymixin B and erythromycin. After the introduction of fluoroquinolones, which inhibit bacterial replication by inhibiting DNA-gyrase and topoisomerase, topical ocular preparations of these antimicrobial agents e.g. ciprofloxacin, levofloxacin, gatifloxacin and moxifloxacin are available and may be employed, considering the cost and bacterial resistance. Topical fluoroquinolones, which have greater corneal penetration and achieve higher ocular concentrations, offer advantage. Considering the activity against both Gram-positive and Gram-negative microorganisms and penetration through inflamed cornea, moxifloxacin holds promise, among the fluoroquinolones [27, 28].

Hyperacute bacterial conjunctivitis is severe condition, which may also involve cornea leading to sight-threatening sequelae. Hyperacute bacterial conjunctivitis due to *N. gonorrhoeae* must be treated aggressively with combined systemic and topical antibiotic therapy [8, 11]. Systemic therapy with cephalosporins such as ceftrioxane and cefixime to eradicate the gonococcal infection is recommended. Chlamydial conjunctivitis is usually associated with concurrent genital or respiratory tract infections, and thus it is better treated with combined systemic and topical antibiotic therapy. In neonates and pregnant women, oral erythromycin combined with erythromycin ointment is usually indicated. In adults, oral teracyclines (tetracycline, doxycycline, minocycline) and as topical ointment are the drugs of choice [8, 11].

Viral infections of conjunctiva, usually by adenoviruses are more common than the bacterial infections and are contagious. Good hygiene to prevent the spread of infection within the community is the most effective strategy in management of viral conjunctival infections. Viral conjunctivitis is self-limiting and usually regresses within 2 weeks without complications [8, 10]. Earlier topical corticosteroids were used for symptomatic relief of inflammation but because their use is associated with serious adverse effects like increase of intraocular pressure, progression of cataract, masking of infection, they have been replaced with topical NSAIDs [4]. Topical anti-virals are not used routinely but in cases of severe conjunctivitis due to herpetic infections, topical therapy with antivirals like acyclovir, ganciclovir, cifdovir may be indicated to prevent corneal infection.

Mycotic infections, though rare are difficult to treat. Combined oral and topical therapy with azole antifungals such as oral ketoconazole, itraconazole, and fluconazole, with topical fluconazole, itraconazole drops and nighttime antibiotics may be useful.

Parasitic conjunctivitis has been treated with mechanical removal of larvae under slit-lamp. In addition, appropriate systemic chemotherapy may be required for severe cases [15].

Management strategies of ocular allergic disorders may be divided into primary, secondary and tertiary line of treatment [3]. Avoidance of allergens, cold compresses and lubrication comprises the first line of treatment. Removing the source of offending allergen or change of occupational venue, if possible, is the first and foremost step, which may alleviate the symptoms and be curative in some cases. Cold compression provides symptomatic relief from itching, while lubricating with artificial tears assists by direct removal or dilution of allergens coming in contact with conjunctival surface.

The second line of treatment of acute and chronic forms of ocular allergy may include the use of topical antihistaminic, decongestants, mast cell stabilizers and NSAIDs. Topical administration of antihistaminics like levocabastine, emedastine effectively controls the H_1 receptor mediated pruritus. Although topical antihistaminics alone can provide the symptomatic relief, combining antihistaminic with vasoconstrictors is more effective than either agent alone [29]. Vasoconstrictors like naphazoline and phenylepherine effectively reduce the erythema. In addition, mast cell stabilizers like sodium chromoglycate, nedocromil, lodoxamide may be used for severe cases. With the availability of second-generation topical antihistaminics having dual- or multiple-actions (i.e., mast cell stabilizing, cytokine synthesis inhibition) like olapatadine, azelastine, ketotifen results similar to combination of different agents can be obtained. PGs like PGI_2 and PGE_2 have been found to be extremely pruritogenic to conjunctiva. Topical NSAIDs like ketorolac, diclofenac and flurbiprofen have been reported to significantly reduce the itching and hyperemia associated with SAC and VKC [30,31]. Since COX 2 is expressed in inflammatory cells, bromfenac, a selective COX 2 inhibitor, appears promising [4].

The tertiary treatment, which includes the use of mild topical corticosteroids and immunomodulators like cyclosporin, tacrolimus are considered in severe cases refractive to secondary line of treatment, to avoid irreversible corneal damage and scarring. Since, the use of corticosteroids is associated with localized ocular complications, modified corticosteroids like rimexolone and loteprednol etabonate (which are rapidly metabolized in the anterior chamber of the eye) have been used effectively. Topical cyclosporin A has been found to be highly effective in severe cases, and may be used as alternative to corticosteroids.

GPC being induced by foreign body may also be considered as iatrogenic conjunctivitis. The first and foremost treatment modality in management of GPC is removal of contact lenses. Usually patients of GPC may resume wearing contact lenses using the lenses made of different materials. Good lens hygiene, lens care and frequent replacement of lenses are also useful. Topical mast cell stabilizers, antihistaminics and NSAIDs are indicated in management of severe cases of GPC.

REFERENCES

[1] Harry, J. & Mission, G. (2001). *Clinical Ophthalmic Pathology, Principles of Diseases of the Eye and Associated Structures*. Oxford, UK: Butterworth Heinemann.

[2] Guidelines on the diagnosis and treatment of conjunctivitis. I. Introduction. *Ocular Immunology and Inflammation. 2(1),* S1.DOI; 10.3109/092739494090739 98.

[3] Bielory, L. (2002). Ocular allergy guidelines: a practical treatment algorithm. *Drugs, 62(11),* 1611-1634.

[4] Ahuja, M., Dhake, A.S., Sharma, S.K. & Majumdar, D.K. (2008). Topical ocular delivery of NSAIDs. *The AAPS Journal.* 10, 229-241

[5] Woodward, D.F., Nieves, A.L, Hawley, S.B., Joseph, R., Merlino, G.F. & Spada, C.S. (1995). The pruritogenic and inflammatory effects of prostanoids in the conjunctiva. *J Ocul Pharmacol Ther. 11(3),* 339-347.

[6] Malhotra, M. & Majumdar, D.K. (2006). Aqueous, oil and ointment formulations of ketorolac: efficacy against prostaglandin E_2-induced ocular inflammation and safety: a technical note. *AAPS PharmSciTech. 7(4),* Article 96, E1-E6.

[7] Guidelines on the diagnosis and treatment of conjunctivitis. II. Clinical signs of conjunctivitis. (1994). *Ocular Immunology and Inflammation, 2(1),* S3-S8. DOI; 10.3109/09273949409074000

[8] Guidelines on the diagnosis and treatment of conjunctivitis. III. Infectious conjunctivitis (1994). *Ocular Immunology and Inflammation, 2(1),* S9-S16. DOI; 10.3109/09273949409074007.

[9] Guidelines on the diagnosis and treatment of conjunctivitis. IV. Non-Infectious conjunctivitis. *Ocular Immunology and Inflammation, 2(1),* S17-S34. DOI; 10.3109/09273949409073999.

[10] Galor, A., & Jeng, B.H. (2008). Red eye for the internist: when to treat, when to refer. *Cleve Clin J Med, 75 (2),* 137-144.

[11] Tarabishy, A.B., & Jeng, B.H., (2008). Bacterial conjunctivitis: a review for internists. *Cleve Clin J Med, 75 (2),* 507-512.

[12] Xuguang, S., Zhixin, W., Zhiqun, W., Shiyun, L. & Ran L. (2007). Ocular fungal isolates and antifungal susceptibility in northern China. *Am J Ophthalmol. 143(1),* 131-133.

[13] John, S.S. & Mohandas, S.G. (2005). Conjunctival oculosporidiosis with scleral thinning and staphyloma formation. *Indian J Ophthalmol. 53(4),* 272-274.

[14] Chen, J.L., Wang, C.C., Sheu, S.J. & Yeh, T.I. (2005). Conjunctival aspergilloma with multiple mulberry nodules: a case report. *Kaohsiung J Med Sci. 21(6),* 286-290.

[15]Kaliaperumal, S., Rao, V.A. & Parija, S.C. (2005). Cysticercosis of the eye in South India--a case series. *Indian J Med Microbiol. 23(4)*, 227-230.

[16]Pandey, A., Madan, M., Asthana, A.K., Das, A., Kumar, S. & Jain, K. (2009) External ophthalmomyiasis caused by Oestrus ovis: a rare case report from India. *Korean J Parasitol. 47(1),* 57-59.

[17]Chowdhary, A., Bansal, R., Singh, K. & Singh V. (2003). Ocular cysticercosis--a profile. *Trop Doct. 33(3)*, 185-188.

[18]Shen, J., Gasser, R.B., Chu, D., Wang, Z., Yuan, X., Cantacessi, C. & Otranto, D. (2006). Human thelaziosis--a neglected parasitic disease of the eye. *J Parasitol. 92(4)*, 872-5.

[19]Blochmichel, E., Helleboid, L. & Corvec, M.L. (1993). Chronic allergic conjunctivitis. *Ocular Immunology & Inflammation, 1 (1)*, 9-12.

[20]Cuvillo, A.D., Sastre, J., Montoro, J., Jáuregui, I., Dávila, I., Ferrer, M., Bartra, J., Mullo, J. & Valero, A. (2009). Allergic conjunctivitis and H_1 antihistamines. *J Investig Allergol Clin Immunol. 19, Suppl. 1*: 11-18.

[21]Kumar, S. (2009). Vernal keratoconjunctivitis: a major review. *Acta Ophthalmol. 87*, 133-147.

[22]Kumaraswami, T.M. (1965). Iatrogenic disorders in ophthalmology. *Indian J Ophthalmol, 13*, 109-113.

[23]Kawasaki, S., Nishida, K., Sotozono, C., Quantock, A.J. & Kinoshita, S. (2000) Conjunctival inflammation in the chronic phase of Stevens–Johnson syndrome. *Br J Ophthalmol, 84*, 1191–1193.

[24]Crosby, S.S., Murray, K.M., Marvin, J.A., Heimbach, D.M. & Tartaglione, T.A. (1986). Management of Stevens-Johnson syndrome. *Clin Pharm. 5(8)*, 682-689.

[25]Rose, P. (2007). Management strategies for acute infective conjunctivitis in primary care: a systematic review. *Expert Opin Pharmacother. 8(12)*, 1903-1921.

[26]Sheikh, A. & Hurwitz, B. (2001). Topical antibiotics for acute bacterial conjunctivitis: a systematic review. *Br J Gen Pract. 51(467)*, 473-477.

[27]Oliveira, A.D., D'Azevedo, P.A. & Francisco, W. (2007). In vitro activity of fluoroquinolones against ocular bacterial isolates in São Paulo, Brazil. *Cornea. 26(2)*, 194-198.

[28]Yağci, R., Oflu, Y., Dinçel, A., Kaya, E., Yağci, S., Bayar, B., Duman, S., Bozkurt, A.(2007). Penetration of second-, third-, and fourth-generation topical fluoroquinolone into aqueous and vitreous humour in a rabbit endophthalmitis model. *Eye. 21(7)*, 990-994. Epub 2006 May 26.

[29]Smith, J.P., Lanier, B.Q., Tremblay, N., Ward, R.L. & DeFaller, J.M. (1982). Treatment of allergic conjunctivitis with ocular decongestants. *Curr Eye Res. 2 (2)*, 141-147.

[30]Schalnus, R. (2003). Topical nonsteroidal anti-inflammatory therapy in ophthalmology. *Ophthalmologica, 217*, 89-98.

[31]Swamy, B. N., Chilov, M., McClellan, K. & Petsoglou, C. (2007). Topical non- steroidal anti-inflammatory drugs in allergic conjunctivitis: meta-analysis of randomized trial data. *Ophthalmic Epidemiology, 14*, 311-319.

INDEX

D

F

G

H

I

M

polymorphonuclear, 16, 46, 196

polysaccharide, 90

polyvinyl alcohol, 80, 88, 95

polyvinylpyrrolidone, 80, 97

poor, ix, 24, 44, 110, 113, 123, 124, 141, 150, 187

poor performance, 187

population, vii, x, 1, 2, 30, 35, 42, 50, 66, 69, 142, 144, 153, 162, 170, 171, 176, 186

porosity, 45

postoperative, 111, 112, 113, 130

potassium, 24, 81

Prednisolone, 28, 99, 112, 143, 151

pregnancy, 77, 78

pregnant women, 200

premature ovarian failure, 77

preservative, 33, 34, 41, 43, 53, 81, 82, 89, 97, 98, 142, 144, 147, 150

preservatives, viii, ix, 55, 80, 81, 82, 141, 142, 144, 153, 154, 155, 200

pressure, x, 26, 27, 29, 54, 90, 109, 111, 113, 144, 145, 195, 201

prevention, 23, 26, 50, 109, 113, 128, 153, 174

primary care, 203

probable cause, 80

probiotic, 65

prodrugs, 110

production, vii, viii, 1, 2, 5, 6, 7, 8, 9, 11, 12, 13, 15, 16, 19, 20, 21, 24, 26, 27, 29, 30, 36, 37, 41, 46, 47, 48, 55, 60, 69, 75, 76, 80, 82, 85, 87, 88, 91, 92, 98, 99, 110, 112, 113, 114, 119, 121, 124, 125, 127, 132, 196, 197

production costs, 75

productivity, 2, 30

progesterone, 36, 61, 137

prognosis, ix, 3, 34, 44, 50, 57, 58, 59, 142, 153, 181

pro-inflammatory, 14, 15, 17, 26, 27, 29

proinflammatory effect, 36

proliferation, 5, 6, 14, 18, 19, 20, 21, 28, 29, 30, 37, 38, 86, 112

promoter, 169, 176

prophylactic, 3, 41, 43, 53, 54, 58, 59

prophylaxis, vii, 1, 24, 34, 43, 112

propionic acid, 113

prostaglandin, 12, 15, 111, 145, 202

prostaglandins, x, 8, 10, 27, 111, 112, 113, 195, 196

prostanoids, 202

prostheses, 44, 45, 46, 62, 199

prosthetics, 45

proteases, 10, 15, 37

protection, viii, 98, 107, 109, 114, 116, 125

protein, 6, 7, 10, 11, 18, 20, 22, 31, 40, 42, 45, 46, 71, 87, 92, 102, 111, 136, 170, 175, 184

proteins, 18, 20, 38, 43, 56, 77, 79, 80, 112, 196

proteoglycans, 10

protocol, 58

protocols, 58

protozoa, 199

provocation, 26, 152, 155

pruritus, 25, 26, 29, 31, 38, 48, 82, 201

pseudo, 179, 180

Pseudomonas, 81

Pseudomonas aeruginosa, 81

Psoriasis, 135

psychosis, 145

ptosis, 52, 112

puberty, 35, 44

pulse, 33, 34, 42, 49, 58

PVA, 74, 95

P-value, 172

pyrimidine, 146, 157

pyrrole, 129, 146

Q

QT interval, 23

quality of life, vii, 1, 2, 30, 59, 69, 75

quaternary ammonium, 81, 143

R

radiation, 187, 193

radiologists, 181

radiotherapy, 187, 193

range, 3, 57, 75, 115, 116, 124, 142

RANTES, 10, 22, 37

rapamycin, 93, 102

reactive oxygen species, 22

reactivity, 36, 65, 144, 146, 147, 153, 157, 158, 166

reading, 147, 148, 149, 152

reagent, 123

REAL classification, 188

receptors, viii, 2, 3, 5, 6, 8, 9, 10, 13, 14, 15, 19, 20, 23, 25, 26, 27, 31, 36, 60, 61, 67, 68, 70, 77, 86, 99, 169, 177, 196

recognition, 5, 14

recovery, x, 82, 195, 200

redness, vii, 1, 10, 15, 22, 25, 28, 31, 34, 36, 38, 67, 108, 142, 152, 196, 197

reflection, 79

T

X

Z